AF771468

VOLUME EIGHTY SIX

ADVANCES IN FOOD AND NUTRITION RESEARCH

Biological Emerging Risks in Foods

SERIES EDITORS

GEORGE F. STEWART	**(1948–1982)**
EMIL M. MRAK	**(1948–1987)**
C. O. CHICHESTER	**(1959–1988)**
BERNARD S. SCHWEIGERT	**(1984–1988)**
JOHN E. KINSELLA	**(1989–1993)**
STEVE L. TAYLOR	**(1995–2011)**
JEYAKUMAR HENRY	**(2011–2016)**
FIDEL TOLDRÁ	**(2016–)**

VOLUME EIGHTY SIX

ADVANCES IN FOOD AND NUTRITION RESEARCH

Biological Emerging Risks in Foods

Edited by

DAVID RODRÍGUEZ-LÁZARO

Microbiology Division,
Department of Biotechnology and Food Science,
University of Burgos, Burgos, Spain

ELSEVIER

ACADEMIC PRESS

An imprint of Elsevier

Academic Press is an imprint of Elsevier
50 Hampshire Street, 5th Floor, Cambridge, MA 02139, United States
525 B Street, Suite 1650, San Diego, CA 92101, United States
The Boulevard, Langford Lane, Kidlington, Oxford OX5 1GB, United Kingdom
125 London Wall, London, EC2Y 5AS, United Kingdom

First edition 2018

Copyright © 2018 Elsevier Inc. All Rights Reserved.

No part of this publication may be reproduced or transmitted in any form or by any means, electronic or mechanical, including photocopying, recording, or any information storage and retrieval system, without permission in writing from the publisher. Details on how to seek permission, further information about the Publisher's permissions policies and our arrangements with organizations such as the Copyright Clearance Center and the Copyright Licensing Agency, can be found at our website: www.elsevier.com/permissions.

This book and the individual contributions contained in it are protected under copyright by the Publisher (other than as may be noted herein).

Notices
Knowledge and best practice in this field are constantly changing. As new research and experience broaden our understanding, changes in research methods, professional practices, or medical treatment may become necessary.

Practitioners and researchers must always rely on their own experience and knowledge in evaluating and using any information, methods, compounds, or experiments described herein. In using such information or methods they should be mindful of their own safety and the safety of others, including parties for whom they have a professional responsibility.

To the fullest extent of the law, neither the Publisher nor the authors, contributors, or editors, assume any liability for any injury and/or damage to persons or property as a matter of products liability, negligence or otherwise, or from any use or operation of any methods, products, instructions, or ideas contained in the material herein.

ISBN: 978-0-12-813977-6
ISSN: 1043-4526

For information on all Academic Press publications
visit our website at https://www.elsevier.com/books-and-journals

ELSEVIER
Book Aid International
Working together
to grow libraries in
developing countries
www.elsevier.com • www.bookaid.org

Publisher: Zoe Kruze
Acquisition Editor: Sam Mahfoudh
Editorial Project Manager: Teresa Pons-Ferrer
Production Project Manager: Denny Mansingh
Cover Designer: Christian J. Bilbow

Typeset by SPi Global, India

CONTENTS

CONTRIBUTORS

Nigel Cook
Jorvik Food and Environmental Virology, York, United Kingdom

Alessandra De Cesare
Department of Agricultural and Food Sciences, University of Bologna, Bologna, Italy

Lucas Domínguez
Foodborne Zoonoses and Antimicrobial Resistance Unit, VISAVET Health Surveillance Center; Department of Animal Health, Veterinary Faculty, Complutense University, Madrid, Spain

Doris H. D'Souza
University of Tennessee, Knoxville, TN, United States

Diego Florez-Cuadrado
Foodborne Zoonoses and Antimicrobial Resistance Unit, VISAVET Health Surveillance Center, Complutense University, Madrid, Spain

Lourdes García-Sánchez
Biotechnology and Food Science Department, University of Burgos, Burgos, Spain

Marta Hernandez
Microbiology Division, Department of Biotechnology and Food Science, University of Burgos, Burgos; Laboratory of Molecular Biology and Microbiology, ITACyL, Valladolid, Spain

Kieran Jordan
Teagasc Food Research Centre, Cork, Ireland

Olivia McAuliffe
Teagasc Food Research Centre, Cork, Ireland

Beatriz Melero
Biotechnology and Food Science Department, University of Burgos, Burgos, Spain

Miguel A. Moreno
Foodborne Zoonoses and Antimicrobial Resistance Unit, VISAVET Health Surveillance Center; Department of Animal Health, Veterinary Faculty, Complutense University, Madrid, Spain

Walter Randazzo
IATA-CSIC; University of Valencia, Valencia, Spain

Lucy J. Robertson
Department of Food Safety and Infection Biology, Norwegian University of Life Sciences, Oslo, Norway

David Rodríguez-Lázaro
Microbiology Division, Department of Biotechnology and Food Science, University of Burgos, Burgos, Spain

Jordi Rovira
Biotechnology and Food Science Department, University of Burgos, Burgos, Spain

Gloria Sanchez
IATA-CSIC, Valencia, Spain

María Ugarte-Ruíz
Foodborne Zoonoses and Antimicrobial Resistance Unit, VISAVET Health Surveillance Center, Complutense University, Madrid, Spain

PREFACE

The promotion of a high level of Food Safety and Quality is a major policy priority worldwide. Food safety is compromised by foodborne diseases, which are one of the most serious problems in public health and one of the main causes of illness and death. It is estimated that around 600 million cases of foodborne diseases occur worldwide each year, which can cause from mild gastroenteritis to syndromes with a fatal outcome. This volume tackles fundamental and practical aspects on emerging biological risks associated to food, from the main aspects of those pathogens, to the current situation and the future perspectives on this relevant food safety issue.

Chapter 1 reviews the impact of foodborne pathogenic microorganisms on public health from a global perspective, emphasizing the role of neglected organisms, such us foodborne viruses and parasites, as well as the zoonotic potential of most of the emerging biological risks with major environmental implication associated mainly to intensive animal production. Chapters 2 and 3 provide a relevant overview of the relevance of enteric viruses in foodborne diseases; while Chapter 2 focuses on human noroviruses providing relevant information on the routes of transmission, their prevalence in different food commodities, and the current procedures for their inactivation, Chapter 3 emphasizes the role of the foodborne transmission in the human infection with hepatitis E virus, and the relevant role of the zoonotic potential of this viral agent. Chapter 4 shows a comprehensive review on foodborne parasites, highlighting their neglected situation and emerging nature, and discusses the most recent efforts on their control. Chapter 5 addresses one of the most relevant issues on public health, the antimicrobial resistance, and the role and impact of the food chain in its dissemination, and describes the genetic mechanisms underpinning this phenomenon. Chapters 6–8 focus on the major bacterial pathogens transmitted by food. Chapters 6 discusses the reemergence of *Salmonella* as a foodborne problem, showing the most important sources and specific actions to restart decreasing the number of human salmonellosis. Chapter 7 highlights the relevance of the occurrence and control of *Listeria monocytogenes* for the food industry and public health, as well as describes novel methods for its control. Chapter 8 provides relevant information on *Campylobacter*, from the relevant mechanisms and strategies to persist in the food chain, to the sources, to the transmission routes and the different strategies to avoid the public health risk associated with this pathogen.

I am grateful for the excellent contributions made by the authors of the chapters, who are international experts on each of the foodborne pathogens described. I am completely confident that this volume will provide accurate and relevant information to readers who wish to know in more detail relevant aspects of the main foodborne pathogens that pose an emerging risk to consumers.

DAVID RODRÍGUEZ-LÁZARO

CHAPTER ONE

Emerging Biological Risks in a Global Context: An Introduction

David Rodríguez-Lázaro[*,1], **Marta Hernandez**[*,†]
[*]Microbiology Division, Department of Biotechnology and Food Science, University of Burgos, Burgos, Spain
[†]Laboratory of Molecular Biology and Microbiology, ITACyL, Valladolid, Spain
[1]Corresponding author: e-mail address: drlazaro@ubu.es

Contents

Abstract

Foodborne diseases are one of the most serious problems in public health and one of the main causes of illness and death. It is estimated that around 600 million cases of gastroenteritis occur worldwide each year. At present, more than 200 foodborne diseases are known, which can cause from mild gastroenteritis to syndromes with a fatal outcome, with the added possibility of chronic complications, and more than 40 agents have been described that can cause foodborne diseases. Some of the most relevant foodborne pathogens are neglected or their impact underestimated such as foodborne viruses and parasites. Most of the foodborne pathogenic microorganisms possess a zoonotic potential with high environmental impact by the intensive animal production, and consequently the environment plays a very important role in their transmission. Consequently, a coordinated approach must be implemented to control emerging foodborne pathogens in primary production (animal health), in the community (human health), and in the environment (environmental health).

Promoting a high level of food safety is a major policy worldwide. Moreover, guaranteeing the safety and quality of food products along the food chain is the principal demand of consumers, as they expect their food to be tasty and wholesome as well as safe. Foodborne diseases are one of the most serious problems in public health and one of the main causes of illness and death (Anonymous, 2010; Scallan, Griffin, Angulo, Tauxe, & Hoekstra, 2011;

Advances in Food and Nutrition Research, Volume 86
ISSN 1043-4526
https://doi.org/10.1016/bs.afnr.2018.04.001
© 2018 Elsevier Inc.
All rights reserved.

Scallan, Hoekstra, et al., 2011; Wallace et al., 2000). Concern for the safety of food products has been increased considerably during the last decades by the rapid globalization of the food market and profound changes in food consumption habits (D'Agostino & Rodriguez-Lazaro, 2009). At present, more than 200 foodborne diseases (Bryan, 1982) are known, which can cause from mild gastroenteritis to syndromes with a fatal outcome, with the added possibility of chronic complications (Mead et al., 1999). More than 40 agents have been described that can cause food diseases (CAST, 1994).

It is estimated that around 600 million cases of gastroenteritis occur worldwide each year (WHO, 2015), causing about 60 million liters of diarrhea per day, which is equivalent to all the water that passes through the Victoria Falls in 1 min. In this sense, a recently published study estimates that every year in the United States, almost 48 million episodes associated with food caused by pathogenic microorganisms (Scallan, Griffin, et al., 2011; Scallan, Hoekstra, et al., 2011), causing annual economic losses associated with medical expenses and working hours of almost 78 billion dollars (Scharff, 2012), equivalent to the European multiannual research program Horizon 2020. Only the 31 most prominent (including bacteria such as *Salmonella* spp. or *Listeria monocytogenes*, viruses such as norovirus or hepatitis A virus, and protozoa such as *Toxoplasma gondii* or *Cryptosporidium* spp.) account for almost 9.5 million episodes that involve almost 56,000 hospitalizations and more than 1000 deaths (Scallan, Griffin, et al., 2011) (Table 1). These include mainly human noroviruses that cause the highest number of cases and the second largest in hospitalizations (Scallan, Griffin, et al., 2011).

Table 1 Estimated Annual Number of Episodes of Foodborne Diseases Produced by the 31 Most Relevant Pathogens in the United States

Organism	Transmission via Food (%)	No. of Foodborne Cases
Bacteria	—	3.645.773 (2.321.468–5.581.290)
Parasites	—	232.705 (161.923–369.893)
Viruses	—	5.509597 (3.273.623–8.355.586)
Norovirus	26	5.461.731 (3.277.078–8.309.480)
Total	—	9.388.075 (6.641.440–12.745.709)

Adapted from Scallan, E., Hoekstra, R. M., Angulo, F. J., Tauxe, R. V., Widdowson, M. A., Roy, S. L., et al. (2011). Foodborne illness acquired in the United States—Major pathogens. *Emerging Infectious Diseases, 17*, 7–15; Scallan, E., Griffin, P. M., Angulo, F. J., Tauxe, R. V., Hoekstra, R. M. (2011). Foodborne illness acquired in the United States—Unspecified agents. *Emerging Infectious Diseases, 17*, 16–22.

Table 2 Number of Foodborne Outbreaks (Including Those Transmitted by Water), Human Cases, Hospitalizations, and Deaths by Causal Agent in the EU Member States, 2015

	Outbreaks		Cases			
Organism	**No.**	**Notification Rate**	**No.**	**Average per Outbreak**	**Hospitalization**	**Deaths**
Bacteria	1470	0.32	9.382	6.4	1.968	8
Bacterial toxins	849	0.18	8.847	10.4	497	3
Parasites	52	0.01	302	5.8	44	0
Viruses	401	0.09	14.754	36.8	531	5
Norovirus	289	0.07	13.536	46.8	352	1
Total	4362	0.95	45.874	10.5	3.892	17

Adapted from EFSA (2016). The European Union summary report on trends and sources of zoonoses, zoonotic agents and food-borne outbreaks in 2015. *EFSA Journal, 14*, 4634.

Similar data are observed in EU (Table 2) and in other countries such as United Kingdom (Adak, Meakins, Yip, Lopman, & O'Brien, 2005) or Australia (Hall et al., 2005). Therefore, the impact of foodborne pathogens in public health systems is very considerable. For example, it has been estimated that diseases caused by pathogenic microorganisms cause 1% of hospitalizations and 0.2% of deaths in the United States (Buzby, Frenzen, & Rasco, 2001).

Humanity has suffered diseases caused by foodborne pathogens since before the dawn of civilization. Only in the last century have technological advances led to a characterization of the etiological agents and their epidemiology. However, most of the epidemiological efforts and data have been directly associated with pathogenic bacteria, but information on viral and parasitic infections is generally more scarce. For example, the first recorded outbreak of foodborne diseases of probable viral etiology occurred at the beginning of the 20th century; in 1914, four cases of paralytic disease occurred in an English community, among children who drank milk from a common source; the mode of contamination of the milk was not determined (Jubb, 1915). Nine additional outbreaks of foodborne poliomyelitis were reported in the United Kingdom and the United States until 1949. The diagnoses in these outbreaks were necessarily clinical—1949 was the year in which the in vitro culture of poliovirus was first announced—so that laboratory diagnostic methods were not yet available. Several studies have been published that provide information on the risk of foodborne viruses (Cook & Rzezutka, 2006; Koopmans & Duizer, 2004; Rodríguez-Lázaro et al., 2012).

However, nowadays, the importance of viral diseases transmitted by food and water is still underestimated largely due to the difficulties in accumulating accurate data on the incidence of outbreaks and isolated cases often occur. However, although there is clear evidence that the data may be clearly underestimated, the incidence of enteric viruses associated with food consumption has increased in recent years in developed countries and has become the main cause of gastroenteritis, causing almost 60% of episodes associated with food (Scallan, Griffin, et al., 2011). Similarly, there is not too much information on foodborne parasitic diseases, and parasites are relatively neglected (Pedrique et al., 2013); 60% of neglected tropical diseases are parasitic, and almost half of them (42%) with potential to be transmitted by food (WHO, 2017). However, although they are largely unknown, there are a wide variety of viruses and parasites of human or animal origin that can spread in the environment and infect people through water and food, mainly by ingestion and occasionally by skin contact. They are released into the environment through various routes, including water runoff and aerosols. In addition, zoonotic viruses and parasites can infect humans exposed to contaminated surface waters. Foods of animal origin may also be contaminated and their consumption may cause human infection if the viruses and parasites (as for bacterial pathogens) are not inactivated during food processing.

Most of those foodborne pathogens (including bacteria, viruses, and parasites) are transmitted by the fecal–oral route. Infected humans can excrete large amounts of human pathogenic agents, and also animals and plants, as well as other excreta and secrets, can also transport high pathogenic loads. Interestingly, enteric viruses, fecal-orally transmitted, are generally not enveloped and therefore are very stable in the environment (Rzeżutka & Cook, 2004) and include important etiological agents, some of which are thought to be emerging zoonotic pathogens. These viruses cannot always be effectively eliminated by current wastewater treatment methods (Thompson et al., 2003; van den Berg, Lodder, van der Poel, Vennema, & de Roda Husman, 2005; Vantarakis & Papapetropoulou, 1999) and can therefore cause viral contamination of the environment through both treated and untreated wastewater.

Other examples of indirect routes of transmission of emerging foodborne pathogens are runoff from manure used in agriculture. It can also produce direct fecal contamination of the environment by humans and animals, for example, by bathers or defecation of wild animals in the soil or in surface waters. The consequent contamination of marine and coastal waters, rivers and other surface waters, groundwater, and plants and fruits is associated with the subsequent risks of the reintroduction of the pathogenic agents in human and animal populations. Individuals with a compromised immune system, including children, the elderly, pregnant women, and people infected with HIV, are more susceptible to these infections and the prognosis of the disease may be more serious. This is the case, for example, of *L. monocytogenes* or rotavirus.

Environmentally transmitted enteric pathogenic microorganisms include important etiologic agents of mild diseases such as gastroenteritis, as well as agents of more serious diseases, such as meningitis and hepatitis. Therefore, most of the foodborne biological pathogens possess a zoonotic potential and can represent an example of the application of the "ONE HEALTH" strategy, since the interests of animal, environmental, and human health can converge.

1. ZOONOTIC TRANSMISSION OF FOODBORNE PATHOGENS: FROM THE ENVIRONMENT TO THE FOOD AND THE CONSUMER

One of the main routes of transmission of foodborne pathogenic microorganisms including bacteria, viruses, and parasites to humans is the zoonotic pathway, either associated with the consumption of contaminated products of animal origin, or during the handling of food by infected handlers. Also, another frequent cause of food contaminated by foodborne pathogens is their contact with water contaminated with feces. The inadequate consumption of drinking water, the consumption of contaminated crops after being irrigated or fertilized with wastewater, and the ingestion of shellfish grown in contaminated waters are, therefore, common causes of infection transmitted by food to humans.

Several factors affect the contamination of foods such as seafood, fruits, and vegetables. Climatic variables such as the season, tidal cycles, rainfall, and floods have been implicated in the microbial contamination of the environment. Similarly, good practices in the primary sector, both in livestock and agriculture, as well as in the subsequent processing of these raw materials are absolutely necessary to minimize the risk of contamination of the food. Improper irrigation practices, wastewater treatment and reuse, wastewater overflows, and wastewater emissions from contaminated sources are direct causes of environmental contamination and sources of foodborne outbreaks. Likewise, shellfish produced in areas close to livestock farms or intensive agriculture, or waste treatment plants, present a high risk of transport of foodborne pathogens, mainly enteric viruses.

There is growing concern about outbreaks of foodborne illness associated with the foods of animal origin, which has led to consumer concerns about safety in the food supply chain. The health risk associated with operations with animals depends on several factors. The most important is related to the animal species that is being raised and the concentration of pathogenic microorganisms in animal manure. In addition, some pathogenic organisms survive for long periods despite the production practices and sanitizing treatments used, maintaining their infectious capacity in the environment until it is ingested by a human or animal host. Enteric pathogenic microorganisms are excreted fecally and, therefore, spread through contaminated soils and waters; therefore, any other animal species that grazes on the same pastures and/or drinks from the same water sources as the infected cattle is likely to be exposed to infection. Consequently, they can be contaminated by the same or closely related pathogenic agent and, therefore, represent a high risk of further dissemination.

Most of the foodborne pathogens that emerge in human populations are of animal origin. There is a wide spectrum of modes of transmission for zoonotic microorganisms through domestic animals or wild reservoirs. These can be direct or indirect and include transmission through contaminated food, water, air, and soil. The meat can be contaminated by excreta during the slaughter of the animals or during their subsequent processing, but it may also have been contaminated before due to the infection of the live animal. The risk of foodborne infection depends on the route of infection, the level of contamination, and the degree of inactivation during the processing of food. Livestock farms produce large amounts of waste that can cause serious environmental problems. In fact, accidental or deliberate spills, excessive use of animal waste as a fertilizer, and releases of animal waste improperly or incompletely treated constitute significant environmental risks of contamination. As expected, the detection of foodborne pathogens in contaminated waters (groundwater, lakes, rivers, estuaries, runoff and irrigation tanks of farms, etc.) is much more frequent in areas of intensive production. However, the modes and levels of environmental contamination differ in the different types of foodborne pathogens and animal species.

2. THE PARTICULAR CASE OF ENTERIC VIRUSES

The importance of enteric viruses in the field of food safety is evidenced by the interest shown by different international organizations. The Codex Alimentarius Commission issued a document on the relevance of viruses in food and the aspects that need to be developed: among other rapid methods of diagnosis, studies to establish the correlation between infectivity and molecular detection and studies on the effectiveness of different food-processing treatments for the inactivation of enteric viruses (FAO/OMS, 2008). In this regard, EFSA has also published several guidelines on the relevance and control of viruses in food (EFSA, 2011, 2012, 2014), in line with the guidelines on general hygiene principles for the control of viruses in foods prepared by the Codex Alimentarius Commission (FAO/OMS, 2012), which stresses that the control of food risks must begin during agricultural or animal production and continue throughout the food chain (from farm to fork).

As indicated earlier, human noroviruses are the main causative agent of gastroenteritis in the United States with almost 5.5 million episodes per year and more than 14,500 hospitalizations (Scallan, Griffin, et al., 2011) (Table 1). In a published economic study, it has been estimated that the US annual expenditure associated with the processes associated with human noroviruses of food origin represents 2000 million dollars and 5000 QALYs—that is, loss of 5000 years with perfect health (Scallan, Hoekstra, et al., 2011). Similar data are obtained in EU (Table 2). In 2015, 9.2% of food outbreaks were associated with enteric viruses (EFSA, 2016). However, this figure is lower than that obtained in 2014, where this organism represented the first cause of food outbreaks with 20.4% (1072 outbreaks) (EFSA, 2015). In 2015, the notification rate of foodborne outbreaks caused by enteric viruses was 0.09 outbreaks per 100,000 inhabitants (Table 2), slightly higher than those observed for *Campylobacter* (EFSA, 2016). It is of special relevance that, although the number of outbreaks was not the highest in 2015, the total number of people affected by gastrointestinal infections of viral origin associated with food was 14,754, and only one causative agent, norovirus, caused 13,436 cases. Noroviruses were also the causative agents associated with the largest outbreaks in terms of total human cases involved and the highest average number of cases per outbreak (Table 2). This agent was involved in three of the five most relevant combinations (combinations of causative agents and food vehicles) that caused the greatest number of human cases in outbreaks with strong evidence: sprouts in combination with tap water, buffet meals, and other foods (EFSA, 2016).

To this remarkable numerical importance, we must add two other important factors: the wide variety of foods that can transmit enteric viruses (Koopmans, von Bonsdorff, Vinjé, de Medici, & Monroe, 2002), as well as the difficulty of being able to be propagated in the laboratory for diagnosis or study (Pintó & Bosch, 2008). Bivalve molluscs, vegetables eaten raw, berry fruits, and prepared foods are the main foods involved in viral infections.

One of the main differences between enteric viruses and foodborne pathogenic is the host specificity. While most of foodborne pathogenic bacteria have a zoonotic capacity, i.e., the origin or source of infection comes from animals and can be transmitted to humans via the ingestion of contaminated food, as in the case of important bacteria such as *Salmonella* spp., *Campylobacter*, or *L. monocytogenes* (see the further specific chapters), most of the enteric viruses associated with food outbreaks only present a unique specificity for the human host. Thus, enteric viruses mainly associated with gastroenteritis can only be transmitted to susceptible humans via the ingestion of food contaminated with human feces containing these viruses, as in the case of caliciviruses (norovirus and sapovirus) and hepatitis A virus, which represent more than 95% of intestinal infections mediated by viruses in humans (Scallan, Griffin, et al., 2011). Until recently, it was thought that all enteric viruses transmitted by food could only originate in humans and, therefore, its transmission was limited to manipulators of contaminated food, cross-contamination of food, and contamination by water. However, several recent outbreaks of the hepatitis E virus have shown that it is a zoonotic virus capable of being transmitted by the consumption of raw or lightly cooked meat products (Mishiro, 2004; Tei et al., 2004).

One of the main characteristics of enteric viruses is that they do not have a lipoprotein envelope, which gives them a high stability in the environment, as well as in food-processing environments. The viruses that are outside a host can be considered as inert particles and, not having intrinsic metabolism, do not require any nutrient to persist. However, they have a degree of robustness that allows them to remain infectious during the different situations and conditions that can be found between one host and another. The longer a virus can survive outside a host, the greater are its chances of transmission. These possibilities will be affected by various environmental conditions and factors such as heat, humidity, and pH; enteric viruses are very resistant to desiccation, to ionizing radiation and at low temperatures, even to freezing. This is illustrated by the number of outbreaks associated with enteric viruses attributable to the transmission of water or food (Lopman et al., 2004; Scallan, Griffin, et al., 2011). In addition, the presence of organic matter and the tendency of viruses to form aggregates increase viral stability. Also, the main conservation conditions used in food processes have a not very relevant virus lethal; they are resistant to acidic and basic pH and to different types of disinfectants and even at high temperatures, especially at temperatures below 90–100°C (Baert, Debevere, & Uyttendaele, 2009). Thus, once in foods such as vegetables, viruses can persist under usual storage conditions between purchase and consumption.

Other characteristics of special relevance in the epidemiology of enteric viral diseases are the very low infective dose—below 100 viral particles, and in some cases, amounts close to 1–5 infectious viral particles (De Roda-Husman & Bouwnegt, 2013)—and the high excretion capacity both in vomiting and in diarrhea of the infected hosts (above 10^5 viral particles per mL). Of special relevance is the low infective dose, in marked contrast, for example, to that observed in the case of relevant foodborne bacterial pathogens such as *L. monocytogenes*, or thermotolerant *Campylobacter*, in which the infective doses exceed 100 and 1000 cfu, respectively (Allos, 2001; ICMSF, 1996). Likewise, the excretion of enteric viruses in certain cases greatly favors their dispersion through the environment; this is the case of projectile vomiting in norovirus infections where the excretions can reach more than 2 m away. These two facts, low infective dose and high excretion, facilitate the dissemination and the possibility of producing outbreaks with a very high number of affected people. Likewise, in the case of caliciviruses, and in particular in human noroviruses, there is no natural immunity, thus not conferring postinfection immunity, and the patients are susceptible to new episodes within a few weeks.

Finally, one of the peculiarities of the enteric viruses of most relevance in food safety is their high difficulty in their detection associated with the fact that they do not multiply ("replicate") in food and that there are no fully established cell lines for the main foodborne pathogenic viruses; they do not exist for human caliciviruses or the hepatitis E virus, and the wild strains of hepatitis A virus associated with food outbreaks adapt very poorly to their replication in cell lines in the laboratory.

3. CONCLUDING REMARKS

The information described earlier points out that foodborne pathogenic microorganisms represent a serious problem in Public Health, both because of the number of cases they cause in developing and industrialized countries and because of the economic cost associated with their treatment. Likewise, the zoonotic potential of most of them also confers them an emergent character.

This high impact on welfare and economy associated with their emerging nature has caused both scientists and institutions in Public Health to focus their efforts on their detection and control. There is clear evidence that existing data on the prevalence of foodborne pathogens may be underestimated. Likewise, it is also necessary to know exactly what is its incidence in the different stages of the food production chain, and especially in that which is dedicated to the transformation of products of animal origin. Finally, it is also necessary to calibrate the current disinfection procedures in the food industry to establish in a reliable manner a quantitative evaluation of the biological risk in foods. As already indicated earlier, most of the pathogenic agents have a zoonotic potential associated with animal species with high environmental impact by its intensive production system, which gives the environment a very important role in their transmission. It is necessary, therefore, to articulate, in a coordinated approach, those three pillars: control in primary production (animal health), in the community (human health), and in the environment (environmental health). The most effective way to do this is to apply a global approach based on a "ONE HEALTH" strategy.

REFERENCES

Adak, G. K., Meakins, S. M., Yip, H., Lopman, B. A., & O'Brien, S. J. (2005). Disease risks from foods, England and Wales, 1996-2000. *Emerging Infectious Diseases*, *11*, 365–372.

Allos, B. M. (2001). Campylobacter jejuni infections: Update on emerging issues and trends. *Clinical Infectious Diseases*, *32*, 1201–1206.

Anonymous. (2010). Surveillance for foodborne disease outbreaks—United States, 2007. *Morbidity and Mortality Weekly Report*, *59*, 973–979.

Baert, L., Debevere, J., & Uyttendaele, M. (2009). The efficacy of preservation methods to inactivate foodborne viruses. *International Journal of Food Microbiology*, *131*, 83–94.

Bryan, F. L. (1982). *Diseases transmitted by foods (a classification and summary)* (2nd ed.). Atlanta: CDC, Center for Professional Development and Training.

Buzby, J. C., Frenzen, P., & Rasco, B. (2001). Product liability and microbial foodborne illness. In *Agricultural economic report No. AER799 food and rural economics division*: Economic Research Service, U.S. Department of Agriculture.

CAST. (1994). *CAST report: Foodborne pathogens: Risks and consequences*. Task Force Report No. 122, Washington, DC: Council for Agricultural Science and Technology.

Cook, N., & Rzezutka, A. (2006). Hepatitis viruses. In Y. Motarjemi & M. Adams (Eds.), *Emerging foodborne pathogens* (pp. 282–308). Cambridge: Woodhead Publishing Limited.

D'Agostino, M., & Rodriguez-Lazaro, D. (2009). Harmonisation and validation of methods in food safety—Dood PCR: A case study. In G. Barbosa-Cánovas, A. Mortimer, D. Lineback, W. Spiees, K. Buckle, & P. Collona (Eds.), *Global issues in food science and technology*: Elsevier.

De Roda-Husman, A. M., & Bouwnegt, M. (2013). Quantitative risk assessment for food- and waterborne viruses. In N. Cook (Ed.), *Viruses in food and water* (pp. 159–176). Woodhead.
EFSA. (2011). Scientific opinion on an update on the present knowledge on the occurrence and control of foodborne viruses. *EFSA Journal, 9*, 2190.
EFSA. (2012). Scientific opinion on norovirus (NoV) in oysters: Methods, limits and control options. *EFSA Journal, 10*, 2500.
EFSA. (2014). Scientific Opinion on the risk posed by pathogens in food of non-animal origin. Part 2 Salmonella and Norovirus in berries. *EFSA Journal, 12*, 3706.
EFSA. (2015). Scientific opinion on the risk posed by pathogens in food of non-animal origin. Part 2. *Salmonella* and Norovirus in berries. *EFSA Journal, 13*, 4329.
EFSA. (2016). The European Union summary report on trends and sources of zoonoses, zoonotic agents and food-borne outbreaks in 2015. *EFSA Journal, 14*, 4634.
FAO/OMS. (2008). *Document CX/FH 08/40/9.*
FAO/OMS. (2012). Doc CAC/GL 79-2012 guidelines on the application of general principles of food hygiene to the control of viruses in food: Meeting report. In *Microbiological risk assessment series. No. 13.*
Hall, G., Kirk, M. D., Becker, N., Gregory, J. E., Unicomb, L., Millard, G., et al. (2005). Estimating foodborne gastroenteritis, Australia. *Emerging Infectious Diseases, 11*, 1257–1264.
ICMSF. (1996). *Microorganisms in foods 5.* Blackie Academic & Professional.
Jubb, G. (1915). The third outbreak of epidemic poliomyelitis at West Kirby. *The Lancet, 1*, 67.
Koopmans, M., & Duizer, E. (2004). Foodborne viruses: An emerging problem. *International Journal of Food Microbiology, 90*, 23–41.
Koopmans, M., von Bonsdorff, C. H., Vinjé, J., de Medici, D., & Monroe, S. (2002). Foodborne viruses. *FEMS Microbiology Reviews, 26*, 187–205.
Lopman, B. A., Reacher, M. H., Vipond, I. B., Hill, D., Perry, C., Halladay, T., et al. (2004). Epidemiology and cost of nosocomial gastroenteritis, Avon, England, 2002–2003. *Emerging Infectious Diseases, 10*, 1827–1834.
Mead, P. S., Slutsker, L., Dietz, V., McCaig, L. F., Bresee, J. S., Shapiro, C., et al. (1999). Food-related illness and death in the United States. *Emerging Infectious Diseases, 5*, 607–625.
Mishiro, S. (2004). Recent topics on hepatitis E virus: Emerging, zoonotic, and animal-to-human transmission in Japan. *Uirusu, 54*, 243–248.
Pedrique, B., Strub-Wourgaft, N., Some, C., Olliaro, P., Trouiller, P., Ford, N., et al. (2013). The drug and vaccine landscape for neglected diseases (2000-11): A systematic assessment. *The Lancet. Global Health, 1*, e371–e379.
Pintó & Bosch. (2008). Rethinking virus detection in food. In M. P. G. Koopmans, D. O. Vliver, & A. Bosch (Eds.), *Foodborne viruses: Progress and challenges.* Washington: ASM Press.
Rodríguez-Lázaro, D., Cook, N., Ruggeri, F. M., Sellwood, J., Nasser, A., Nascimento, M. S., et al. (2012). Virus hazards from food, water and other contaminated environments. *FEMS Microbiology Reviews, 36*, 786–814.
Rzeżutka & Cook. (2004). Survival of human enteric viruses in the environment and food. *FEMS Microbiology Reviews, 28*, 441–453.
Scallan, E., Griffin, P. M., Angulo, F. J., Tauxe, R. V., & Hoekstra, R. M. (2011). Foodborne illness acquired in the United States—Unspecified agents. *Emerging Infectious Diseases, 17*, 16–22.
Scallan, E., Hoekstra, R. M., Angulo, F. J., Tauxe, R. V., Widdowson, M. A., Roy, S. L., et al. (2011). Foodborne illness acquired in the United States—Major pathogens. *Emerging Infectious Diseases, 17*, 7–15.
Scharff, R. L. (2012). Economic burden from health losses due to foodborne illness in the United States. *Journal of Food Protection, 75*, 123–131.

Tei, S., Kitajima, N., Ohara, S., Inoue, Y., Miki, M., Yamatani, T., et al. (2004). Consumption of uncooked deer meat as a risk factor for hepatitis E virus infection: An age- and sex-matched case-control study. *Journal of Medical Virology*, *74*, 67–70.

Thompson, S. S., Jackson, J. L., Suva-Castillo, M., Yanko, W. A., El Jack, Z., Kuo, J., et al. (2003). Detection of infectious human adenoviruses in tertiary-treated and ultraviolet-disinfected wastewater. *Water Environment Research*, *75*, 163–170.

van den Berg, H., Lodder, W., van der Poel, W., Vennema, H., & de Roda Husman, A. M. (2005). Genetic diversity of noroviruses in raw and treated sewage water. *Research in Microbiology*, *156*, 532–540.

Vantarakis, A., & Papapetropoulou, M. (1999). Detection of enteroviruses, adenoviruses and hepatitis A viruses in raw sewage and treated effluents by nested-PCR. *Water, Air, and Soil Pollution*, *114*, 85–93.

Wallace, D. J., Van Gilder, T., Shallow, S., Fiorentino, T., Segler, S. D., Smith, K. E., et al. (2000). Incidence of foodborne illnesses reported by the foodborne diseases active surveillance network (FoodNet)-1997. FoodNet Working Group. *Journal of Food Protection*, *63*, 807–809.

WHO. (2015). *WHO estimates of the global burden of foodborne diseases*. Geneve: WHO. http://apps.who.int/iris/bitstream/handle/10665/199350/9789241565165_eng.pdf?sequence=1.

WHO. (2017). *Neglected tropical diseases*. Geneve: WHO. www.who.int/neglected_diseases/diseases/en/.

CHAPTER TWO

Norovirus: The Burden of the Unknown

Walter Randazzo*,†, Doris H. D'Souza‡, Gloria Sanchez*,1
*IATA-CSIC, Valencia, Spain
†University of Valencia, Valencia, Spain
‡University of Tennessee, Knoxville, TN, United States
[1]Corresponding author: e-mail address: gloriasanchez@iata.csic.es

Contents

Abstract

Human noroviruses (HNoVs) are primarily transmitted by the fecal–oral route, either by person-to-person contact, or by ingestion of contaminated food or water as well as by aerosolization. Moreover, HNoVs significantly contribute to foodborne diseases being the causative agent of one-fifth of acute gastroenteritis worldwide. As a consequence of globalization, transnational outbreaks of foodborne infections are reported with increasing frequency. Therefore, in this review, state-of-the-art information regarding

Advances in Food and Nutrition Research, Volume 86
ISSN 1043-4526
https://doi.org/10.1016/bs.afnr.2018.02.005
© 2018 Elsevier Inc.
All rights reserved.

molecular procedures for human norovirus detection in food as well common food processing technologies have been summarized. Besides, the purpose of this chapter is to consolidate basic information on various aspects of HNoVs and to summarize food processing technologies that can potentially be applied in the food industry.

1. INTRODUCTION

1.1 Classification and Structure

Human noroviruses (HNoVs) of the *Caliciviridae* family and classified under the *Norovirus* genus, are responsible for sporadic cases and outbreaks of acute gastroenteritis (AGE) (Greening & Cannon, 2016). HNoVs are small round structured, 28–35 nm viruses with a linear, positive-sense, single-stranded RNA genome of about 7.4–7.7 kb in length. The HNoV genome is organized into three open reading frames (ORFs). ORF1 encodes a polyprotein that is posttranslationally cleaved into seven nonstructural mature proteins (NS1–NS7), that functions in viral replication; ORF2 encodes the major capsid protein (VP1) that maintains the virus structure together with ORF3 that encodes the minor capsid protein (VP2) (Vinjé, 2015). The viral capsid VP1 has 90 dimers that consist of a shell domain (S) and a protruding (P) domain. The P domain includes P1 and P2 subregions, where P2 subdomain which is highly variable is reported to contain the putative neutralization sites and interacts with the putative human norovirus cellular receptors called histoblood group antigens (HBGA) (Prasad et al., 1999). Nevertheless, some HNoV strains have been found not to bind any HBGA ligand, suggesting potential additional cofactors (Almand, Moore, & Jaykus, 2017).

HNoVs are currently classified into seven genogroups (G), three of which (GI, GII, and GIV) are responsible for human outbreaks. Furthermore, GI and GII are responsible for the vast majority of clinical cases (Vinjé, 2015).

1.2 Features of Norovirus Infection

Common symptoms associated with HNoV infection are diarrhea, vomiting, nausea, and stomach cramps, together with low-grade fever, headache, chills, muscle aches, and fatigue (Lopman et al., 2015). People with norovirus illness usually develop symptoms of gastroenteritis within 12–48 h after the exposure, and most otherwise healthy people feel better after 1 or 3 days, with symptoms resolving on their own, and are not known to experience any long-term health effects (Teunis et al., 2008).

1.3 Route of Transmission

The main routes of transmission of infectious particles occur due to diarrheal and/or vomiting episodes that release viral particles at high infectious doses/levels, which are main concerns in closed environments such as nursing homes, long-term care and healthcare facilities, concerts, events, and cruise-ships (Marsh et al., 2017; Sánchez, Randazzo, & D'Souza, 2018). For the latter, the majority (97%) of AGE outbreaks that were reported and diagnosed on cruise ships in the United States during 2008–14 were caused by HNoVs (Mouchtouri et al., 2017). Infected foodhandlers, food service workers, sewage treatment workers have all been identified as contributing to HNoV outbreaks. Ready-to-eat foods that do not undergo further processing, fresh leafy greens, fresh and frozen vegetables and fruits, sliced deli meats, ice (Cheng et al., 2017), and bakery items have all been implicated in HNoV outbreaks (D'Souza, Moe, & Jaykus, 2007; Sánchez et al., 2018).

1.4 Epidemiology

In spite of the increasing rate of reported outbreaks caused by HNoVs, their incidence has been challenging to estimate due to the technical limitations associated with their diagnosis and also because of the mild and self-limiting nature of the disease. In fact, HNoV cases are very often not reported to public authorities since it rarely requires medical care or hospitalization, though sometimes, it is needed and occurs for the elderly or immunocompromised (Atmar et al., 2014; Teunis et al., 2008). Given this fact of underreporting of HNoV outbreaks, HNoVs are still reported to remain the leading causative agents of foodborne infections and AGE worldwide, having epidemic as well as sporadic incidences (WHO, 2015). Globally, there are an estimated 120 million illnesses, with over 35,000 deaths attributed to HNoV foodborne illness each year (WHO, 2015) and an annual estimated cost of $64.5 billion (Bartsch, Lopman, Ozawa, Hall, & Lee, 2016). According to the latest epidemiological data available, HNoVs are the cause of 9%–20% of foodborne outbreaks reported in Europe (EFSA, 2015a, 2016a), with 12,591 cases, 349 hospitalizations, and 1 death in 2015. In the United States, the incidence of foodborne outbreaks caused by HNoV during 1998–2015 was 5362 outbreaks, 140,101 illnesses, 1431 hospitalizations, and 13 deaths (assessed online 10/10/2017 at https://wwwn.cdc.gov/foodborneoutbreaks).

HNoV outbreak incidences do not appear to vary much among low-, middle-, and high-income settings, thus making them the leading cause of diarrheal diseases even in high-income countries with about 18 cases per 100 persons (Lopman et al., 2015). Additionally, it has been predicted that a person will experience an average of three to eight episodes of HNoV gastroenteritis in their lifetime, of which at least one will occur under the age of 5 years (Patel, 2008). A seasonal variation of reported outbreaks has been observed in high-income countries with higher rates in winter, although it seems to depend more on healthcare infections rather than foodborne infections (McLeod, Polo, Le Saux, & Le Guyader, 2017).

1.5 Norovirus in Food

Contamination of a food item with HNoVs can occur at any point from the farm to fork. Examples of food items implicated in outbreaks have been reported earlier. In the past, most of the outbreaks have been linked to shellfish, though most food items (leaf greens, fresh and frozen berries, and mixed in smoothies or juices, fresh and frozen vegetables, herbs as ingredients in food preparations), sliced deli meats, bakery items, are all known to be implicated depending on handling, processing, and storage conditions. As reported earlier, closed setting environments and restaurants, hotels, and catering services are most common places of HNoV outbreaks (Chen, Hall, & Kirk, 2017; EFSA, 2016a; Hall, Wikswo, Pringle, Gould, & Parashar, 2014).

Approximately 14% of all HNoV outbreaks worldwide can be attributed to contaminated food (Verhoef et al., 2015), in the same order of magnitude as the 36% reported in the United States and 9.8% in the European Union as estimated from outbreak surveillance data (CDC, 2017; EFSA, 2017; Hall et al., 2014). Globally, foodborne hazards cause approximately 600 million illnesses annually, mainly due to infectious agents causing diarrheal diseases, with HNoVs being responsible for 120 million cases attributed to water and food (WHO, 2015).

2. ADVANCES IN THE CULTIVATION OF HUMAN NOROVIRUS

One of the most important breakthroughs in HNoV research has been the successful cultivation of multiple HNoV strains (including four GII.4 variants and GII.3, GII.17, and GI.1) in human jejuna enteroid monolayers (Ettayebi et al., 2016). Although, differences exist among the HNoV strains depending on the varying contents of the intestine (bile as an example) that promote HNoV replication. While further strides need to be made to increase the propagation and infection levels of this system (currently at

~1200 and ~2.0×10^4 genome equivalents/well depending on the strain), this breakthrough should enable research that has been previously hindered (Ettayebi et al., 2016). These numerous challenges in the successful propagation of HNoVs reproducibly and high titer that have continued to prevail has hindered the study of understanding HNoV–host interactions, transmission and control mechanisms (Knight, Li, Uyttendaele, & Jaykus, 2013).

In the past (since the 1970s), numerous studies to better understand the infection and pathology of HNoVs were undertaken by infecting healthy volunteers (Atmar & Estes, 2001; Dolin et al., 1972; Frenck et al., 2012; Hutson, Atmar, Graham, & Estes, 2002; Lindesmith et al., 2003; Lindesmith et al., 2005; Richards, 2012). Thus ethical issues were a natural concern, along with study reproducibility. More recent studies then focused on using laboratory studies with animal models including chimpanzees (Bok et al., 2011), mice (Taube et al., 2013), calves (Souza, Azevedo, Jung, Cheetham, & Saif, 2008), and pigs. The animal rights issues, ethics, handling, and expense of these models continue to remain a concern.

As reported earlier (Sánchez et al., 2018), more suitable then would be cell lines, primary cultures, as well as three-dimensional cultures simulating intestinal tissues for in vitro replication of HNoVs which were not very successful in obtaining reproducible or infectious titers at high levels (Duizer et al., 2004; Lay et al., 2010; Papafragkou, Hewitt, Park, Greening, & Vinjé, 2013). HNoV cultivation in B cells was reported recently but the limitation was replication for only a single HNoV strain at limited levels (Jones et al., 2015, 2014). Thus, currently though expensive with much needed expertise, the human jejuna enteroid monolayers lay the foundation for future in vitro studies with HNoVs.

3. NOROVIRUS DETECTION IN FOOD

Despite accounting for approximately one-fifth of all AGE cases worldwide, HNoV has received comparatively less attention than other foodborne pathogens (Bartsch et al., 2016). So far, routine methods are not available for cultivation of HNoV isolated from food matrices. Because of the increasing number of HNoV foodborne outbreaks, it has become even more important to have reliable and widely applicable techniques for the detection and quantification of HNoV in food. Moreover, since the infectious dose of HNoV is very low (18–2,800 genomic equivalents) (Teunis et al., 2008), sensitive methods are therefore needed when screening food products for HNoV. HNoV detection has basically been tackled by using the detection of viral genomes by molecular amplification techniques such as reverse transcriptase polymerase chain reaction (RT-PCR) or real-time quantitative PCR (RT-qPCR). Though, traditional sequencing and whole genome sequencing seem to be the trend to detect and classify HNoV strains in outbreak tracking (Yang et al., 2017).

3.1 Virus Extraction From Food

Extraction of HNoV from food can be defined as the separation and concentration of HNoV particles from the food matrix. Such methodologies usually consist of a virus elution step, following by virus concentration and purification designed to reduce sample volume and remove at least some of the matrix compounds while simultaneously recovering most of the contaminating viruses. The type of food, its composition, and the route of contamination determine how to release viruses from food before nucleic acid extraction (Bosch et al., 2011), and therefore many different methods have been developed (Stals, Baert, Van Coillie, & Uyttendaele, 2012).

Usually, an elution buffer is used to release HNoV from food. Many virus concentration procedures use manipulation of pH and/or ionic conditions to facilitate virus adsorption to, or elution from the food matrix. Beef extract and glycine are commonly added to the elution buffers in order to reduce nonspecific virus adsorption to the food matrix (Stals et al., 2012). Moreover, the high protein concentration of beef extract facilitates flocculation of viruses during polyethylene glycol (PEG) precipitation. However, beef extract might also interfere with molecular detection methods, which may result in false-negative results. PEG precipitation is then followed by relatively low speed centrifugation after which the virus precipitate is recovered for further purification.

Quality control checks including internal amplification controls and process controls are essential to monitor any issue that can result in false-negative results (D'Agostino, Cook, Rodriguez-Lazaro, & Rutjes, 2011). With regard to this issue, the ISO 15216-1:2017 includes the use of a titrated mengovirus suspension as a process control, that is added during the initial step of the extraction and is assayed and quantified by RT-qPCR at the end of the procedure (Costafreda, Bosch, & Pintó, 2006). This provides an accurate estimation of the performance of the whole procedure. As there does not seem to a universal extraction protocol to efficiently recover human enteric viruses from all types of foods, the ISO 15216-1:2017 proposes different virus elution and concentration methods depending on the sample, i.e., treatment of the digestive glands with proteinase K for shellfish, precipitation with PEG for soft fruits and leafy vegetables, and adsorption on to positively charged membranes followed by ultrafiltration for bottled water (as described in Sanchez et al., 2018). Even though concentration methods applied to a contaminated food are known to have a great impact on the performance of the procedures, comparatively little attention has been given to this area (Butot, Zuber, & Baert, 2014).

Once the virus is extracted, either infectivity assays when available could be used and/or molecular methods for detection. For molecular detection, RNA has to be first released or extracted by disruption of the viral capsid. The standard Boom protocol that uses chaotropic reagents followed by adsorption of RNA to silica particles (Boom et al., 1990) or commercial kits can be used to obtain purified and high yield of RNA.

Alternatively, nucleic acid aptamers, short ssDNA sequences having binding affinity for HNoV, have been used as binding ligands to capture and concentrate HNoV from lettuce (Escudero-Abarca, Suh, Moore, Dwivedi, & Jaykus, 2014).

Currently, different international institutions such as the US CDC (https://www.cdc.gov/norovirus/lab-testing/diagnostic.htmland) and Health Canada (http://www.hc-sc.gc.ca/fn-an/res-rech/analy-meth/microbio/volume5-eng.php#share) have published procedures for HNoV detection in food samples. Moreover, a standardized RT-qPCR-based procedure has recently been issued for HNoV GI and GII in several food matrices, including shellfish, berries, vegetables, and bottled water (ISO 15216-1:2017), including an international validation study involving 18 laboratories from 11 countries (Lowther et al., 2017).

3.2 Molecular Detection Methods

Traditional means for microbial detection cannot be applied for HNoV detection in food, however, molecular methodologies can provide timely and accurate information about the presence of HNoV in food. So far, several newer molecular procedures have been applied to detect and quantify HNoVs in food such as nucleic acid sequence-based amplification, NASBA (Houde et al., 2006; Kou, Wu, Zhang, & Fan, 2006; Moore et al., 2004), and reverse-transcriptase loop-mediated isothermal amplification techniques, RT-LAMP (Fukuda, Takao, Kuwayama, Shimazu, & Miyazaki, 2006). However, RT-qPCR remains the current gold standard for HNoV detection, due to its sensitivity, specificity, speed, and ability to deliver quantitative data (as also described in Sanchez et al., 2018).

During the development of molecular assays, highly conserved primers–probe set should be targeted to increase the ability to detect the varying strains of HNoV among the genogroups that affect humans. The ORF1/ORF2 junction is reportedly the best genome region target for HNoV detection (Höhne & Schreier, 2004; Kageyama et al., 2003; Katayama et al., 2002; Loisy et al., 2005; Nishida et al., 2003). Yet currently, a single assay to simultaneously detect all HNoV genotypes remains elusive.

Although the current gold standard, RT-qPCR methodologies have drawbacks in detecting the viral RNA of both infectious and inactivated HNoV, potentially overestimating the amount of infectious viruses. In fact, the persistence of viral RNA in food and in the environment may be much greater than that of the corresponding infectious viruses (Baert, Uyttendaele, Van Coillie, & Debevere, 2008; Butot, Putallaz, Amoroso, & Sánchez, 2009; Butot, Putallaz, & Sánchez, 2008; Hewitt & Greening, 2004). To enable differentiation between infectious and inactivated viral particles, different approaches based on capsid integrity have been reported (DiCaprio, 2017; Sanchez et al., 2018), including: (i) pretreatment with nucleases and/or proteolytic enzymes prior to nucleic acid extraction in order to remove any signal form damaged or exposed genomes (Lamhoujeb, Fliss, Ngazoa, & Jean, 2008; Nowak et al., 2011); (ii) use of binding of HNoV (with intact binding site) to porcine gastric mucin (PGM) (Tan & Jiang, 2005; Tang et al., 2010) which allows for selective recovery of potentially infectious HNoVs in foods (Dancho, Chen, & Kingsley, 2012; DiCaprio et al., 2016), and (iii) pretreatment of nucleic acid with conventional and newly developed intercalating dyes (i.e., propidium monoazide, PMA and ethidium monoazide, EMA; PMAxx and PEMAX, respectively) (Elizaquível, Aznar, & Sánchez, 2014; Randazzo, López-Gálvez, Allende, Aznar, & Sánchez, 2016). This approach is based on the ability of intercalating dyes to penetrate only damaged or altered capsids and intercalates covalently into the viral genome after exposure to strong visible light, thus preventing and interfering with PCR amplification. Until now, intercalating dyes combined with RT-qPCR have successfully been applied to virus suspensions in order to discriminate between infectious and inactivated HNoV (Table 1), and additionally these pretreatments have been already applied to detect potentially infectious HNoVs in water samples, sewage, vegetables, and shellfish and discriminate between infectious and noninfectious virions (Randazzo et al., 2018; Randazzo, López-Gálvez, et al., 2016). Interestingly, this approach

Table 1 Application of Intercalating Dyes for the Detection of Potentially Infectious Human Noroviruses

Inactivation Process	Dye/Surfactant	Matrix	Successful Discrimination	References
Heat (72°C, 5 min)	PMA		Yes by RT-PCR but not by RT-qPCR	Parshionikar, Laseke, and Fout (2010)
Heat (90°C, 5 min)	PMA	Stool suspension	Yes (SYBR green RT-qPCR)	Escudero-Abarca, Rawsthorne, Goulter, Suh, and Jaykus (2014)
Heat	PMA		No (by RT-PCR)	Karim, Fout, Johnson, White, and Parshionikar (2015)
Chlorine				
Chlorine	PMA/sodium lauroylsarcosinate		Yes	Lee, Lee, Yoon, Kim, and Ha (2018)
Heat (65–85°C, 2 min)	PMA	Stool and spinach	Yes	Jeong, Park, and Ha (2017)
Heat (99°C, 5 min)	PMAxx/Triton	Stool, lettuce, and spinach	Yes	Randazzo, López-Gálvez, et al. (2016)
		Mussels, oysters, and cockles	Yes	Randazzo et al. (2018)

proved to reduce false-positive RT-qPCR signals for HNoV in naturally contaminated water samples (Blanco et al., 2017; Randazzo et al., 2018; Randazzo, López-Gálvez, et al., 2016). On the other hand, some downsides with this approach have been noted, particularly to achieve complete suppression of RT-qPCR signal from the inactivated viruses present in some particular food matrices, e.g., shellfish (Randazzo et al., 2018). As mentioned earlier, whole genome sequencing of viruses from outbreak and food samples are being pursued for simultaneous detection and confirmation of HNoV strains in outbreak tracking, though significant progress needs to be made for routing food sample testing to link to clinical settings.

4. PREVALENCE OF HUMAN NOROVIRUS IN FOODS

Additionally as mentioned earlier (Sanchez et al., 2018), shellfish and all ready-to-eat foods have been implicated in HNoV outbreaks indicating HNoV prevalence in them. Shellfish contamination by HNoVs has been and continues to be an important health and economic problem (Bellou, Kokkinos, & Vantarakis, 2013). Last year, the European Commission launched a monitoring program to estimate the European prevalence of HNoV contamination in oysters collected from representative monitoring points at production areas and dispatch centers using the ISO 15216-1:2017 (EFSA, 2016b; ISO 15216-1:2017). Moreover, the health risks associated with the consumption of raw oysters are not sufficiently reduced by current commercial depuration procedures applied to reduce microbiological contamination (McLeod et al., 2017). High levels of HNoV in oysters have been reported to date, with markedly varying levels between sites in Europe, with some sites scoring consistently over 1000 copies/g during the winter while others rarely or never exceeding 100 copies/g (EFSA Panel on Biological Hazards, 2012; Polo et al., 2016; Schaeffer, Le Saux, Lora, Atmar, & Le Guyader, 2013).

Belgium, Canada, and France were the first countries to provide data about the prevalence of HNoV on more than 1000 samples of leafy greens. HNoV genomes were frequently detected (28.2%, 33.3%, and 50%, in Canadian, Belgian, and French samples, respectively); however, sequence confirmation was not successful for the majority of the samples tested (Baert et al., 2011). In salad vegetables from European countries, samples were positive in 2% and 2.95% for HNoV GI and HNoV GII, respectively (Kokkinos et al., 2012). In samples from Mexico, HNoV was present in 32.6% samples (Felix-Valenzuela, Resendiz-Sandoval, Burgara-Estrella,

Hernández, & Mata-Haro, 2012) while in Turkey, from 525 samples analyzed, HNoV GII was detected in 1 green onion sample and 1 tomato sample by both SYBR Green and TaqMan RT-qPCR assays (Yilmaz et al., 2011). A recent study performed on salad greens from the Nile Delta showed the validity of the ISO 15216-1:2017 procedure in products naturally contaminated with HNoVs detecting HNoV GI in 20.8%–34.0% of naturally contaminated samples including green onions, watercress, radish, leek, and lettuce with genome copy numbers of around 10^2 per gram (El-Senousy, Costafreda, Pintó, & Bosch, 2013). In 2016, following an outbreak alert in Europe (Rapid Alert System for Food and Feed, RASFF, expedient 2017/0469), Blanco et al. (2017) determined drinking bottled water as the possible source of HNoV transmission. The study estimated the concentration of HNoV GI and GII in two of the four samples as around 10^3–10^4 genome copies per liter of water.

5. APPROACHES TO CONTROL HUMAN NOROVIRUSES IN FOOD PRODUCTS

As nonenveloped viruses, HNoVs tend to be more resistant to inactivation than foodborne bacteria to traditional food manufacturing processes. Most studies to determine the efficacy of different processing technologies as well as the antiviral activity of different compounds have been performed by artificially adding a known amount of virus to a given material, determining the reduction in the infectious titer after subjecting the spiked material to designated conditions, and applying statistical procedures to determine the significance of virus decay (Sánchez & Bosch, 2016). Evidently, this implies the use of virus strains that may be propagated in cell culture and enumerated through infectivity, thus greatly restricting the range of strains that are able to be included in these studies due to the difficulties in developing in vitro cultivation systems to replicate HNoVs. Thus, the infectivity of HNoVs has mainly been inferred through culturable surrogates, such as feline calicivirus (FCV), murine norovirus (MNV), and Tulane virus (TV) (Hirneisen & Kniel, 2013a). Even though these virus models have largely been used to study the survival rate of HNoVs exposed to different inactivation processes, it remains unclear whether HNoVs could be inactivated by the inactivation conditions established for its surrogates (Bae & Schwab, 2008; Knight et al., 2016; NACMCF, 2016). As reported earlier, the environmental persistence of HNoV depends on many physical, biological, and chemical factors such as temperature, ionic strength, chemical constituents, microbial antagonism, the status of the virus (such as virus bound to organic matter or virus aggregation), and the type of virus (Cook, Knight, & Richards, 2016; Knight et al., 2016; Sánchez et al., 2018). Different genotypes of HNoVs have been reported to show different behavior and inactivation rates.

5.1 Norovirus Inactivation by Thermal Processing

Thermal processing remains one of the most important and common methods of food preservation in the food industry (Micali, Fiorino, & Parisi, 2016). Thermal processing has been proven to be a very effective technology for the inactivation of bacteria and yeast. However, until recently heat inactivation of enteric viruses, particularly HNoVs in food, had been poorly explored. It is clearly known that inactivation of HNoVs or any microorganism by heat is influenced by factors such as the presence of organic matter, such as fecal material, the food matrix (e.g., high content of fats or proteins), the initial level of contamination, and the process time–temperature (Li, Predmore, Divers, & Lou, 2012). Understanding the thermal resistance and properties of a target pathogen remains crucial in order to design effective thermal treatment processes for their inactivation and control, which is determined using the *D*-value, defined as the time at a given temperature to cause a 1 log reduction of the target (Bozkurt, D'Souza, & Davidson, 2015). This section focuses on studies using HNoV while information from studies involving only surrogates is not included.

HNoV GI on basil after heating at 75 and 95°C had *D*-values of 5.2 and 4.9 min, on chives of <0.83 min and <0.83 min, on mint of 2.57 min and < 0.83 min, and on parsley of 1.56 and 1.58 min, respectively, when analyzed by RT-qPCR (Butot et al., 2009). While HNoV GII after analysis by RT-qPCR after heating at 75 and 95°C showed *D*-values of 1.71 and 1.55 min on basil, 1.85 and 1.08 min on chives, 1.58 and <0.83 min on mint, 1.64 and 0.89 min on parsley, respectively (Butot et al., 2009). The effect of common cooking procedures on HNoV GII.3 inoculated onto various food products was investigated by RT-qPCR, where spiced tomato sauce treated at 74°C for 1 min, minced meat roasted at 200°C for 30 min, and frozen pizza baked at 200°C for 12 min showed reduction of 0.4, 1.6, and >4 log HNoV genome copies (Mormann, Dabisch, & Becker, 2010). Additionally, spinach, lettuce, and lamb's lettuce have been used as food matrices to assess HNoVs infectivity after heat treatments by applying different intercalating dyes pretreatment coupled with RT-qPCR (Jeong et al., 2017; Randazzo, López-Gálvez, et al., 2016).

The occurrence of HNoV outbreaks associated with the consumption of fried, grilled, stewed, and steamed shellfish indicates that standard cooking procedures do not guarantee complete inactivation of HNoV (McDonnell et al., 1997). Initial studies were performed using HNoV surrogates while more recent studies focused on HNoV using RT-qPCR alone or combined with PGM or intercalating dye pretreatments, where HNoVs in mussels heated at 100°C showed *D*-values of 1.3 min by RT-qPCR (Hewitt & Greening, 2006) and HNoVs in mussels heated at 60°C showed *D*-values of 25 min by RT-qPCR (Croci, Suffredini, Di Pasquale, & Cozzi, 2012). Similarly, Randazzo et al. (2018) assessed the fate of HNoVs GI and GII in bioaccumulated and naturally contaminated oysters after being heat treated. Applying a PMAxx pretreatment before the RT-qPCR to predict HNoVs infectivity, the authors reported reductions of 1.61 and 2.18, and 2.99 and 1.93 log RT-PCRU/100 μL for HNoVs GI and GII in bioaccumulated and naturally contaminated oysters, respectively. Moreover, in bioaccumulated oysters, differences in reduction values between nondye pretreatment and dye-pretreatments increased gradually along with the stepwise increase in temperature, even these results may underestimate the real rate of HNoV inactivation as reported before.

In general, cooking procedures in which an internal temperature of the shellfish reaches at least 90°C for 1.5 min have been considered adequate treatments to eliminate viral infectivity (Codex Alimentarius, 2012; NACMCF, 2008), though recent EFSA publications indicate higher times may be needed (EFSA, 2015b).

5.2 Norovirus Inactivation by Nonthermal Processing

In recent years, the interest for high-quality food products is constantly increasing due to consumer demand. Thus, developments in nonthermal technologies have been advanced by both industry and academia in an attempt to meet the challenge of producing safe processed food of a high quality, although some concerns as to current consumer acceptability and regulation have limited their applications.

5.2.1 High-Pressure Processing (HPP)

HPP is a nonthermal, cold processing technique in which the food in its final flexible packaging is subjected to high levels of hydrostatic pressure, inactivating microorganisms, extending the shelf life, and guaranteeing the food safety of the product (Rodrigo, van Loey, & Hendrickx, 2007). Effects of HNoV by HPP have mainly been investigated using HNoV surrogates while little information is available on HNoVs (Table 2; adapted

Table 2 Effect of HPP Treatments on Human Noroviruses Applied to Food Samples

HNoV Genotype	Pressure (MPa)	Processing Conditions (Time, Temperature)	Food Type	Inactivation (Log Reduction)	References
GI	650	2 min, 0°C	Raspberries	2.5	Huang et al. (2016)
	600	5 min, 6°C	Oysters	4.0	Leon et al. (2011)
		2 min, 1°C	Green onions	>3.0	Sido, Huang, Liu, and Chen (2017)
		2 min, 0°C	Strawberry quarters	1.9	Huang et al. (2016)
	550	2 min, 0°C	Strawberry puree	>3.0	Huang et al. (2016)
			Blueberry puree	2.9	
			Raspberry puree	2.9	
	500	2 min, 1°C	Salsa (mainly tomatoes)	>3.0	Sido et al. (2017)
		2 min, 0°C	Blueberry	>3.2	Huang et al. (2016)
			Oysters	>4.3	Ye et al. (2015)
		5 min, 1°C	Clam's homogenate	4.0	Ye, Li, Kingsley, Jiang, and Chen (2014)
	450			4.1	
	400			2.8	

GII	650	2 min, 0°C	Strawberry quarters	3.1	Huang et al. (2016)
	550	2 min, 0°C	Blueberry puree	>4.4	Huang et al. (2016)
			Raspberry	>4.1	
	500	2 min, 1°C	Green onions	>3.0	Sido et al. (2017)
		5 min, 1°C	Oyster's homogenate	4.0	Ye et al. (2014)
	450			4.3	
	400			2.9	
		2 min, 0°C	Strawberry puree	>4.2	Huang et al. (2016)
		5 min, 25°C	Oyster	1.87–1.99	Imamura et al. (2017)
	350	2 min, 0°C	Raspberry puree	>4.2	Huang et al. (2016)
			Oysters	>4.2	Ye et al. (2015)
	300	2 min, 1°C	Salsa (mainly tomatoes)	>3.0	Sido et al. (2017)
		2 min, 0°C	Blueberries	>4.1	Huang et al. (2016)

Adapted from Sánchez, G., Randazzo, W., & D'Souza, Ḋ. H. (2018). Chapter 10: Human Noroviruses. In D. Liu (Ed.), Handbook of foodborne diseases. Taylor & Francis.

from Sánchez et al., 2018), showing that different processing factors (pressure, holding temperature, and time) and food properties (pH, fat, salt, sugar, or protein content) are key factors that need to be considered during the design of effective HPP treatments (reviewed by Kingsley, 2013; Lou, Neetoo, Chen, & Li, 2015; Sanchez et al., 2018). For instance, higher inactivation of HNoV and its surrogates are reported at neutral than at acidic pH when applying HPP (Chen, Hoover, & Kingsley, 2005; Kingsley & Chen, 2008; Li, Chen, & Kingsley, 2013; Lou et al., 2016; Lou, Neetoo, Chen, & Li, 2011), which was confirmed for HNoV GI and GII using a PGM capture method (Li, Chen, & Kingsley, 2013). Low temperatures also enhanced the HPP effect on HNoV surrogates (Kingsley, Holliman, Calci, Chen, & Flick, 2007; Lou et al., 2011; Sánchez, Aznar, Martínez, & Rodrigo, 2011) and HNoVs GII (Lou et al., 2016). A baroprotective effect was observed with $CaCl_2$, NaCl, and sucrose using HNoV surrogates (Kingsley & Chen, 2008; Sánchez et al., 2011), which were also reported by Lou et al. (2016) for HNoV GII in PBS and DMEM in comparison to water. HPP of artificially contaminated foods including vegetables, purees, clams, and oysters have been summarized in Table 2 (adapted from Sánchez et al., 2018). HNoV GI was reported to be inactivated at 600 MPa for 5 min at 6°C in a human volunteer study, while 400 MPa at 6°C for 5 min did not protect all volunteers (Leon et al., 2011). HNoV genotype GII.4 is reported to be more sensitive to pressure treatments than GI.1 (Huang et al., 2016; Li, Chen, & Kingsley, 2013; Lou et al., 2016; Ye et al., 2014).

5.2.2 High-Pressure Homogenization (HPH)

HPH is a purely mechanical and continuous process with relatively lower pressure (<400 MPa) and shorter exposure time (s), ideal for liquid foods. There are not many studies reported in literature as of date using this approach. HPH at 300 MPa for <2 s showed reduction of 3 log for FCV-F9 in buffer, milk, and juices, while MNV-1 was more resistant and showed much lower titer reduction (D'Souza, Su, Roach, & Harte, 2009; Horm & D'Souza, 2011; Horm, Davidson, Harte, & D'Souza, 2012; Horm, Harte, & D'Souza, 2012).

5.2.3 Atmospheric Pressure Plasma (APP)

APP is an innovative approach which uses a neutral ionized gas that contains highly reactive species of ions, molecules, and photons (Wan, Coventry,

Swiergon, Sanguansri, & Versteeg, 2009). As summarized by Sanchez et al. (2018), cold APP (CAPP) treatment on HNoV GII.4 has shown that increased plasma treatment times led to decreased genome copies of HNoV on inoculated surfaces (Ahlfeld et al., 2015). Similarly, the CAP plasma generation power, the feed gas mixture, the exposure time and distance, and the virus suspension medium affected FCV-F9 inactivation (Aboubakr et al., 2015). Alshraiedeh, Alkawareek, Gorman, Graham, and Gilmore (2013) used a nonthermal plasma jet that showed rapid reduction of 3 log after 3 min and more than 7 log after 9 min for MS2 bacteriophage. Nonthermal plasma treatments of stainless steel surfaces were reported to show reductions for HNoV surrogates, with ranking of reduction being FCV-F9 > MS2 > MNV-1 (D'Souza, 2013). With respect to treatment of foods, APP jet treatment after 5 min on fresh meats caused >2 log reduction in MNV infectivity without changing meat quality (Bae, Park, Choe, & Ha, 2015), while dielectric barrier discharge APP reportedly reduced TV by only 0.7 log in packaged lettuce (Min et al., 2016).

5.2.4 High-Power Ultrasound (HPU)

HPU has shown to effectively inactivate bacteria in liquid foods and fresh produce at low frequencies arranging from 20 to 100 kHz (Bilek & Turantaş, 2013). HPU at 0.56 kW/L, 20 kHz for 60 min was reported to be ineffective for MNV-1 reduction in lettuce wash water (Sánchez, Elizaquível, Aznar, & Selma, 2015), though 1.5 log reduction of MNV-1 after 30 min in orange juice was reported earlier (Su, Zivanovic, & D'Souza, 2010). Furthermore, steam ultrasound as well showed that this technology currently as set does not appear to be adequate for foodborne viral decontamination until further optimization of parameters can be achieved (Schultz, Uhrbrand, NØrrung, & Dalsgaard, 2012).

5.2.5 Radiation

Ionizing radiations for food safety purposes indicate doses of 10 kGy by WHO, 4 kGy for fresh iceberg lettuce and spinach, and 5.5 kGy in fresh seafood products by the FDA (Food and Drug Administration, 2012; Goodburn & Wallace, 2013; and as described in Sanchez et al., 2018). HNoV surrogates are reported to be more resistant to irradiation (ionizing) than bacterial pathogens, and this technology does not seem to be adequately effective against HNoV strains (Sánchez et al., 2018). After 5.0 kGy X-ray treatment, MNV-1 internalized in whole-shell oysters showed 2.0 log

PFU/g reduction (Wu et al., 2017), 2.6 log PFU/g reduction in tuna salad, and >3.5 log PFU/g in half-shell oysters and salmon sushi (Wu et al., 2016). While at 5.6 kGy, 1.7–2.4 log MNV-1 reduction were reported in fresh produce (Feng, Divers, Ma, & Li, 2011).

E-beam irradiation at 4 kGy decreased TV by 1.4 and 1.3 log in strawberries and lettuce, respectively (Predmore et al., 2015), and MNV-1 by 0.4 and 0.7 log in strawberries and cabbage, respectively (Sanglay, Li, Uribe, & Lee, 2011). Gamma irradiation showed better performance than e-beam against HNoV GII.4 (DiCaprio et al., 2016), though the PGM-MB binding assay showed that doses of 22.4 kGy greater than the currently approved levels in whole strawberries were needed to abolish receptor-binding activity. In a very recent study, e-beam at 1, 3, 5, 7, and 10 kGy decreased MNV infectivity by 0.31, 0.6, 0.9, 1.1, and 1.4 log in shellfish meat, respectively, while the sensory parameters evaluated were not significantly modified (Kim, Park, Rui, & Ha, 2017).

The wavelength range for ultraviolet (UV) light for food processing varies from 100 to 400 nm and is categorized as UV-A (320–400 nm), UV-B (280–320 nm), and UV-C (200–280 nm).

UV-C has received FDA approval to control microorganisms on surfaces of food products (Food and Drug Administration, 2007; Li et al., 2011; Park, Kim, Lee, & Ha, 2015). UV-C treatment after 5 min was shown to decrease MNV-1 titers by less than 1 log on fresh-cut lettuce, though 3 log reduction was observed on stainless steel discs, indicating that surface topography, dose, distance, time, matrix are all factors that play a role in the treatment efficacy and that coupling with vaporized hydrogen peroxide can increase its effects (Li et al., 2011). MNV-1 was completely inactivated (>4 log) when blueberries were immersed in agitated water during 12 J/cm^2 of water-assisted UV treatment, with lower 2.5 log reduction with dry UV treatment (Liu, Li, & Chen, 2015).

Pulsed UV light is applicable for food and food-contact surface decontamination by using a xenon lamp emitting wavelengths between 200 and 1000 nm, and pulse durations not exceeding 2 ms, and cumulative intensity not exceeding 12 J/cm^2 (Food and Drug Administration, 2013). MNV-1 was reported to be completely inactivated with pulsed UV light operated at 59 mWs/cm^2 that caused virus structure alterations, with greater reduction on fomites than in liquid, with expected lower efficacy in the presence of organic matter (Jean, Morales-Rayas, Anoman, & Lamhoujeb, 2011; Vimont, Fliss, & Jean, 2015).

5.3 Shellfish Depuration

Shellfish depuration is a commercial processing technology used worldwide, where shellfish are placed in tanks containing clean seawater and allowed to purge the contaminants for several days. Shellfish depuration rapidly removes bacterial pathogens and indicator microorganisms, however the scientific community agrees on the inadequacy of commercial shellfish depuration processes for HNoVs, since there have been many HNoV outbreaks from depurated oysters containing around 10^3 genome copies/g oyster tissue (Le Mennec et al., 2017; McLeod et al., 2017). In addition, half of the publications showed no decrease in HNoV titers during depuration, and in the remaining studies, it took between 9 and 45.5 days for a 1 log reduction, significantly longer than commercial depuration timeframes (reviewed by McLeod et al., 2017). Furthermore, a human volunteer study involving shellfish depuration concluded that the depuration was not successful (Grohmann, Murphy, Christopher, Auty, & Greenberg, 1981).

5.4 Efficacy of Washing Procedures to Eliminate or Inactivate HNoVs on Food Products

Produce and in particular leafy green vegetables and berries that are consumed raw, have gained much recognition as important vehicles for the transmission of foodborne viral pathogens. HNoVs can contaminate produce through contact with incorrectly treated sewage or sewage-polluted water in the fields, as well through contamination irrigation water and irrigation systems, and during processing, storage, distribution, or final preparation. This might occur because HNoV-infected people, contaminated water, or fomites come into contact with foods (Xiao, Tang, & Li, 2017). In fact, experimental studies have shown that approximately 1% of HNoV can be transferred to cucumber from contaminated latex gloves (Rönnqvist et al., 2014). Therefore, improved sanitation and decontamination strategies continue to be researched.

5.4.1 Chlorine and Chlorine Dioxide

The use of chlorine-based sanitizers is widespread throughout the fresh produce industry, with the intention of maintaining microbial safety of produce, avoiding cross-contamination, and recycling water. The mechanism of action of chlorine and chlorine-releasing compounds against viruses is hypothesized to be through destruction of the capsid by oxidation that results in exposure of RNA to degradation by the environment

(Fraisse et al., 2011; Lim, Kim, & Ko, 2010; Tian, Yang, Quigley, Chou, & Jiang, 2013). Many studies have reported on the ability of chlorine and chlorine-based sanitizers to inactivate HNoV and its surrogates (Doultree, Druce, Birch, Bowden, & Marshall, 1999; D'Souza & Su, 2010; Fraisse et al., 2011; Hirneisen & Kniel, 2013a; Lim et al., 2010; Tian et al., 2013) while less information is available on their application in produce. For instance, FCV-F9 infectivity was shown to be reduced by 2.9 log after washing leafy vegetables with 200 ppm chlorine for 2 min (Allwood, Malik, Hedberg, & Goyal, 2004). Butot et al. (2008) explored the efficacy of washing different types of berries and leafy greens with 200 ppm free chlorine, showing that FCV-F9 infectivity was reduced to undetectable levels. Additionally, HNoV inactivation varied according to food type and HNoV genotype, with a maximum of more than 3 log reduction for HNoV GI in blueberries, strawberries, and basil (Butot et al., 2008).

Washing with sodium hypochlorite at 200 mg/L for 15 s was reported to reduce FCV-F9 infectivity on lettuce and jalapeno peppers by less than 1.4 log PFU/mL and to undetectable levels, respectively (Su & D'Souza, 2011). The combination of surfactants (sodium dodecyl sulfate) and polysorbates (Tween 20 at 50 ppm) along with the traditional chlorine (200 ppm) washes, reduced MNV-1 infectivity by 3 log PFU/mL after 1 h in fresh produce (Predmore & Li, 2011). HNoV GI genome copies were reduced by 2.0 log in whole leaf and chopped romaine after chlorine washes at 1.5 and 0.9 mg min/L, respectively, while higher concentrations were needed for HNoV GII inactivation (Dunkin, Weng, Jacangelo, & Schwab, 2017). Free chlorine at 33 and 189 ppm for 1 min using a PGM MB assay was shown to decrease binding of HNoV by 1.4 and 4.1 log, respectively (Kingsley, Vincent, Meade, Watson, & Fan, 2014).

Chlorine dioxide has emerged as an alternative to chlorine as its efficacy is little affected by organic matter and pH, and at 10 ppm for 10 min could inactivate FCV-F9 by less than 1.5 log in raspberries and parsley, and reduced HNoV GI and GII genome copies by less than 1 log (Butot et al., 2008).

5.4.2 Electrostatic Sprays/Electrolyzed Water

Electrolyzed water (EOW)'s exact mechanism of antiviral action remains unclear (Tian, Yang, & Mandrell, 2011). Acidic EOW wash was shown to incrase the binding of HNoV to raspberries and lettuce, causing removal of only ~7.5% and ~4%, respectively (Kingsley & Chen, 2008). A recent study showed that neutral EOW at 250 ppm free available chlorine caused a 4.8 and 0.4 log reduction in HNoV genome copy numbers after 1 min in suspension and on stainless steel, respectively (Moorman, Montazeri, & Jaykus, 2017).

5.4.3 Ozone

Ozone has been used as a strong disinfectant against microorganisms in the environment and on surfaces that can destroy the capsid protein and the viral genome (Kim, Yousef, & Dave, 1999). So far, three studies have reported the effect of gaseous ozone on HNoV surrogates on food matrices (i.e., lettuce, raspberries, strawberries, and green onions) (Hirneisen, Markland, & Kniel, 2011; Predmore, Sanglay, Li, & Lee, 2015). Spraying green onion plants with ozone at 6.25 ppm for 10 min reduced MNV-1 titers by 2.0 log PFU/plant (Hirneisen et al., 2011). Additionally, 6.25 ppm ozone for 4 min reduced FCV-F9 infectivity by more than 6 log $TCID_{50}$/mL in water and by 2 log $TCID_{50}$/mL on lettuce and green onions (Hirneisen & Kniel, 2013b). Comparable inactivation was also obtained for MNV and TV on lettuce and strawberries (Predmore, Sanglay, Li, & Lee, 2015). Very recently, 3 ppm gas ozone for 1 min was shown to reduce MNV-1 infectivity by more than 3.3 log on fresh raspberry (Brié et al., 2018).

5.4.4 Acids/Alkali

Acidic (such as gallic acid and peroxyacetic acid, PAA) as well as alkaline sanitizers have been evaluated against HNoVs or their cultivable surrogates (Cliver, 2009). Though, PAA at 195 ppm reduced HNoV binding by less than 1 log (Kingsley et al., 2014) and at 250 mg/L reduced MNV-1 infectivity by 1 log on shredded lettuce, even in the presence of organic matter (Baert et al., 2009). While washing of lettuce with a PAA-based biocide (100 ppm) for 2 min was reported to cause 3.2 and 2.3 log reduction of FCV-F9 and MNV-1, respectively (Fraisse et al., 2011). Alkaline trisodium phosphate (TSP, pH ~12) at 2% after 30 s was reported to reduce FCV-F9 to nondetectable levels (Su et al., 2010), and when applied at 2% and 5% for 30 s on lettuce and peppers reduced MNV-1 titers by 3 log PFU/mL and to undetectable levels, respectively (Su & D'Souza, 2011). However, the potential disadvantages of TSP to the environment need to be considered.

5.4.5 Natural Compounds

The food industry is driven to seek natural alternate strategies to control pathogens due to the increasing consumer demand for "natural" and "clean" labeled products. To this extent, numerous plant and animal-origin natural compounds have been tested against HNoV surrogates (reviewed by D'Souza, 2014; Li, Baert, & Uyttendaele, 2013; Ryu et al., 2015; Seo & Choi, 2017), with only few reports that have used HNoV strains, i.e., grape seed extract (GSE), green tea extract (GTE) (Falcó et al., 2018; Randazzo, Falcó, Aznar, & Sánchez, 2017), and (−)-epigallocatechin gallate (Falcó et al., 2017; Li et al., 2012) as reported earlier (Sánchez et al., 2018) and summarized in Table 3. Li, Baert, and Uyttendaele (2013) and Li, Baert, et al. (2012) combined a cell-binding RT-qPCR with a saliva-binding ELISA and showed the antiviral effect of GSE on HNoV GII.4. Moreover, recent studies indicated marine algae as novel sources of bioactive compounds that showed in vitro antiviral activity against HNoV surrogates (Choi et al., 2014; Eom et al., 2015). As with any inactivation method, food matrices including proteins and fat decreased the efficacy of bioactives and antimicrobials by protecting or coating viral particles (Li, Baert, et al., 2012). Carvacrol and raspberry juice (Gilling, Kitajima, Torrey, & Bright, 2014; Oh et al., 2012) showed antiviral activity against HNoV surrogates.

Natural compounds that act as photosensitizers include curcumin, a polyphenolic compound extracted from turmeric rhizomes (*Curcuma longa* L.) that has been shown to reduce FCV-F9 and MNV-1 infectivity in solutions using photodynamic inactivation (Randazzo, Aznar, & Sánchez, 2016) and in oysters (Wu et al., 2015; and as reported in Sanchez et al., 2018). The few reports for their use in food applications as mentioned earlier is summarized in Table 3. For example, GSE was reported to be effective in decreasing FCV-F9, MNV-1, and HAV titers on lettuce, jalapeño peppers, apple juice and milk (Joshi et al., 2015; Su & D'Souza, 2013) as well as carvacrol could reduce MNV-1 and FCV-9 levels on lettuce and lettuce wash water (Sánchez, Aznar, & Sánchez, 2015). GTE has also been successfully applied to reduce MNV-1 titers on inoculated lettuce and spinach leaves (Randazzo et al., 2017) and on food contact surfaces (Falcó et al., 2018). Additionally, the enhanced antiviral activity of GTE was related to the change in the amount of catechin derivatives, as a function of pH and storage time (Falcó et al., 2018). Improvements in encapsulation efficiencies and/or release of bioactives in foods is a research needed (Gómez-Mascaraque, Soler, & Lopez-Rubio, 2016).

5.5 Antiviral Polymers for Food Packaging

There is an increasing interest in the application of antimicrobial coatings and films in the food industry, motivated by the increasing consumer

Table 3 Effect of Natural Compounds Against Norovirus Surrogates and HNoV in Food Applications

Natural Compound	Virus (Initial Concentration)	Food Application	Concentration and Test Conditions	Inactivation (Log Reduction)	Reference
Aloe vera extract	MNV (5 log PFU)	Washing cabbage	1 mg/mL at 25°C for 60 min	0.8	Ng et al. (2017)
Carvacrol	FCV (6 log $TCID_{50}$)	Lettuce wash water	0.5% at 37°C for 2 h	3.1	Sánchez, Aznar, and Sánchez (2015)
	MNV (6 log $TCID_{50}$)			4.5	
	FCV (4 log $TCID_{50}$)	Washing lettuce	1% at RT for 30 min	Nondetectable levels	
	MNV (4 log $TCID_{50}$)			1.8	
Cinnamaldehyde	MNV (5 log $TCID_{50}$)	Antimicrobial films	2.60 mg/cm^2 at 37°C, ON, 100% RH	2.7	Fabra et al. (2016)
	FCV (6 log $TCID_{50}$)			Nondetectable levels	
Curcumin	MNV (4 log PFU)	Oysters	20 μM Photoactivation 3.6 J/cm^2, 0.06 W/cm^2 for 60 s	1.15	Wu et al. (2015)
Eriobotryae folium extract	MNV (5 log PFU)	Washing cabbage	1 mg/mL at 25°C for 60 min	0.4	Ng et al. (2017)

Continued

Table 3 Effect of Natural Compounds Against Norovirus Surrogates and HNoV in Food Applications—cont'd

Natural Compound	Virus (Initial Concentration)	Food Application	Concentration and Test Conditions	Inactivation (Log Reduction)	Reference
Grape seed extract	HNoV GII.4 (7 log genomic copies)	0.1% milk	2 mg/mL at 37°C for 60 min	1.2	Li, Baert, et al. (2012)
	MNV (5 log PFU)			1.0	
	HNoV GII.4 (7 log genomic copies)	Lettuce extract		1.2	
	MNV (5 log PFU)			Nondetectable levels	
	FCV (7 log PFU)	Washing lettuce	0.25 and 1 mg/mL at RT for 1 min	2.71; nondetectable levels	Su and D'Souza (2013)
	MNV (5 log PFU)		1 mg/mL at RT for 5 min	1.09	
	FCV (7 log PFU)	Washing peppers	0.25 and 1 mg/mL at RT for 1 min	3.0; nondetectable levels	
	MNV (5 log PFU)		1 mg/mL at RT for 5 min	1.2	

	FCV (4 log PFU)	Apple juice	1 mg/mL at 37°C 5 min	Nondetectable levels	Joshi, Su, and D'Souza (2015)
	MNV (5 log PFU)		15 min	Nondetectable levels	
	FCV (5 log PFU)	2% milk	4 mg/mL at 37°C for 24 h	1.1	
	MNV (6 log PFU)	Chitosan films	5; 10; 15% at 23 °C for 24 h	1.9; 3.2; 4.0	Amankwaah (2013)
	MNV (6 log $TCID_{50}$)	Alginate edible films	0.50 g extract/g alginate at 37°C, ON	1.0	Fabra, Falcó, Randazzo, Sánchez, and López (2018)
			0.75 g extract/g alginate at 37°C, ON	1.7	
Green tea extract	MNV (6 log PFU)	Washing strawberries	10 mg/mL[a] at RT for 10 min	1.08	Marti, Ferrary-Américo, and Barardi (2017)
		Washing lettuce		1.34	
		Washing green onions		0.58	
	MNV (6 log $TCID_{50}$)	Disinfection of stainless steel and glass surfaces	10 mg/mL at RT for 30 min	1.79–3.46	Randazzo et al. (2017)
	HAV (6 log $TCID_{50}$)			Nondetectable levels	

Continued

Table 3 Effect of Natural Compounds Against Norovirus Surrogates and HNoV in Food Applications—cont'd

Natural Compound	Virus (Initial Concentration)	Food Application	Concentration and Test Conditions	Inactivation (Log Reduction)	Reference
	MNV (6 log $TCID_{50}$)	Disinfection of stainless steel and glass surfaces	5 mg/mL (24 h storage and pH 7.2) at RT for 15 min	1.75–1.27	Falcó et al. (2018)
	HAV (5 log $TCID_{50}$)			1.92–1.54	
	MNV (6 log PFU)	Chitosan films	5; 10; 15% at 23 °C for 24 h	1.6; 4.5; 4.2	Amankwaah (2013)
	MNV (6 log $TCID_{50}$)	Alginate edible films	0.50 g extract/g alginate for 37°C, ON	2.0	Fabra et al. (2018)
			0.75 g extract/g alginate for 37°C, ON	1.9	

[a]Polyphenon 60, compounds from GTE, with a minimum of 60% of catechins.
RT: room temperature; ON: overnight; RH: relative humidity; PFU: plaque forming units; $TCID_{50}$: tissue culture infectious dose.
Modified from Sánchez, G., Randazzo, W., & D'Souza, D. H. (2018). Chapter 10: Human Noroviruses. In D. Liu (Ed.), Handbook of foodborne diseases. Taylor & Francis.

demand for safe and stable foods. Extensive research has been conducted to include in the film or coating, antimicrobials such as essential oils and phenolic compounds. However, although their bactericide and fungicide properties have been broadly investigated, little information is available in the literature about how biopolymers could act as carriers of antiviral compounds.

As metals, silver nanoparticles (as well as copper) have been reported to show antiviral properties in polyhydroxyalkanoates based films (Castro Mayorga, Fabra Rovira, Cabedo Mas, Sánchez Moragas, & Lagarón Cabello, 2018; Castro-Mayorga et al., 2017; Warnes, Summersgill, & Keevil, 2015) and magnetic hybrid colloids (Park et al., 2014). The only current report on food applications is using 1.0% silver ions incorporated into polylactide films decreased FCV-F9 to non-detectable levels on lettuce at 4°C, without any significant antiviral effect on paprika (Martínez-Abad, Ocio, Lagarón, & Sánchez, 2013). One of the most promising strategies is the inclusion of the natural antiviral compounds within packaging materials or coating films. As summarized in Table 3, cinnamaldehyde, GTE and GSE showed interesting antiviral properties when included into films developed for food packaging purposes.

6. CONCLUSIONS AND FUTURE PERSPECTIVES

Food contamination by HNoVs is a growing, serious health and economic problem. Currently, without having a robust routing method of cell culture for assessing HNoV infectivity in food, RT-qPCR procedures still remain the gold standard for HNoV detection and quantification, even if these procedures cannot discriminate between inactivated from infectious viruses. To overcome this limitation, different strategies have been evaluated to predict infectivity using RT-PCR-based PGM assays and the use of intercalating dyes in RT-PCR, which seem to be promising tools especially for the discrimination of potentially infectious and noninfectious HNoVs in foods (Sanchez et al., 2018). Furthermore, adopting these procedures in routine monitoring will allow for more accurate quantification of potentially infectious HNoV in food, constituting a useful tool for future risk assessment studies. As recently suggested, application of next-generation sequencing is also a promising technology for both detection and sequence identification of HNoVs (Yang et al., 2017). Furthermore, after identification of contamination or as a preventive measure, decontamination, sanitation, and control measures need to be implicated that are effective against HNoVs.

Future studies should screen for novel bioactives and, especially, the effectiveness of natural compounds in food as antiviral additives and also in food-related application as sanitizing agents mimicking practical scenarios in terms of experimental design. With this increased knowledge of HNoVs, public health and food safety can be improved.

REFERENCES

Aboubakr, H. A., Williams, P., Gangal, U., Youssef, M. M., El-Sohaimy, S. A. A., Bruggeman, P. J., et al. (2015). Virucidal effect of cold atmospheric gaseous plasma on feline calicivirus, a surrogate for human norovirus. *Applied and Environmental Microbiology*, *81*(11), 3612–3622. https://doi.org/10.1128/AEM.00054-15.

Ahlfeld, B., Li, Y., Boulaaba, A., Binder, A., Schotte, U., Zimmermann, J. L., et al. (2015). Inactivation of a foodborne norovirus outbreak strain with nonthermal atmospheric pressure plasma. *mBio*, *6*(1), 1–5. https://doi.org/10.1128/mBio.02300-14.

Allwood, P. B., Malik, Y. S., Hedberg, C. W., & Goyal, S. M. (2004). Effect of temperature and sanitizers on the survival of feline calicivirus, Escherichia coli, and F-specific coliphage MS2 on leafy salad vegetables. *Journal of Food Protection*, *67*(7), 1451–1456.

Almand, E. A., Moore, M. D., & Jaykus, L. A. (2017). Norovirus binding to ligands beyond histo-blood group antigens. *Frontiers in Microbiology*, *8*, 2549. https://doi.org/10.3389/fmicb.2017.02549.

Alshraiedeh, N. H., Alkawareek, M. Y., Gorman, S. P., Graham, W. G., & Gilmore, B. F. (2013). Atmospheric pressure, nonthermal plasma inactivation of MS2 bacteriophage: Effect of oxygen concentration on virucidal activity. *Journal of Applied Microbiology*, *115*(6), 1420–1426. https://doi.org/10.1111/jam.12331.

Amankwaah, C. (2013). *Incorporation of selected plant extracts into edible chitosan films and the effect on the antiviral, antibacterial and mechanical properties of the material*. The Ohio State University.

Atmar, R. L., & Estes, M. K. (2001). Diagnosis of noncultivatable gastroenteritis viruses, the human caliciviruses. *Clinical Microbiology Reviews*, *14*(1), 15–37. https://doi.org/10.1128/CMR.14.1.15-37.2001.

Atmar, R. L., Opekun, A. R., Gilger, M. A., Estes, M. K., Crawford, S. E., Neill, F. H., et al. (2014). Determination of the 50% human infectious dose for norwalk virus. *Journal of Infectious Diseases*, *209*(7), 1016–1022. https://doi.org/10.1093/infdis/jit620.

Bae, S., Park, S. Y., Choe, W., & Ha, S.-D. (2015). Inactivation of murine norovirus-1 and hepatitis A virus on fresh meats by atmospheric pressure plasma jets. *Food Research International*, *76*, 342–347.

Bae, J., & Schwab, K. J. (2008). Evaluation of murine norovirus, feline calicivirus, poliovirus, and MS2 as surrogates for human norovirus in a model of viral persistence in surface water and groundwater. *Applied and Environmental Microbiology*, *74*(2), 477–484. https://doi.org/10.1128/AEM.02095-06.

Baert, L., Mattison, K., Loisy-Hamon, F., Harlow, J., Martyres, A., Lebeau, B., et al. (2011). Review: Norovirus prevalence in Belgian, Canadian and French fresh produce: A threat to human health? *International Journal of Food Microbiology*, *151*(3), 261–269. https://doi.org/10.1016/j.ijfoodmicro.2011.09.013.

Baert, L., Uyttendaele, M., Van Coillie, E., & Debevere, J. (2008). The reduction of murine norovirus 1, B. fragilis HSP40 infecting phage B40-8 and E. coli after a mild thermal pasteurization process of raspberry puree. *Food Microbiology*, *25*(7), 871–874. https://doi.org/10.1016/j.fm.2008.06.002.

Baert, L., Vandekinderen, I., Devlieghere, F., Van, E. C., Debevere, J., & Uyttendaele, M. (2009). Efficacy of sodium hypochlorite and peroxyacetic acid to reduce murine

norovirus 1, B40-8, Listeria monocytogenes, and Escherichia coli 0157:H7 on shredded iceberg lettuce and in residual wash water. *Journal of Food Protection*, *72*(5), 1047–1054.
Bartsch, S. M., Lopman, B. A., Ozawa, S., Hall, A. J., & Lee, B. Y. (2016). Global economic burden of norovirus gastroenteritis. *PLoS One*, *11*(4), 1–16. https://doi.org/10.1371/journal.pone.0151219.
Bellou, M., Kokkinos, P., & Vantarakis, A. (2013). Shellfish-borne viral outbreaks: A systematic review. *Food and Environmental Virology*, *5*(1), 13–23. https://doi.org/10.1007/s12560-012-9097-6.
Bilek, S. E., & Turantaş, F. (2013). Decontamination efficiency of high power ultrasound in the fruit and vegetable industry, a review. *International Journal Food Microbiology*, *166*(1), 155–162.
Blanco, A., Guix, S., Fuster, N., Fuentes, C., Bartolomé, R., Cornejo, T., et al. (2017). Norovirus in bottled water associated with gastroenteritis outbreak, Spain, 2016. *Emerging Infectious Diseases*, *23*(9), 1531–1534. https://doi.org/10.3201/eid2309.161489.
Bok, K., Parra, G. I., Mitra, T., Abente, E., Shaver, C. K., Boon, D., et al. (2011). Chimpanzees as an animal model for human norovirus infection and vaccine development. *Proceedings of the National Academy of Sciences*, *108*(1), 325–330.
Boom, R., Sol, C. J. A., Salimans, M. M. M., Jansen, C. L., Wertheim-Van Dillen, P. M. E., & Van Der Noordaa, J. (1990). Rapid and simple method for purification of nucleic acids. *Journal of Clinical Microbiology*, *28*(3), 495–503.
Bosch, A., Sánchez, G., Abbaszadegan, M., Carducci, A., Guix, S., Le Guyader, F. S., et al. (2011). Analytical methods for virus detection in water and food. *Food Analytical Methods*, *4*(1), 4–12. https://doi.org/10.1007/s12161-010-9161-5.
Bozkurt, H., D'Souza, D. H., & Davidson, P. M. (2015). Thermal inactivation of foodborne enteric viruses and their viral surrogates in foods. *Journal of Food Protection*, *78*(8), 1597–1617. https://doi.org/10.4315/0362-028X.JFP-14-487.
Brié, A., Boudaud, N., Mssihid, A., Loutreul, J., Bertrand, I., & Gantzer, C. (2018). Inactivation of murine norovirus and hepatitis A virus on fresh raspberries by gaseous ozone treatment. *Food Microbiology*, *70*, 1–6. https://doi.org/10.1016/j.fm.2017.08.010.
Butot, S., Putallaz, T., Amoroso, R., & Sánchez, G. (2009). Inactivation of enteric viruses in minimally processed berries and herbs. *Applied and Environmental Microbiology*, *75*(12), 4155–4161. https://doi.org/10.1128/AEM.00182-09.
Butot, S., Putallaz, T., & Sánchez, G. (2008). Effects of sanitation, freezing and frozen storage on enteric viruses in berries and herbs. *International Journal of Food Microbiology*, *126*(1-2), 30–35. https://doi.org/10.1016/j.ijfoodmicro.2008.04.033.
Butot, S., Zuber, S., & Baert, L. (2014). Sample preparation prior to molecular amplification: Complexities and opportunities. *Current Opinion in Virology*, *4*, 66–70. https://doi.org/10.1016/j.coviro.2013.12.004.
Castro Mayorga, J. L., Fabra Rovira, M. J., Cabedo Mas, L., Sánchez Moragas, G., & Lagarón Cabello, J. M. (2018). Antimicrobial nanocomposites and electrospun coatings based on poly(3-hydroxybutyrate-co-3-hydroxyvalerate) and copper oxide nanoparticles for active packaging and coating applications. *Journal of Applied Polymer Science*, *135*(2), 45673. https://doi.org/10.1002/app.45673.
Castro-Mayorga, J. L., Randazzo, W., Fabra, M. J., Lagaron, J. M., Aznar, R., & Sánchez, G. (2017). Antiviral properties of silver nanoparticles against norovirus surrogates and their efficacy in coated polyhydroxyalkanoates systems. *LWT—Food Science and Technology*, *79*, 503–510. https://doi.org/10.1016/j.lwt.2017.01.065.
CDC. (2017). *Surveillance for foodborne disease outbreaks, United States, 2015, annual report*. Retrieved from Atlanta, Georgia https://www.cdc.gov/foodsafety/pdfs/2015FoodBorneOutbreaks_508.pdf.
Chen, Y., Hall, A. J., & Kirk, M. D. (2017). Norovirus disease in older adults living in long-term care facilities: Strategies for management. *Current Geriatrics Reports*, *6*(1), 26–33. https://doi.org/10.1007/s13670-017-0195-z.

Chen, H., Hoover, D. G., & Kingsley, D. H. (2005). Temperature and treatment time influence high hydrostatic pressure inactivation of feline calicivirus, a norovirus surrogate. *Journal of Food Protection*, *68*(11), 2389–2394.
Cheng, H. Y., Hung, M. N., Chen, W. C., Lo, Y. C., Su, Y. S., Wei, H. Y., et al. (2017). Ice-associated norovirus outbreak predominantly caused by GII.17 in Taiwan, 2015. *BMC Public Health*, *17*(1), 870. https://doi.org/10.1186/s12889-017-4869-4.
Choi, Y., Kim, E., Moon, S., Choi, J.-D., Lee, M.-S., & Kim, Y.-M. (2014). Phaeophyta extracts exhibit antiviral activity against feline calicivirus. *Fisheries and Aquatic Sciences*, *17*(1), 155–158.
Cliver, D. O. (2009). Capsid and infectivity in virus detection. *Food and Environmental Virology*, *1*(3), 123. https://doi.org/10.1007/s12560-009-9020-y.
Codex Alimentarius. (2012). *Guidelines on the application of general principles of food hygiene to the control of viruses in food* (p. 13). Codex Committee on Food Hygiene. Vol. CAC/GL 79-2012.
Cook, N., Knight, A., & Richards, G. P. (2016). Persistence and elimination of human norovirus in food and on food contact surfaces: A critical review. *Journal of Food Protection*, *79*(7), 1273–1294. https://doi.org/10.4315/0362-028X.JFP-15-570.
Costafreda, M. I., Bosch, A., & Pintó, R. M. (2006). Development, evaluation, and standardization of a real-time TaqMan reverse transcription-PCR assay for quantification of hepatitis A virus in clinical and shellfish samples. *Applied and Environmental Microbiology*, *72*(6), 3846–3855. https://doi.org/10.1128/AEM.02660-05.
Croci, L., Suffredini, E., Di Pasquale, S., & Cozzi, L. (2012). Detection of norovirus and feline calicivirus in spiked molluscs subjected to heat treatments. *Food Control*, *25*(1), 17–22. https://doi.org/10.1016/j.foodcont.2011.10.004.
D'Souza, D. H., Moe, C., Jaykus, L., Doyle, M., & Beuchat, L. (2007). Foodborne viral pathogens. In *Food microbiology: Fundamentals and frontiers* (pp. 581–607). Washington, DC: ASM Press.
D'Agostino, M., Cook, N., Rodriguez-Lazaro, D., & Rutjes, S. (2011). Nucleic acid amplification-based methods for detection of enteric viruses: Definition of controls and interpretation of results. *Food and Environmental Virology*, *3*(2), 55–60. https://doi.org/10.1007/s12560-011-9063-8.
Dancho, B. A., Chen, H., & Kingsley, D. H. (2012). Discrimination between infectious and non-infectious human norovirus using porcine gastric mucin. *International Journal of Food Microbiology*, *155*(3), 222–226. https://doi.org/10.1016/j.ijfoodmicro.2012.02.010.
DiCaprio, E. (2017). Recent advances in human norovirus detection and cultivation methods. *Current Opinion in Food Science*, *14*, 93–97. https://doi.org/10.1016/j.cofs.2017.02.007.
DiCaprio, E., Phantkankum, N., Culbertson, D., Ma, Y., Hughes, J. H., Kingsley, D., et al. (2016). Inactivation of human norovirus and tulane virus in simple media and fresh whole strawberries by ionizing radiation. *International Journal of Food Microbiology*, *232*, 43–51. https://doi.org/10.1016/j.ijfoodmicro.2016.05.013.
Dolin, R., Blacklow, N. R., Dupont, H., Buscho, R. F., Wyatt, R. G., Kasel, J. A., et al. (1972). Biological properties of norwalk agent of acute infectious nonbacterial gastroenteritis. *Proceedings of the Society for Experimental Biology and Medicine*, *140*(2), 578–583. https://doi.org/10.3181/00379727-140-36508.
Doultree, J., Druce, J., Birch, C., Bowden, D., & Marshall, J. (1999). Inactivation of feline calicivirus, a Norwalk virus surrogate. *Journal of Hospital Infection*, *41*(1), 51–57.
D'Souza, D. H. (2013). In *Inactivation of human enteric virus surrogates on stainless steel surfaces by non-thermal plasma. Paper presented at the 2013 annual meeting (July 28–31, 2013).*
D'Souza, D. H. (2014). Phytocompounds for the control of human enteric viruses. *Current Opinion in Virology*, *4*, 44–49. https://doi.org/10.1016/j.coviro.2013.12.006.
D'Souza, D. H., & Su, X. (2010). Efficacy of chemical treatments against murine norovirus, feline calicivirus, and MS2 bacteriophage. *Foodborne Pathogens and Disease*, 7(3), 319–326.

D'Souza, D. H., Su, X., Roach, A., & Harte, F. (2009). High-pressure homogenization for the inactivation of human enteric virus surrogates. *Journal of Food Protection, 72*(11), 2418–2422.

Duizer, E., Schwab, K. J., Neill, F. H., Atmar, R. L., Koopmans, M. P. G., & Estes, M. K. (2004). Laboratory efforts to cultivate noroviruses. *Journal of General Virology, 85*(1), 79–87. https://doi.org/10.1099/vir.0.19478-0.

Dunkin, N., Weng, S.-C., Jacangelo, J. G., & Schwab, K. J. (2017). Inactivation of human norovirus GI, GII, and surrogates by free chlorine in postharvest leafy green wash water. *Applied and Environmental Microbiology, 83*(22), e01457-17. https://doi.org/10.1128/aem.01457-17.

EFSA. (2015a). The European Union summary report on trends and sources of zoonoses, zoonotic agents and food-borne outbreaks in 2014. *EFSA Journal, 13*(12), 4329.

EFSA. (2015b). Panel on Biological Hazards. Evaluation of heat treatments, different from those currently established in the EU legislation, that could be applied to live bivalve molluscs from B and C production areas, that have not been submitted to purification or relaying, in order to eliminate pathogenic microorganisms. *EFSA Journal, 13*(12), 4332. https://doi.org/10.2903/j.efsa.2015.4332.

EFSA. (2016a). The European Union summary report on trends and sources of zoonoses, zoonotic agents and food-borne outbreaks in 2015. *EFSA Journal, 14*(12), 4634.

EFSA. (2016b). Technical specifications for a European baseline survey of norovirus in oysters. *EFSA Journal, 14*(3), 4414. https://doi.org/10.2903/j.efsa.2016.4414.

EFSA. (2017). The European Union summary report on trends and sources of zoonoses, zoonotic agents and food-borne outbreaks in 2016. *EFSA Journal, 15*(12), e05077. https://doi.org/10.2903/j.efsa.2017.5077.

EFSA Panel on Biological Hazards. (2012). Scientific opinion on norovirus (NoV) in oysters: Methods, limits and control options. *EFSA Journal, 10*(1), 2500. https://doi.org/10.2903/j.efsa.2012.2500.

Elizaquível, P., Aznar, R., & Sánchez, G. (2014). Recent developments in the use of viability dyes and quantitative PCR in the food microbiology field. *Journal of Applied Microbiology, 116*(1), 1–13. https://doi.org/10.1111/jam.12365.

El-Senousy, W. M., Costafreda, M. I., Pintó, R. M., & Bosch, A. (2013). Method validation for norovirus detection in naturally contaminated irrigation water and fresh produce. *International Journal of Food Microbiology, 167*(1), 74–79. https://doi.org/10.1016/j.ijfoodmicro.2013.06.023.

Eom, S. H., Moon, S. Y., Lee, D. S., Kim, H. J., Park, K., Lee, E. W., et al. (2015). In vitro antiviral activity of dieckol and phlorofucofuroeckol-A isolated from edible brown alga Eisenia bicyclis against murine norovirus. *Algae, 30*(3), 241–246. https://doi.org/10.4490/algae.2015.30.3.241.

Escudero-Abarca, B. I., Rawsthorne, H., Goulter, R. M., Suh, S. H., & Jaykus, L. A. (2014). Molecular methods used to estimate thermal inactivation of a prototype human norovirus: More heat resistant than previously believed? *Food Microbiology, 41*, 91–95. https://doi.org/10.1016/j.fm.2014.01.009.

Escudero-Abarca, B. I., Suh, S. H., Moore, M. D., Dwivedi, H. P., & Jaykus, L.-A. (2014). Selection, characterization and application of nucleic acid aptamers for the capture and detection of human norovirus strains. *PLoS One, 9*(9), e106805. https://doi.org/10.1371/journal.pone.0106805.

Ettayebi, K., Crawford, S. E., Murakami, K., Broughman, J. R., Karandikar, U., Tenge, V. R., et al. (2016). Replication of human noroviruses in stem cell-derived human enteroids. *Science, 353*(6306), 1387–1393. https://doi.org/10.1126/science.aaf5211.

Fabra, M., Castro-Mayorga, J., Randazzo, W., Lagarón, J., López-Rubio, A., Aznar, R., et al. (2016). Efficacy of cinnamaldehyde against enteric viruses and its activity after incorporation into biodegradable multilayer systems of interest in food packaging. *Food and Environmental Virology*, *8*(2), 125–132.

Fabra, M. J., Falcó, I., Randazzo, W., Sánchez, G., & López, A. (2018). Antiviral and antioxidant properties of active alginate edible films containing phenolic extracts. *Food Hydrocolloids*. (in press). https://doi.org/10.1016/j.foodhyd.2018.02.026.

Falcó, I., Randazzo, W., Gómez-Mascaraque, L., Aznar, R., López-Rubio, A., & Sánchez, G. (2017). Effect of (-)-epigallocatechin gallate at different pH conditions on enteric viruses. *LWT—Food Science and Technology*, *81*, 250–257. https://doi.org/10.1016/j.lwt.2017.03.050.

Falcó, I., Randazzo, W., Gómez-Mascaraque, L. G., Aznar, R., López-Rubio, A., & Sánchez, G. (2018). Fostering the antiviral activity of green tea extract for sanitizing purposes through controlled storage conditions. *Food Control*, *84*(Suppl. C), 485–492. https://doi.org/10.1016/j.foodcont.2017.08.037.

Felix-Valenzuela, L., Resendiz-Sandoval, M., Burgara-Estrella, A., Hernández, J., & Mata-Haro, V. (2012). Quantitative detection of hepatitis A, rotavirus and genogroup I norovirus by RT-qPCR in fresh produce from packinghouse facilities. *Journal of Food Safety*, *32*(4), 467–473. https://doi.org/10.1111/jfs.12009.

Feng, K., Divers, E., Ma, Y., & Li, J. (2011). Inactivation of a human norovirus surrogate, human norovirus virus-like particles, and vesicular stomatitis virus by gamma irradiation. *Applied and Environmental Microbiology*, 77(10), 3507–3517. https://doi.org/10.1128/AEM.00081-11.

Food and Drug Administration. (2007). Code of federal regulations, 3, 439–440. Irradiation in the production, processing and handling of food: 21CFR. Part 179.39.

Food and Drug Administration. (2012). Irradiation in the production, processing, and handling of food. Final rule. *Federal Register*, 77(112), 34212.

Food and Drug Administration. (2013). Code of federal regulations. 2013. Title 21. Food and drugs. Chapter I. Food and drug administration. Subchapter B. Food for human consumption. Part 179.41. Pulsed light for the treatment of food. 21 CFR 179.41.

Fraisse, A., Temmam, S., Deboosere, N., Guillier, L., Delobel, A., Maris, P., et al. (2011). Comparison of chlorine and peroxyacetic-based disinfectant to inactivate feline calicivirus, murine norovirus and hepatitis A virus on lettuce. *International Journal of Food Microbiology*, *151*(1), 98–104. https://doi.org/10.1016/j.ijfoodmicro.2011.08.011.

Frenck, R., Bernstein, D. I., Xia, M., Huang, P., Zhong, W., Parker, S., et al. (2012). Predicting susceptibility to norovirus GII. 4 by use of a challenge model involving humans. *Journal of Infectious Diseases*, *206*, 1386–1393.

Fukuda, S., Takao, S., Kuwayama, M., Shimazu, Y., & Miyazaki, K. (2006). Rapid detection of norovirus from fecal specimens by real-time reverse transcription-loop-mediated isothermal amplification assay. *Journal of Clinical Microbiology*, *44*(4), 1376–1381. https://doi.org/10.1128/JCM.44.4.1376-1381.2006.

Gilling, D. H., Kitajima, M., Torrey, J. R., & Bright, K. R. (2014). Antiviral efficacy and mechanisms of action of oregano essential oil and its primary component carvacrol against murine norovirus. *Journal of Applied Microbiology*, *116*(5), 1149–1163. https://doi.org/10.1111/jam.12453.

Gómez-Mascaraque, L. G., Soler, C., & Lopez-Rubio, A. (2016). Stability and bioaccessibility of EGCG within edible micro-hydrogels. Chitosan vs. gelatin, a comparative study. *Food Hydrocolloids*, *61*, 128–138.

Goodburn, C., & Wallace, C. A. (2013). The microbiological efficacy of decontamination methodologies for fresh produce: A review. *Food Control*, *32*(2), 418–427. https://doi.org/10.1016/j.foodcont.2012.12.012.

Greening, G. E., & Cannon, J. L. (2016). Human and animal viruses in food (including taxonomy of enteric viruses). In *Viruses in foods* (pp. 5–57). Springer.

Grohmann, G. S., Murphy, A. M., Christopher, P. J., Auty, E., & Greenberg, H. B. (1981). Norwalk virus gastroenteritis in volunteers consuming depurated oysters. *The Australian Journal of Experimental Biology and Medical Science*, *59*(Pt. 2), 219–228.

Hall, A. J., Wikswo, M. E., Pringle, K., Gould, L. H., & Parashar, U. D. (2014). Vital Signs: Foodborne norovirus outbreaks—United States, 2009–2012. *Morbidity and mortality weekly report. Surveillance summaries*, *63*(22), 491–495. https://doi.org/10.1007/s12560-016-9235-7.

Hewitt, J., & Greening, G. E. (2004). Survival and persistence of norovirus, hepatitis A virus, and feline calicivirus in marinated mussels. *Journal of Food Protection*, *67*(8), 1743–1750.

Hewitt, J., & Greening, G. E. (2006). Effect of heat treatment on hepatitis A virus and norovirus in New Zealand Greenshell mussels (Perna canaliculus) by quantitative real-time reverse transcription PCR and cell culture. *Journal of Food Protection*, *69*(9), 2217–2223.

Hirneisen, K. A., & Kniel, K. E. (2013a). Comparing human norovirus surrogates: Murine norovirus and tulane virus. *Journal of Food Protection*, *76*(1), 139–143. https://doi.org/10.4315/0362-028X.JFP-12-216.

Hirneisen, K. A., & Kniel, K. E. (2013b). Inactivation of internalized and surface contaminated enteric viruses in green onions. *International Journal of Food Microbiology*, *166*(2), 201–206. https://doi.org/10.1016/j.ijfoodmicro.2013.07.013.

Hirneisen, K. A., Markland, S. M., & Kniel, K. E. (2011). Ozone inactivation of norovirus surrogates on fresh produce. *Journal of Food Protection*, *74*(5), 836–839. https://doi.org/10.4315/0362-028X.JFP-10-438.

Höhne, M., & Schreier, E. (2004). Detection and characterization of norovirus outbreaks in Germany: Application of a one-tube RT-PCR using a fluorogenic real-time detection system. *Journal of Medical Virology*, *72*(2), 312–319. https://doi.org/10.1002/jmv.10573.

Horm, K. M., & D'Souza, D. H. (2011). Survival of human norovirus surrogates in milk, orange, and pomegranate juice, and juice blends at refrigeration (4 C). *Food Microbiology*, *28*(5), 1054–1061.

Horm, K. M., Davidson, P. M., Harte, F. M., & D'Souza, D. H. (2012). Survival and inactivation of human norovirus surrogates in blueberry juice by high-pressure homogenization. *Foodborne Pathogens and Disease*, *9*(11), 974–979.

Horm, K. M., Harte, F. M., & D'Souza, D. H. (2012). Human norovirus surrogate reduction in milk and juice blends by high pressure homogenization. *Journal of Food Protection*, *75*(11), 1984–1990.

Houde, A., Leblanc, D., Poitras, E., Ward, P., Brassard, J., Simard, C., et al. (2006). Comparative evaluation of RT-PCR, nucleic acid sequence-based amplification (NASBA) and real-time RT-PCR for detection of noroviruses in faecal material. *Journal of Virological Methods*, *135*(2), 163–172.

Huang, R., Ye, M., Li, X., Ji, L., Karwe, M., & Chen, H. (2016). Evaluation of high hydrostatic pressure inactivation of human norovirus on strawberries, blueberries, raspberries and in their purees. *International Journal of Food Microbiology*, *223*, 17–24. https://doi.org/10.1016/j.ijfoodmicro.2016.02.002.

Hutson, A. M., Atmar, R. L., Graham, D. Y., & Estes, M. K. (2002). Norwalk virus infection and disease is associated with ABO histo-blood group type. *Journal of Infectious Diseases*, *185*(9), 1335–1337. https://doi.org/10.1086/339883.

Imamura, S., Kanezashi, H., Goshima, T., Suto, A., Ueki, Y., Sugawara, N., et al. (2017). Effect of high-pressure processing on human noroviruses in laboratory-contaminated oysters by bio-accumulation. *Foodborne Pathogens and Disease*, *14*(9), 518–523. https://doi.org/10.1089/fpd.2017.2294.

ISO 15216-1. (2017). Microbiology of food and animal feed—Horizontal method for determination of Hepatitis A Virus and norovirus in food using real-time RT-PCR—Part 1.

In *Method for quantification*: *Vol. 15216-1*. Geneva, Switzerland: International Organization for Standardization.

Jean, J., Morales-Rayas, R., Anoman, M. N., & Lamhoujeb, S. (2011). Inactivation of hepatitis A virus and norovirus surrogate in suspension and on food-contact surfaces using pulsed UV light (pulsed light inactivation of food-borne viruses). *Food Microbiology*, *28*(3), 568–572. https://doi.org/10.1016/j.fm.2010.11.012.

Jeong, M. I., Park, S. Y., & Ha, S. D. (2017). Thermal inactivation of human norovirus on spinach using propidium or ethidium monoazide combined with real-time quantitative reverse transcription-polymerase chain reaction. *Food Control*, *78*, 79–84. https://doi.org/10.1016/j.foodcont.2017.02.026.

Jones, M. K., Grau, K. R., Costantini, V., Kolawole, A. O., de Graaf, M., Freiden, P., et al. (2015). Human norovirus culture in B cells. *Nature Protocols*, *10*(12), 1939–1947. https://doi.org/10.1038/nprot.2015.121.

Jones, M. K., Watanabe, M., Zhu, S., Graves, C. L., Keyes, L. R., Grau, K. R., et al. (2014). Enteric bacteria promote human and mouse norovirus infection of B cells. *Science*, *346*(6210), 755–759. https://doi.org/10.1126/science.1257147.

Joshi, S. S., Su, X., & D'Souza, D. H. (2015). Antiviral effects of grape seed extract against feline calicivirus, murine norovirus, and hepatitis A virus in model food systems and under gastric conditions. *Food Microbiology*, *52*, 1–10. https://doi.org/10.1016/j.fm.2015.05.011.

Kageyama, T., Kojima, S., Shinohara, M., Uchida, K., Fukushi, S., Hoshino, F. B., et al. (2003). Broadly reactive and highly sensitive assay for Norwalk-like viruses based on real-time quantitative reverse transcription-PCR. *Journal of Clinical Microbiology*, *41*(4), 1548–1557. https://doi.org/10.1128/JCM.41.4.1548-1557.2003.

Karim, M. R., Fout, G. S., Johnson, C. H., White, K. M., & Parshionikar, S. U. (2015). Propidium monoazide reverse transcriptase PCR and RT-qPCR for detecting infectious enterovirus and norovirus. *Journal of Virological Methods*, *219*, 51–61. https://doi.org/10.1016/j.jviromet.2015.02.020.

Katayama, K., Shirato-Horikoshi, H., Kojima, S., Kageyama, T., Oka, T., Hoshino, F. B., et al. (2002). Phylogenetic analysis of the complete genome of 18 norwalk-like viruses. *Virology*, *299*(2), 225–239. https://doi.org/10.1006/viro.2002.1568.

Kim, S. E., Park, S. Y., Rui, M.-l., & Ha, S.-D. (2017). Effects of electron beam irradiation on murine norovirus-1 in abalone (Haliotis discus hannai) meat and viscera. *LWT—Food Science and Technology*, *86*, 611–618. https://doi.org/10.1016/j.lwt.2017.08.058.

Kim, J.-G., Yousef, A. E., & Dave, S. (1999). Application of ozone for enhancing the microbiological safety and quality of foods: A review. *Journal of Food Protection*, *62*(9), 1071–1087.

Kingsley, D. (2013). High pressure processing and its application to the challenge of virus-contaminated foods. *Food and Environmental Virology*, *5*(1), 1–12.

Kingsley, D., & Chen, H. (2008). Aqueous matrix compositions and pH influence feline calicivirus inactivation by high pressure processing. *Journal of Food Protection*, *71*(8), 1598–1603.

Kingsley, D., Holliman, D. R., Calci, K. R., Chen, H., & Flick, G. J. (2007). Inactivation of a norovirus by high-pressure processing. *Applied and Environmental Microbiology*, *73*(2), 581–585. https://doi.org/10.1128/AEM.02117-06.

Kingsley, D., Vincent, E. M., Meade, G. K., Watson, C. L., & Fan, X. (2014). Inactivation of human norovirus using chemical sanitizers. *International Journal of Food Microbiology*, *171*, 94–99. https://doi.org/10.1016/j.ijfoodmicro.2013.11.018.

Knight, A., Haines, J., Stals, A., Li, D., Uyttendaele, M., Knight, A., et al. (2016). A systematic review of human norovirus survival reveals a greater persistence of human norovirus RT-qPCR signals compared to those of cultivable surrogate viruses.

International Journal of Food Microbiology, 216, 40–49. https://doi.org/10.1016/j.ijfoodmicro.2015.08.015.

Knight, A., Li, D., Uyttendaele, M., & Jaykus, L. A. (2013). A critical review of methods for detecting human noroviruses and predicting their infectivity. *Critical Reviews in Microbiology, 39*(3), 295–309. https://doi.org/10.3109/1040841X.2012.709820.

Kokkinos, P., Kozyra, I., Lazic, S., Bouwknegt, M., Rutjes, S., Willems, K., et al. (2012). Harmonised investigation of the occurrence of human enteric viruses in the leafy green vegetable supply chain in three European countries. *Food and Environmental Virology, 4*(4), 179–191. https://doi.org/10.1007/s12560-012-9087-8.

Kou, X., Wu, Q., Zhang, J., & Fan, H. (2006). Rapid detection of noroviruses in fecal samples and shellfish by nucleic acid sequence-based amplification. *Journal of Microbiology, 44*(4), 403–408.

Lamhoujeb, S., Fliss, I., Ngazoa, S. E., & Jean, J. (2008). Evaluation of the persistence of infectious human noroviruses on food surfaces by using real-time nucleic acid sequence-based amplification. *Applied and Environmental Microbiology, 74*(11), 3349–3355. https://doi.org/10.1128/AEM.02878-07.

Lay, M. K., Atmar, R. L., Guix, S., Bharadwaj, U., He, H., Neill, F. H., et al. (2010). Norwalk virus does not replicate in human macrophages or dendritic cells derived from the peripheral blood of susceptible humans. *Virology, 406*(1), 1–11. https://doi.org/10.1016/j.virol.2010.07.001.

Le Mennec, C., Parnaudeau, S., Rumebe, M., Le Saux, J. C., Piquet, J. C., & Le Guyader, S. F. (2017). Follow-up of norovirus contamination in an oyster production area linked to repeated outbreaks. *Food and Environmental Virology, 9*(1), 54–61. https://doi.org/10.1007/s12560-016-9260-6.

Lee, H. W., Lee, H. M., Yoon, S. R., Kim, S. H., & Ha, J. H. (2018). Pretreatment with propidium monoazide/sodium lauroyl sarcosinate improves discrimination of infectious waterborne virus by RT-qPCR combined with magnetic separation. *Environmental Pollution, 233*, 306–314. https://doi.org/10.1016/j.envpol.2017.10.081.

Leon, J. S., Kingsley, D. H., Montes, J. S., Richards, G. P., Lyon, G. M., Abdulhafid, G. M., et al. (2011). Randomized, double-blinded clinical trial for human norovirus inactivation in oysters by high hydrostatic pressure processing. *Applied and Environmental Microbiology, 77*(15), 5476–5482. https://doi.org/10.1128/AEM.02801-10.

Li, D., Baert, L., de Jonghe, M., van Coillie, E., Ryckeboer, J., Devlieghere, F., et al. (2011). Inactivation of murine norovirus 1, coliphage φ{symbol}X174, and Bacillus fragilis phage b40-8 on surfaces and fresh-cut iceberg lettuce by hydrogen peroxide and UV light. *Applied and Environmental Microbiology, 77*(4), 1399–1404. https://doi.org/10.1128/AEM.02131-10.

Li, D., Baert, L., & Uyttendaele, M. (2013). Inactivation of food-borne viruses using natural biochemical substances. *Food Microbiology, 35*(1), 1–9. https://doi.org/10.1016/j.fm.2013.02.009.

Li, D., Baert, L., Zhang, D., Xia, M., Zhong, W., Van Coillie, E., et al. (2012). Effect of grape seed extract on human norovirus GII.4 and murine norovirus 1 in viral suspensions, on stainless steel discs, and in lettuce wash water. *Applied and Environmental Microbiology, 78*(21), 7572–7578. https://doi.org/10.1128/AEM.01987-12.

Li, X., Chen, H., & Kingsley, D. H. (2013). The influence of temperature, pH, and water immersion on the high hydrostatic pressure inactivation of GI.1 and GII.4 human noroviruses. *International Journal of Food Microbiology, 167*(2), 138–143. https://doi.org/10.1016/j.ijfoodmicro.2013.08.020.

Li, J., Predmore, A., Divers, E., & Lou, F. (2012). New interventions against human norovirus: Progress, opportunities, and challenges. *Annual Review of Food Science and Technology, 3*(1), 331–352. https://doi.org/10.1146/annurev-food-022811-101234.

Lim, M. Y., Kim, J. M., & Ko, G. (2010). Disinfection kinetics of murine norovirus using chlorine and chlorine dioxide. *Water Research, 44*(10), 3243–3251. https://doi.org/10.1016/j.watres.2010.03.003.

Lindesmith, L., Moe, C., LePendu, J., Frelinger, J. A., Treanor, J., & Baric, R. S. (2005). Cellular and humoral immunity following snow mountain virus challenge. *Journal of Virology, 79*(5), 2900–2909. https://doi.org/10.1128/JVI.79.5.2900-2909.2005.

Lindesmith, L., Moe, C., Marionneau, S., Ruvoen, N., Jiang, X., Lindblad, L., et al. (2003). Human susceptibility and resistance to Norwalk virus infection. *Nature Medicine, 9*(5), 548–553. https://doi.org/10.1038/nm860.

Liu, C., Li, X., & Chen, H. (2015). Application of water-assisted ultraviolet light processing on the inactivation of murine norovirus on blueberries. *International Journal of Food Microbiology, 214*, 18–23. https://doi.org/10.1016/j.ijfoodmicro.2015.07.023.

Loisy, F., Atmar, R. L., Guillon, P., Le Cann, P., Pommepuy, M., & Le Guyader, F. S. (2005). Real-time RT-PCR for norovirus screening in shellfish. *Journal of Virological Methods, 123*(1), 1–7. https://doi.org/10.1016/j.jviromet.2004.08.023.

Lopman, B., Atmar, R., Baric, R., Estes, M., Hall, A., Iturriza-Gómara, M., et al. (2015). Global burden of norovirus and prospects for vaccine development. *Centers for Disease Control and Prevention*. https://www.cdc.gov/norovirus/downloads/global-burden-report.pdf.

Lou, F., DiCaprio, E., Li, X., Dai, X., Ma, Y., Hughes, J., et al. (2016). Variable high-pressure-processing sensitivities for genogroup II human noroviruses. *Applied and Environmental Microbiology, 82*(19), 6037–6045.

Lou, F., Neetoo, H., Chen, H., & Li, J. (2011). Inactivation of a human norovirus surrogate by high-pressure processing: Effectiveness, mechanism, and potential application in the fresh produce industry. *Applied and Environmental Microbiology*, 77(5), 1862–1871. https://doi.org/10.1128/AEM.01918-10.

Lou, F., Neetoo, H., Chen, H., & Li, J. (2015). High hydrostatic pressure processing: A promising nonthermal technology to inactivate viruses in high-risk foods. *Annual Review of Food Science and Technology, 6*, 389–409.

Lowther, J. A., Bosch, A., Butot, S., Ollivier, J., Made, D., Rutjes, S. A., et al. (2017). Validation of ISO method 15216 part 1—Quantification of hepatitis A virus and norovirus in food matrices. *International Journal of Food Microbiology*. (in press). https://doi.org/10.1016/j.ijfoodmicro.2017.11.014.

Marsh, Z. A., Grytdal, S. P., Beggs, J. C., Leshem, E., Gastanaduy, P. A., Rha, B., et al. (2017). The unwelcome houseguest: Secondary household transmission of norovirus. *Epidemiology and Infection*, 1–9. https://doi.org/10.1017/s0950268817002783.

Marti, E., Ferrary-Américo, M., & Barardi, C. R. M. (2017). Viral disinfection of organic fresh produce comparing polyphenon 60 from green tea with chlorine. *Food Control, 79*(Suppl. C), 57–61. https://doi.org/10.1016/j.foodcont.2017.03.021.

Martínez-Abad, A., Ocio, M. J., Lagarón, J. M., & Sánchez, G. (2013). Evaluation of silver-infused polylactide films for inactivation of Salmonella and feline calicivirus in vitro and on fresh-cut vegetables. *International Journal of Food Microbiology, 162*(1), 89–94. https://doi.org/10.1016/j.ijfoodmicro.2012.12.024.

McDonnell, S., Kirkland, K. B., Hlady, W. G., Aristeguieta, C., Hophins, R. S., Monroe, S. S., et al. (1997). Failure of cooking to prevent shellfish-associated viral gastroenteritis. *Archives of Internal Medicine, 157*(1), 111–116.

McLeod, C., Polo, D., Le Saux, J. C., & Le Guyader, F. S. (2017). Depuration and relaying: A review on potential removal of norovirus from oysters. *Comprehensive Reviews in Food Science and Food Safety, 16*(4), 692–706. https://doi.org/10.1111/1541-4337.12271.

Micali, M., Fiorino, M., & Parisi, S. (2016). *The chemistry of thermal food processing procedures*. Springer International Publishing.

Min, S. C., Roh, S. H., Niemira, B. A., Sites, J. E., Boyd, G., & Lacombe, A. (2016). Dielectric barrier discharge atmospheric cold plasma inhibits Escherichia coli O157:H7, Salmonella, Listeria monocytogenes, and tulane virus in Romaine lettuce. *International Journal of Food Microbiology*, *237*, 114–120. https://doi.org/10.1016/j.ijfoodmicro.2016.08.025.

Moore, C., Clark, E. M., Gallimore, C. I., Corden, S. A., Gray, J. J., & Westmoreland, D. (2004). Evaluation of a broadly reactive nucleic acid sequence based amplification assay for the detection of noroviruses in faecal material. *Journal of Clinical Virology*, *29*(4), 290–296. https://doi.org/10.1016/S1386-6532(03)00170-7.

Moorman, E., Montazeri, N., & Jaykus, L. A. (2017). Efficacy of neutral electrolyzed water for inactivation of human norovirus. *Applied and Environmental Microbiology*, *83*(16). https://doi.org/10.1128/AEM.00653-17.

Mormann, S., Dabisch, M., & Becker, B. (2010). Effects of technological processes on the tenacity and inactivation of norovirus genogroup II in experimentally contaminated foods. *Applied and Environmental Microbiology*, *76*(2), 536–545. https://doi.org/10.1128/AEM.01797-09.

Mouchtouri, V. A., Verykouki, E., Zamfir, D., Hadjipetris, C., Lewis, H. C., Hadjichristodoulou, C., et al. (2017). Gastroenteritis outbreaks on cruise ships: Contributing factors and thresholds for early outbreak detection. *Eurosurveillance*, *22*(45), 1–8. https://doi.org/10.2807/1560-7917.ES.2017.22.45.16-00576.

NACMCF. (2008). National Advisory Committee on Microbiological Criteria for Foods (NACMCF). Response to the questions posed by the food and drug administration and the national marine fisheries service regarding determination of cooking parameters for safe seafood for consumers. *Journal of Food Protection*, *71*(6), 1287–1308. https://doi.org/10.4315/0362-028X-71.6.1287.

NACMCF. (2016). Response to the questions posed by the food safety and inspection service, the Centers for Disease Control and Prevention, the National Marine Fisheries Service, and the Defense Health Agency, veterinary services activity regarding control strategies for reducing foodborne norovirus infections. *Journal of Food Protection*, *79*(5), 843–889. https://doi.org/10.4315/0362-028X.JFP-15-215.

Ng, Y. C., Kim, Y. W., Ryu, S., Lee, A., Lee, J. S., & Song, M. J. (2017). Suppression of norovirus by natural phytochemicals from Aloe vera and Eriobotryae folium. *Food Control*, *73*, 1362–1370. https://doi.org/10.1016/j.foodcont.2016.10.051.

Nishida, T., Kimura, H., Saitoh, M., Shinohara, M., Kato, M., Fukuda, S., et al. (2003). Detection, quantitation, and phylogenetic analysis of noroviruses in Japanese oysters. *Applied and Environmental Microbiology*, *69*(10), 5782–5786. https://doi.org/10.1128/AEM.69.10.5782-5786.2003.

Nowak, P., Topping, J. R., Fotheringham, V., Gallimore, C. I., Gray, J. J., Iturriza-Gómara, M., et al. (2011). Measurement of the virolysis of human GII.4 norovirus in response to disinfectants and sanitisers. *Journal of Virological Methods*, *174*(1-2), 7–11. https://doi.org/10.1016/j.jviromet.2011.03.004.

Oh, M., Bae, S. Y., Lee, J. H., Cho, K. J., Kim, K. H., & Chung, M. S. (2012). Antiviral effects of black raspberry (Rubus coreanus) juice on foodborne viral surrogates. *Foodborne Pathogens and Disease*, *9*(10), 915–921. https://doi.org/10.1089/fpd.2012.1174.

Papafragkou, E., Hewitt, J., Park, G. W., Greening, G., & Vinjé, J. (2013). Challenges of culturing human norovirus in three-dimensional organoid intestinal cell culture models. *PLoS One*, *8*(6), 1–7. https://doi.org/10.1371/journal.pone.0063485.

Park, S. Y., Kim, A.-N., Lee, K.-H., & Ha, S.-D. (2015). Ultraviolet-C efficacy against a norovirus surrogate and hepatitis A virus on a stainless steel surface. *International Journal of Food Microbiology*, *211*, 73–78. https://doi.org/10.1016/j.ijfoodmicro.2015.07.006.

Park, S. Y., Park, H. H., Kim, S. Y., Kim, S. J., Woo, K., & Ko, G. (2014). Antiviral properties of silver nanoparticles on a magnetic hybrid colloid. *Applied and Environmental Microbiology*, *80*(8), 2343–2350. https://doi.org/10.1128/AEM.03427-13.

Parshionikar, S., Laseke, I., & Fout, G. S. (2010). Use of propidium monoazide in reverse transcriptase PCR to distinguish between infectious and noninfectious enteric viruses in water samples. *Applied and Environmental Microbiology*, *76*(13), 4318–4326. https://doi.org/10.1128/AEM.02800-09.

Patel, M. M. (2008). Systematic literature review of role of noroviruses in sporadic gastroenteritis. *Emerging Infectious Disease Journal—CDC*, *14*(8), 1224–1231, August 2008.

Polo, D., Schaeffer, J., Fournet, N., Le Saux, J. C., Parnaudeau, S., McLeod, C., et al. (2016). Digital PCR for quantifying norovirus in oysters implicated in outbreaks, France. *Emerging Infectious Diseases*, *22*(12), 2189–2191. https://doi.org/10.3201/eid2212.160841.

Prasad, B. V., Hardy, M. E., Dokland, T., Bella, J., Rossmann, M. G., & Estes, M. K. (1999). X-ray crystallographic structure of the Norwalk virus capsid. *Science*, *286*(5438), 287–290.

Predmore, A., & Li, J. (2011). Enhanced removal of a human norovirus surrogate from fresh vegetables and fruits by a combination of surfactants and sanitizers. *Applied and Environmental Microbiology*, 77(14), 4829–4838. https://doi.org/10.1128/AEM.00174-11.

Predmore, A., Sanglay, G. C., DiCaprio, E., Li, J., Uribe, R. M., & Lee, K. (2015). Electron beam inactivation of tulane virus on fresh produce, and mechanism of inactivation of human norovirus surrogates by electron beam irradiation. *International Journal of Food Microbiology*, *198*, 28–36. https://doi.org/10.1016/j.ijfoodmicro.2014.12.024.

Predmore, A., Sanglay, G., Li, J., & Lee, K. (2015). Control of human norovirus surrogates in fresh foods by gaseous ozone and a proposed mechanism of inactivation. *Food Microbiology*, *50*, 118–125. https://doi.org/10.1016/j.fm.2015.04.004.

Randazzo, W., Aznar, R., & Sánchez, G. (2016). Curcumin-mediated photodynamic inactivation of norovirus surrogates. *Food and Environmental Virology*, *8*, 244–250.

Randazzo, W., Falcó, I., Aznar, R., & Sánchez, G. (2017). Effect of green tea extract on enteric viruses and its application as natural sanitizer. *Food Microbiology*, *66*, 150–156. https://doi.org/10.1016/j.fm.2017.04.018.

Randazzo, W., Khezri, M., Ollivier, J., Le Guyader, F. S., Rodríguez-Díaz, J., Aznar, R., et al. (2018). Optimization of PMAxx pretreatment to distinguish between human norovirus with intact and altered capsids in shellfish and sewage samples. *International Journal of Food Microbiology*, *266*, 1–7. https://doi.org/10.1016/j.ijfoodmicro.2017.11.011.

Randazzo, W., López-Gálvez, F., Allende, A., Aznar, R., & Sánchez, G. (2016). Evaluation of viability PCR performance for assessing norovirus infectivity in fresh-cut vegetables and irrigation water. *International Journal of Food Microbiology*, *229*, 1–6. https://doi.org/10.1016/j.ijfoodmicro.2016.04.010.

Richards, G. P. (2012). Critical review of norovirus surrogates in food safety research: Rationale for considering volunteer studies. *Food and Environmental Virology*, *4*(1), 6–13. https://doi.org/10.1007/s12560-011-9072-7.

Rodrigo, D., van Loey, A., & Hendrickx, M. (2007). Combined thermal and high pressure colour degradation of tomato puree and strawberry juice. *Journal of Food Engineering*, *79*(2), 553–560. https://doi.org/10.1016/j.jfoodeng.2006.02.015.

Rönnqvist, M., Aho, E., Mikkelä, A., Ranta, J., Tuominen, P., Rättö, M., et al. (2014). Norovirus transmission between hands, gloves, utensils, and fresh produce during simulated food handling. *Applied and Environmental Microbiology*, *80*(17), 5403–5410. https://doi.org/10.1128/AEM.01162-14.

Ryu, S., You, H. J., Kim, Y. W., Lee, A., Ko, G. P., Lee, S. J., et al. (2015). Inactivation of norovirus and surrogates by natural phytochemicals and bioactive substances. *Molecular Nutrition & Food Research*, *59*(1), 65–74. https://doi.org/10.1002/mnfr.201400549.

Sánchez, G., Aznar, R., Martínez, A., & Rodrigo, D. (2011). Inactivation of human and murine norovirus by high-pressure processing. *Foodborne Pathogens and Disease*, *8*(2), 249–253. https://doi.org/10.1089/fpd.2010.0667.

Sánchez, C., Aznar, R., & Sánchez, G. (2015). The effect of carvacrol on enteric viruses. *International Journal of Food Microbiology*, *192*, 72–76. https://doi.org/10.1016/j.ijfoodmicro.2014.09.028.

Sánchez, G., & Bosch, A. (2016). Survival of enteric viruses in the environment and food. In S. M. Goyal & J. L. Cannon (Eds.), *Viruses in foods* (pp. 367–392). Cham: Springer International Publishing.

Sánchez, G., Elizaquível, P., Aznar, R., & Selma, M. V. (2015). Virucidal effect of high power ultrasound combined with a chemical sanitizer containing peroxyacetic acid for water reconditioning in the fresh-cut industry. *Food Control*, *52*, 126–131. https://doi.org/10.1016/j.foodcont.2014.12.021.

Sánchez, G., Randazzo, W., & D'Souza, D. H. (2018). Chapter 10: Human noroviruses. In D. Liu (Ed.), *Handbook of foodborne diseases*. Taylor & Francis.

Sanglay, G. C., Li, J., Uribe, R. M., & Lee, K. (2011). Electron-beam inactivation of a norovirus surrogate in fresh produce and model systems. *Journal of Food Protection*, *74*(7), 1155–1160. https://doi.org/10.4315/0362-028X.JFP-10-405.

Schaeffer, J., Le Saux, J.-C., Lora, M., Atmar, R. L., & Le Guyader, F. S. (2013). Norovirus contamination on French marketed oysters. *International Journal of Food Microbiology*, *166*(2), 244–248. https://doi.org/10.1016/j.ijfoodmicro.2013.07.022.

Schultz, A. C., Uhrbrand, K., NØrrung, B., & Dalsgaard, A. (2012). Inactivation of norovirus surrogates on surfaces and raspberries by steam-ultrasound treatment. *Journal of Food Protection*, *75*(2), 376–381. https://doi.org/10.4315/0362-028X.JFP-11-271.

Seo, D. J., & Choi, C. (2017). Inhibition of murine norovirus and feline calicivirus by edible herbal extracts. *Food and Environmental Virology*, *9*(1), 35–44. https://doi.org/10.1007/s12560-016-9269-x.

Sido, R. F., Huang, R., Liu, C., & Chen, H. (2017). High hydrostatic pressure inactivation of murine norovirus and human noroviruses on green onions and in salsa. *International Journal of Food Microbiology*, *242*, 1–6. https://doi.org/10.1016/j.ijfoodmicro.2016.11.003.

Souza, M., Azevedo, M. S. P., Jung, K., Cheetham, S., & Saif, L. J. (2008). Pathogenesis and immune responses in gnotobiotic calves after infection with the genogroup II.4-HS66 strain of human norovirus. *Journal of Virology*, *82*(4), 1777–1786. https://doi.org/10.1128/JVI.01347-07.

Stals, A., Baert, L., Van Coillie, E., & Uyttendaele, M. (2012). Extraction of food-borne viruses from food samples: A review. *International Journal of Food Microbiology*, *153*(1-2), 1–9. https://doi.org/10.1016/j.ijfoodmicro.2011.10.014.

Su, X., & D'Souza, D. H. (2011). Trisodium phosphate for foodborne virus reduction on produce. *Foodborne Pathogens and Disease*, *8*(6), 713–717. https://doi.org/10.1089/fpd.2010.0763.

Su, X., & D'Souza, D. H. (2013). Grape seed extract for foodborne virus reduction on produce. *Food Microbiology*, *34*(1), 1–6. https://doi.org/10.1016/j.fm.2012.10.006.

Su, X., Zivanovic, S., & D'Souza, D. H. (2010). Inactivation of human enteric virus surrogates by high-intensity ultrasound. *Foodborne Pathogens and Disease*, 7(9), 1055–1061. https://doi.org/10.1089/fpd.2009.0515.

Tan, M., & Jiang, X. (2005). Norovirus and its histo-blood group antigen receptors: An answer to a historical puzzle. *Trends in Microbiology*, *13*(6), 285–293. https://doi.org/10.1016/j.tim.2005.04.004.

Tang, Q., Li, D., Xu, J., Wang, J., Zhao, Y., Li, Z., et al. (2010). Mechanism of inactivation of murine norovirus-1 by high pressure processing. *International Journal of Food Microbiology, 137*(2-3), 186–189. https://doi.org/10.1016/j.ijfoodmicro.2009.10.033.

Taube, S., Kolawole, A. O., Höhne, M., Wilkinson, J. E., Handley, S. A., Perry, J. W., et al. (2013). A mouse model for human norovirus. *mBio, 4*(4), 1–8. https://doi.org/10.1128/mBio.00450-13.

Teunis, P. F. M., Moe, C. L., Liu, P., Miller, S. E., Lindesmith, L., Baric, R. S., et al. (2008). Norwalk virus: How infectious is it? *Journal of Medical Virology, 80*(8), 1468–1476. https://doi.org/10.1002/jmv.21237.

Tian, P., Yang, D., & Mandrell, R. (2011). Differences in the binding of human norovirus to and from Romaine lettuce and raspberries by water and electrolyzed waters. *Journal of Food Protection®, 74*(8), 1364–1369.

Tian, P., Yang, D., Quigley, C., Chou, M., & Jiang, X. (2013). Inactivation of the tulane virus, a novel surrogate for the human norovirus. *Journal of Food Protection, 76*(4), 712–718. https://doi.org/10.4315/0362-028X.JFP-12-361.

Verhoef, L., Hewitt, J., Barclay, L., Ahmed, S. M., Lake, R., Hall, A. J., et al. (2015). Norovirus genotype profiles associated with foodborne transmission, 1999–2012. *Emerging Infectious Diseases, 21*(4), 592–599. https://doi.org/10.3201/eid2104.141073.

Vimont, A., Fliss, I., & Jean, J. (2015). Efficacy and mechanisms of murine norovirus inhibition by pulsed-light technology. *Applied and Environmental Microbiology, 81*(8), 2950–2957. https://doi.org/10.1128/AEM.03840-14.

Vinjé, J. (2015). Advances in laboratory methods for detection and typing of norovirus. *Journal of Clinical Microbiology, 53*(2), 373–381. https://doi.org/10.1128/JCM.01084-13.

Wan, J., Coventry, J., Swiergon, P., Sanguansri, P., & Versteeg, C. (2009). Advances in innovative processing technologies for microbial inactivation and enhancement of food safety—Pulsed electric field and low-temperature plasma. *Trends in Food Science and Technology, 20*(9), 414–424. https://doi.org/10.1016/j.tifs.2009.01.050.

Warnes, S. L., Summersgill, E. N., & Keevil, C. W. (2015). Inactivation of murine norovirus on a range of copper alloy surfaces is accompanied by loss of capsid integrity. *Applied and Environmental Microbiology, 81*(3), 1085–1091. https://doi.org/10.1128/aem.03280-14.

WHO. (2015). WHO estimates of the global burden of foodborne diseases. In *Foodborne diseases burden epidemiology reference group 2007–2015.* WHO Press.

Wu, Y., Chang, S., Nannapaneni, R., Coker, R., Haque, Z., & Mahmoud, B. S. M. (2016). The efficacy of X-ray doses on murine norovirus-1 (MNV-1) in pure culture, half-shell oyster, salmon sushi, and tuna salad. *Food Control, 64*, 77–80. https://doi.org/10.1016/j.foodcont.2015.12.018.

Wu, Y., Chang, S., Nannapaneni, R., Zhang, Y., Coker, R., & Mahmoud, B. S. M. (2017). The effects of X-ray treatments on bioaccumulated murine norovirus-1 (MNV-1) and survivability, inherent microbiota, color, and firmness of Atlantic oysters (Crassostrea virginica) during storage at 5°C for 20 days. *Food Control, 73*(Pt. B), 1189–1194. https://doi.org/10.1016/j.foodcont.2016.10.036.

Wu, J., Hou, W., Cao, B., Zuo, T., Xue, C., Leung, A. W., et al. (2015). Virucidal efficacy of treatment with photodynamically activated curcumin on murine norovirus bio-accumulated in oysters. *Photodiagnosis and Photodynamic Therapy, 12*(3), 385–392. https://doi.org/10.1016/j.pdpdt.2015.06.005.

Xiao, S., Tang, J. W., & Li, Y. (2017). Airborne or fomite transmission for norovirus? A case study revisited. *International Journal of Environmental Research and Public Health, 14*(12), 1571. https://doi.org/10.3390/ijerph14121571.

Yang, Z., Mammel, M., Papafragkou, E., Hida, K., Elkins, C. A., & Kulka, M. (2017). Application of next generation sequencing toward sensitive detection of enteric viruses isolated from celery samples as an example of produce. *International Journal of Food Microbiology, 261*, 73–81. https://doi.org/10.1016/j.ijfoodmicro.2017.07.021.

Ye, M., Li, X., Kingsley, D. H., Jiang, X., & Chen, H. (2014). Inactivation of human norovirus in contaminated oysters and clams by high hydrostatic pressure. *Applied and Environmental Microbiology*, *80*(7), 2248–2253.

Ye, M., Lingham, T., Huang, Y., Ozbay, G., Ji, L., Karwe, M., et al. (2015). Effects of high-hydrostatic pressure on inactivation of human norovirus and physical and sensory characteristics of oysters. *Journal of Food Science*, *80*(6), M1330–M1335. https://doi.org/10.1111/1750-3841.12899.

Yilmaz, A., Bostan, K., Altan, E., Muratoglu, K., Turan, N., Tan, D., et al. (2011). Investigations on the frequency of norovirus contamination of ready-to-eat food items in Istanbul, Turkey, by using real-time reverse transcription PCR. *Journal of Food Protection*, *74*(5), 840–843. https://doi.org/10.4315/0362-028X.JFP-10-475.

CHAPTER THREE

Hepatitis E Virus: A New Foodborne Zoonotic Concern

David Rodríguez-Lázaro[*,1], **Marta Hernandez**[*,†], **Nigel Cook**[‡]
[*]Microbiology Division, Department of Biotechnology and Food Science, University of Burgos, Burgos, Spain
[†]Laboratory of Molecular Biology and Microbiology, ITACyL, Valladolid, Spain
[‡]Jorvik Food and Environmental Virology, York, United Kingdom
[1]Corresponding author: e-mail address: drlazaro@ubu.es

Contents

Abstract

Hepatitis E virus (HEV) is an enteric nonenveloped single-stranded RNA virus. Among the mammalian lineages, four genotypes are associated to human infection: genogroups 1 and 2 infect only humans and are mainly found in developing countries, while genogroups 3 and 4 are zoonotic, being found in a variety of animal species including pigs, and are autochthonous in developed countries. HEV infection can result in liver damage and with genotypes 1 and 2 symptoms can be particularly severe in pregnant women, with a high lethality ratio. Several cases of foodborne transmission of hepatitis E have been reported, often involving consumption of meat, especially raw or undercooked. Information is lacking on the exact extent of foodborne transmission of HEV.

1. INTRODUCTION

Hepatitis E is a major cause of acute hepatitis, particularly associated with contact with contaminated water in developing countries (Rodríguez-Lázaro et al., 2012). The disease is endemic in parts of the world with poor sanitation and hygiene, where it can occur in large outbreaks. Infection with the

Advances in Food and Nutrition Research, Volume 86
ISSN 1043-4526
https://doi.org/10.1016/bs.afnr.2018.04.002
© 2018 Elsevier Inc.
All rights reserved.

hepatitis E virus (HEV) can cause liver damage, and the symptoms can be particularly severe in pregnant women. This virus is also found in a variety of animal species, including pigs, and is now recognized as a zoonotic agent (Rodríguez-Lázaro et al., 2012). Several cases of hepatitis E transmission transmitted by food have been reported, often associated with consumption of meat, especially raw or undercooked. Consequently, HEV has captured the attention of both scientist and public health professionals during the last two decades, reflected by the annual number of publications devoted to their study, which has increased threefold since 2000 (Fig. 1).

The discovery of HEV was somewhat bizarre. The virus was discovered by the Soviet doctor Mikhail Balayan in 1983 (Balayan et al., 1983), while investigating several cases of non-A and non-E hepatitis among Soviet soldiers in the Afghanistan war. Although he wanted to continue the investigation in Moscow, refrigeration systems were not available, and he prepared a yogurt with the fecal samples of nine infected soldiers, drank it, then returned to Moscow, and waited for symptoms. After 35 days, he developed an acute hepatitis and he started to collect and analyze his own fecal samples, where found a new virus producing liver damage in laboratory animals which could be observed by electron microscopy.

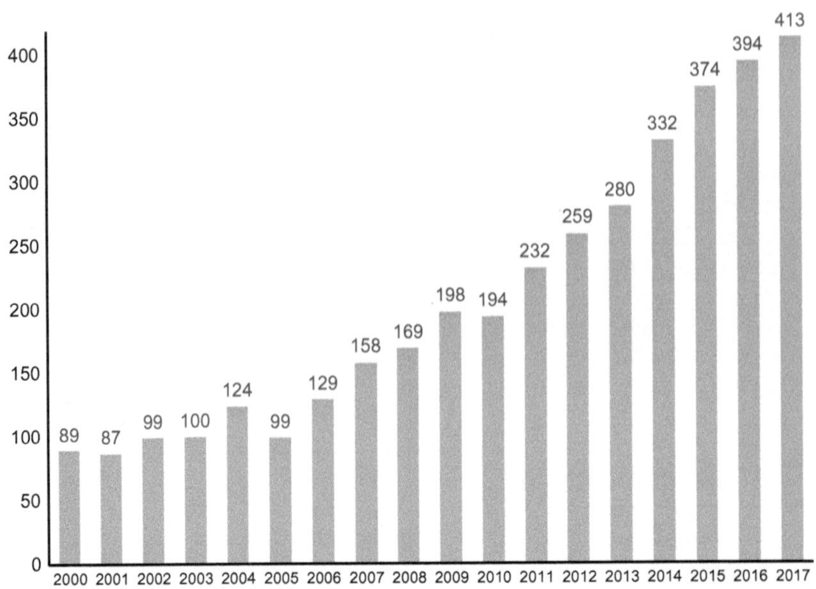

Fig. 1 Increase in the number of publications associated with hepatitis E since 2000. *PubMed.*

The first reported outbreak of hepatitis E occurred in Delhi, India, in 1955 and 1956, although it was not recognized as such until the 1990s, when advances in molecular diagnostics and immunodiagnostics made it possible to identify the viral agent. In developed countries, the disease was initially thought to be related only to travel to endemic areas. However, over the past few years, several cases of locally acquired hepatitis E have been reported in Europe, United States, and Japan, and evidence of animal reservoirs has been discovered. Routes of transmission of hepatitis E in developed countries are still not fully elucidated, but several cases of foodborne transmission have been reported.

2. CHARACTERISTICS OF HEV

HEV is a nonenveloped single-stranded RNA. Virion particles are approximately 27–34 nm diameter, with an icosahedral protein shell or capsid, which encloses a 7.5 kb linear RNA genome (Tam et al., 1991). Its genome has three open reading frames (ORFs): the ORF1 that encodes the nonstructural polyprotein (nsp), the ORF2 that encodes the viral capsid protein, and the ORF3 that encodes a small regulatory phosphoprotein (Chandra, Kar-Roy, Kumari, Mayor, & Jameel, 2008).

Propagation of HEV by cell culture is very difficult. PLC/PRF/5 cells, derived from human hepatocellular carcinoma, and A549 cells, derived from human lung cancer, have been used as cell propagation lines and some wild strains, mainly of genotypes 3 and 4, have been cultured in vitro, but results have been inconsistent, and to date there is no cell line which has been validated for routine use for HEV propagation (Cook, D'Agostino, & Johne, 2017).

The HEV is classified in a separate genus, *Hepevirus*, within the family *Hepeviridae* (Emerson & Purcell, 2003). This family contains viruses that infect mammals, including humans, as well as birds and fish. The avian HEV (Payne, Ellis, Plant, Gregory, & Wilcox, 1999) and HEV infecting trout (Batts, Yun, Hedrick, & Winton, 2011) share about 50% of the nucleotide sequence of the strains of mammalian HEV and have not been associated with human cases. Recent data based on complete genome sequences of human and animal strains and amino acid partial sequences ORF1/ORF2 indicate the existence of three groups in mammals (Smith, Purdy, & Simmonds, 2013). The first group corresponds to viruses that infect humans, pigs, wild boars, deer, and rabbits. This group contains the four main genotypes and new genotypes

Table 1 HEV Genotypes, Natural Hosts, and Zoonotic Infection to Humans

Genus	Species	Genotype	Natural Host	Human Infection
Orthohepevirus	*Orthohepevirus* A	1	Human	Yes
		2	Human	Yes
		3	Human, pig, wild board, rabbit, mongoose	Yes
		4	Human, pig, wild board, yak	Yes
		5	Wild board	Unknown
		6	Wild board	Unknown
		7	Camel	Yes
	Orthohepevirus B		Poultry	No
	Orthohepevirus C	C1	Rat	No
		C2	Ferret	No
	Orthohepevirus D		Bat	No
Piscihepevirus			Trouch	No

Adapted from Nan, Y., & Zhang, Y. J. (2016). Molecular biology and infection of hepatitis E virus. *Frontiers in Microbiology*, 7, 1419.

of wild boar (Takahashi et al., 2011) and rabbit (Zhao et al., 2009). The second group corresponds to viruses that infect rats and ferrets (Johne et al., 2010; Raj et al., 2012), and the third group corresponds to viruses that infect bats (Drexler et al., 2012) (Table 1). Recently, four tentative genera have been proposed: *Orthohepevirus*, including strains of mammals except those of bat; *Chiropteran hepevirus*, including bat strains; *Avihepevirus*, including avian strains; and *Piscihepevirus*, including trout virus (Meng, 2013).

All identified strains of HEV infecting humans have been classified into four genotypes (1–4), but there is only one serotype (Lu, Li, & Hagedorn, 2006). Within the four genotypes associated with human infections, several subtypes have been suggested based upon complete or partial virus genome sequences. The lineages within genotypes 1 and 2 are less divergent and seem to be more conserved in comparison to strains of genotypes 3 and 4. More importantly, genotypes 1 and 2 only seem to affect humans, whereas genotypes 3 and 4 have been isolated in a wide range of animals, indicating a zoonotic potential for strains of these HEV genotypes. Viruses of genotype 1 are predominantly isolated from outbreaks and sporadic cases in Asia and Africa, while strains of genotype 2 have been observed in outbreaks in Mexico and Africa. Genotype 3 occurs worldwide, but genotype 4 mainly in Asia. The autochthonous infections observed in the United States and Europe to date are almost exclusively caused by strains of genotype 3, with a likelihood of mainly zoonotic transmission, although due to its long incubation period it has been very difficult to identify the actual transmission routes.

Recent studies of genetic variability indicate that no coherent criteria can be defined for the assignment of subgenotypes within each genotype (Oliveira-Filho, Konig, & Thiel, 2013; Smith et al., 2013). However, several studies based on full-length genome sequences have provided very interesting epidemiological molecular data, dividing the 4 major genotypes into 24 subgenotypes (5 for genotype 1, 2 for genotype 2, 10 for genotype 3, and 7 for genotype 4) (Lu et al., 2006; Purdy & Khudyakov, 2011). In developing countries, subgenotypes 1a, 1b, and 1c are prevalent in Asia, while subgenotypes 1d and 1e are found in Africa (Lu et al., 2006). Subgenotypes 3a and 3b are circulating in the United States and Japan and can be clearly distinguished from subgenotypes 3f, 3c, and 3e, which circulate in Europe (Bouquet et al., 2011; Izopet et al., 2012; Legrand-Abravanel et al., 2009). Phylogenetic and coalescence analyses based on numerous complete sequences of genotype 3 strains of patients with acute hepatitis, and domestic pigs and wild boars, provide evidence that strains of subgenotype 3e were introduced from Europe into Japan through the importation of pigs into the 1960s, where it subsequently spread from pigs to wild boars (Nakano et al., 2013).

3. PATHOGENESIS

The infectious dose of HEV is unknown. After entry via oral ingestion, the virus passes through the intestinal tract, where it probably replicates. The virus then passes to the liver, and after replication there, is released into the bile and blood by mechanisms that are not yet fully understood. It is assumed that hepatocytes are the primary target cells in which the virus replicates in the cytoplasm. On the basis of the lack of an efficient cell culture system, the mechanism by which HEV enters the hepatic cells and how the virion is released from the cells is not yet fully understood (Ippagunta, Naik, Jameel, Ramana, & Aggarwal, 2011). HEV replication in the liver results in damage to that organ, but the pathogenesis and mechanisms of liver injury during HEV infection are still not clearly understood; however, immune mechanisms may be involved.

In humans, HEV infections often occur asymptomatically, but after an incubation period ranging from 15 to 60 days, the disease may manifest as an acute icteric viral hepatitis. Viral particles can be found in the bile and feces of the infected person during the late incubation phase, and up to 2 weeks after the onset of clinical disease. The clinical symptoms in most cases are very similar to those reported during hepatitis A and include anorexia, nausea, jaundice, fever, and abdominal pain (Aggarwal, Kini, Sofat, Naik, & Krawczynski, 2000) (Table 2). During acute infection with HEV genotypes 1 and 2, the case fatality rate in the general population is 0.2%–1%. The case fatality rate in developing countries is higher, ranging from 8% to 11%. The most susceptible individuals in developing countries are young adults and pregnant women and the case fatality rate during pregnancy approaches 15%–25%. In developed countries, disease resulting from autochthonous infection, mainly by genotype 3, seems to be more prevalent in middle aged and elderly men and is normally lethal only in patients with underlying chronic liver disease.

Table 2 Clinical Features of the HEV in Developing and Developed Countries

	Description or Value	
	Hepatitis E in Developing Countries	**Hepatitis E in Developed Countries**
Age (years)	15–30	>50
Gender (ratio M:F)	2:1	>3:1
Clinical course	Self-limiting hepatitis	Self-limiting hepatitis
Neurological complications	Yes	Yes
Deaths in pregnant females	Yes; 20%–25% in final trimester	No
Outcome in patients with underlying chronic liver disease	Poor	Poor
Chronic infection	No	Yes; only genotype 3
Prevalence	3.4 million cases/year, 70,000 deaths, 3000 stillbirths	Unknown

Adapted from Kamar, N., Dalton, H. R., Abravanel, F., & Izopet, J. (2014). Hepatitis E virus infection. *Clinical Microbiology Reviews, 27*, 116–138.

HEV is excreted by the fecal route; up to 10^8 copies of the viral genome can be excreted per milligram of feces for several days before the onset of symptoms (Li, Kamili, & Krawczynski, 2006). RNA of HEV has also been detected in pig urine and it has been suggested that this may play a relevant role in its transmission in this animal reservoir (Rodríguez-Lázaro et al., 2012). However, the transmission of HEV via aerosol has not been described, but should not be ruled out as it can be excreted through urine.

4. EPIDEMIOLOGY

The most common route of transmission of hepatitis E is consumption of contaminated drinking water, with person-to-person transmission being uncommon. The occurrence of hepatitis E is highest in Central and South-East Asia, North and West Africa, and Mexico, areas where fecal contamination of water is common, and seroprevalence in populations from endemic regions ranges between 3% and 26%. Outbreaks involving several thousand cases have been recorded in countries such as India, Myanmar, and China. In North America and Europe, cases of hepatitis E are uncommon, although seroprevalence ranges from 1% to 5%; most of the cases of HEV genotypes 1 and 2 infection are travel related via visits to endemic areas, but several cases of autochthonous hepatitis E have been reported.

In developing countries, where HEV genotypes 1 and 2 can be disseminated via contaminated water, the fecal excretion of HEV by humans assists the endemicity of the disease (Aggarwal et al., 2000; Ippagunta et al., 2011; Li et al., 2006, Kumar, Beniwal, Kar, Sharma, & Murthy, 2004; Nicand et al., 2005). Genotypes 1 and 2 HEV particles can be found in water, demonstrating that environmental dissemination plays a key role in HEV epidemiology (Ippagunta, Naik, Sharma, & Aggarwal, 2007). However, in developed countries, where most of the HEV infections are locally acquired and associated with genotypes 3 and 4, the relevance of animal reservoirs is evident. The full range of mammalian species that can act as reservoirs is unknown. The strains infecting mammals such as domestic pigs, wild boars, deer, and rabbits are the etiological agents of zoonotic HEV infection in humans (Dalton, Bendall, Ijaz, & Banks, 2008; Pavio et al., 2010; Tei, Kitajima, Takahashi, & Mishiro, 2003). There are a range of animal species that can act as HEV reservoirs: anti-HEV antibodies have been identified in several animals including chickens, pigs, wild boars, deer, cats, dogs, mongooses, horses, cattle, sheep, and rodents.

However, variants that infect rats (Johne et al., 2010), ferrets (Raj et al., 2012), mongoos (Nakamura et al., 2006), and bats (Drexler et al., 2012) have not been found in humans. The main animal reservoir is the domestic pig, with high levels of HEV infection being reported from several countries all over the world, although the infection in pigs appears to be asymptomatic (Pavio et al., 2010; Van der Poel et al., 2001). HEV strains with very similar RNA sequences have been detected in pigs and humans, which prompts concern over the potential extent of zoonotic transmission of the virus through consumption of contaminated pork products (Di Bartolo et al., 2012). HEV genotype 3 has a global distribution (Dalton et al., 2008). On the contrary, genotype 4 is found mainly in China and Japan (Lu et al., 2006), but recently, it has also been detected in Europe, both in pigs (Hakze-van der Honing, van Coillie, Antonis, & van der Poel, 2011) and in humans (Colson et al., 2012; Garbuglia et al., 2013; Tesse et al., 2012). Genotypes 3 and 4 are also detected in wild boar and deer, but the prevalence is low compared to that of domestic pigs (Pavio et al., 2010).

Direct contact with infected animals is another possible route of HEV transmission (Colson, Borentain, et al., 2007; Colson, Coze, et al., 2007; Di Bartolo et al., 2012; Meng et al., 2002). Seroprevalence studies show that veterinarians and pig handlers are more likely than the general population to be anti-HEV IgG positive (Renou et al., 2007). The route of infection transmitted by water may also be important for genotypes 3 and 4. Genotype 3 has been detected in untreated wastewater, pig manure, pig slurry storage facilities, and river water (Clemente-Casares et al., 2003; Galiana, Fernandez-Barredo, Garcia, Gomez, & Perez-Gracia, 2008; Kasorndorkbua et al., 2005; La Rosa, Pourshaban, Iaconelli, Vennarucci, & Muscillo, 2010). It has also been detected in mussels and oysters (McCreary et al., 2008; Rutjes et al., 2009; Song et al., 2010). However, the relative importance of the environmental transmission of genotypes 3 and 4 remains unknown.

Finally, HEV infection has been described via blood transfusion in several countries (Haïm-Boukobza et al., 2012; Hewitt et al., 2014; Matsubayashi et al., 2004, 2008). For example, a study in the United Kingdom found (Hewitt et al., 2014) that 1 out of 2848 blood donors tested positive to genotype 3, and 43% of the recipients of blood components were infected, developing a chronic disease in 25% of the cases. HEV has also been detected in blood derivatives (Adlhoch et al., 2009; Baylis, Gartner, Nick, Ovemyr, & Blumel, 2012; Baylis, Koc, Nick, & Blumel, 2012; Ijaz, Szypulska, Tettmar, Kitchen, & Tedder, 2012).

5. ZOONOTIC TRANSMISSION OF HEV

Foodborne transmission of HEV was first demonstrated in clusters of Japanese patients after eating raw or undercooked meat from swine, wild boar, or Sika deer (Tei et al., 2003). The genomic sequences of HEVs identified from the infected patients were identical to those recovered from the frozen leftover meat (Jiménez-Clavero et al., 2003; Tei et al., 2003). Through either detection of HEV sequences or epidemiological study, more hepatitis E cases have been linked to the consumption of food products contaminated with the virus. This includes infection via locally produced meat products (Colson, Borentain, et al., 2007; Colson, Coze, et al., 2007) but also from game meat and processed pork (Legrand-Abravanel et al., 2009). Eating raw or undercooked pork products has been identified as a higher risk factor of HEV infection (Colson, Borentain, et al., 2007; Colson, Coze, et al., 2007) with the possibility of several thousand people being infected each year. RNA sequences of HEV have been found in various tissues and organs of swine (Purcell & Emerson, 2008) deer and boar (Dalton et al., 2007; Kamar et al., 2012). Pork livers purchased from local supermarkets may be contaminated with the virus (Colson et al., 2008; Sinha, Jha, Lakhtakia, & Narayan, 2003; Thapa, Biswas, Mallick, & Ghosh, 2009), and some of these contaminated commercial pork livers may contain infectious viruses (Colson et al., 2008). Bivalve molluscs are known transmitters of enteric viruses and oysters especially are eaten raw worldwide; HEV has been detected in mussels, shellfish, and other bivalves (Colson, Borentain, et al., 2007; Colson, Coze, et al., 2007; Crossan et al., 2012; Diez-Valcarce et al., 2012). More recently, HEV sequences have been detected on soft fruits and vegetables, with irrigation water as the suspected contamination origin (Brassard, Gagné, Généreux, & Côté, 2012; Kokkinos et al., 2012; Maunula et al., 2013), and in cow and goat milk (Huang et al., 2016; Long et al., 2017).

6. PREVALENCE OF HEV IN PORK PRODUCTS AND OTHER FOOD MATRICES

HEV has been detected in pork products (liver, sausages) sold at retail, in several countries including Czech Republic, Germany, Italy, Spain, and United Kingdom (Berto, Martelli, Grierson, & Banks, 2012;

Di Bartolo et al., 2012). HEV RNA detection rates ranging from 4% to 6.5% have been reported for commercially available pig liver (Bouwknegt, Lodder-Verschoor, van der Poel, Rutjes, & de Roda Husman, 2007; Wenzel et al., 2011), but more recent studies elevate those percentages over 20% in Spain. In pig liver sausages and raw sausages from Germany, HEV RNA detection rates between 20% and 22% have been described (Szabo et al., 2015). Especially high detection rates (>57%) have been reported for a local liver sausage from France called "Figatelli" (Martin-Latil, Hennechart-Collette, Guillier, & Perelle, 2014; Pavio et al., 2010).

Recently, an episode of confirmed zoonotic transmission has occurred in Andalusia, Spain, that offers very relevant information (Rivero-Juarez et al., 2017). A patient infected with HIV was diagnosed with an acute hepatitis E infection at the Reina Sofia University Hospital in Córdoba in October 2015. The patient was negative to the immunological tests, but HEV RNA was detected in his blood serum. The patient reported that his family traditionally hunted wild boar for consumption and that the whole family had consumed boar meat stewed, roasted, or prepared on the grill during the previous month. The eight members of the family were positive for the presence of virus RNA, but without presenting clinical symptoms. Two samples of wild boar meat which the family had kept were analyzed, and HEV genotype 3 RNA was detected. There was 100% homology between the HEV isolates from the members of the family and the meat. Finally, the prevalence of HEV infection among wild boars in the same hunting area was also evaluated: HEV RNA identical to that identified in the family members and the analyzed meat was detected in serum samples from nine wild boars. This is very interesting because it shows that the boar is an important reservoir of the virus and can be a very important route of transmission. In wild boar hunting areas such as Andalusia, HEV is very prevalent in these animals (De Deus et al., 2008). It also highlights a specific potential a public health issue, since the south of Spain is the most important exporter worldwide of wild boar meat. Finally, the study highlights the importance of adequate culinary treatments at home to guarantee the total elimination of the virus in meat products. There have been a very limited range of studies on the heat resistance of HEV, but the information has raised questions regarding what may be the most effective cooking procedure to inactivate the virus. HEV remains infectious after heating at 56°C for 1 h (Emerson, Arankalle, & Purcell, 2005), and cooking hamburger pate at 71°C for at least 5 min is necessary to eliminate contaminating HEV infectivity (Barnaud, Rogee, Garry, Rose, & Pavio, 2012).

7. INFORMATION LACKING

The discovery in pigs of HEV strains related to human strains is significant as regards the issue of interspecies transfer and zoonotic infection. Even if pork products are hitherto thoroughly cooked at temperatures which should inactivate viruses, a potential for zoonotic foodborne transfer of HEV may remain via environmental contamination via manure from infected pigs. HEV may be widespread in the general pig population, and if so, it is possible that much of the pig manure which is stored on farms and subsequently spread onto agricultural land as fertilizer could contain infectious HEV particles. This could result in exposure of the human population. It may be informative to study prevalence and survival of HEV in the environment and on crops and foods, and also to develop methods to detect interspecies transfer at an early stage (van der Poel et al., 2001). The tests used for HEV RNA detection are based on the reverse transcription-polymerase chain reaction (RT-PCR), targeting specific sequences of the HEV genome, for example, the conserved region of the ORF3 locus. Nonstandardized protocols for the homogenization and virus extraction from pork products prior to RT-PCR analysis have been developed. This lack of harmonization implies that the diverse prevalence studies have used different detection methodologies, and consequently the results obtained in those studies cannot be compared easily. In addition, one of the main technology barriers is the poor detection limit, which probably underestimates real HEV prevalence in both pig and other animal herds, and in the derived food products and the environment. There is currently no standard method for detection of HEV in foods, although at the time of writing one is under consideration by the European Committee for Standardisation (CEN).

There are significant gaps in our knowledge regarding the survival of HEV in foods and the environment (including food contact surfaces), and also regarding the effect of elimination procedures used in food supply chain settings. The lack of a reliable infectivity assay has hampered extensive study. It has been recommended that studies be undertaken to develop an efficient propagation system (based on in vitro cell culture), to facilitate the acquisition of extensive information on the potential risk posed by of HEV foodstuffs and the environment, and its response to disinfection and elimination procedures.

In conclusion, the main research priorities for HEV include the virus dynamic in pig herds and how animal husbandry practices can affect it, the development and validation of methodologies for HEV inactivation in foods, the development of harmonized methods for HEV detection in meat and meat products and for evaluating HEV infectivity, the characterization of the HEV burden in humans, and the phylogenetic relationships between strains from humans, pigs, food products, food chains, and the environment. This list of research needs reflects the significant challenge of zoonotic HEV, which will require a committed effort by various national and international stakeholders—government, research bodies, and the farming and processing sectors—to address.

REFERENCES

Adlhoch, C., Wolf, A., Meisel, H., Kaiser, M., Ellerbrok, H., & Pauli, G. (2009). High HEV prevalence in four different wild boar populations in East and West Germany. *Veterinary Microbiology*, *139*, 270–278.

Aggarwal, R., Kini, D., Sofat, S., Naik, S. R., & Krawczynski, K. (2000). Duration of viraemia and faecal viral excretion in acute hepatitis E. *The Lancet*, *356*, 1081–1082.

Balayan, M. S., Andjaparidze, A. G., Savinskaya, S. S., Ketiladze, E. S., Braginsky, D. M., Savinov, A. P., et al. (1983). Evidence for a virus in non-A, non-B hepatitis transmitted via the fecal-oral route. *Intervirology*, *20*, 23–31.

Barnaud, E., Rogee, S., Garry, P., Rose, N., & Pavio, N. (2012). Thermal inactivation of infectious hepatitis E virus in experimentally contaminated food. *Applied and Environmental Microbiology*, *78*, 5153–5159.

Batts, W., Yun, S., Hedrick, R., & Winton, J. (2011). A novel member of the family Hepeviridae from cutthroat trout (Oncorhynchus clarkii). *Virus Research*, *158*, 116–123.

Baylis, S. A., Gartner, T., Nick, S., Ovemyr, J., & Blumel, J. (2012). Occurrence of hepatitis E virus RNA in plasma donations from Sweden, Germany and the United States. *Vox Sanguinis*, *103*, 89–90.

Baylis, S. A., Koc, O., Nick, S., & Blumel, J. (2012). Widespread distribution of hepatitis E virus in plasma fractionation pools. *Vox Sanguinis*, *102*, 182–183.

Berto, A., Martelli, F., Grierson, S., & Banks, M. (2012). Hepatitis E virus in pork food chain, United Kingdom, 2009-2010. *Emerging Infectious Diseases*, *18*, 1358–1360.

Bouquet, J., Tesse, S., Lunazzi, A., Eloit, M., Rose, N., Nicand, E., et al. (2011). Close similarity between sequences of hepatitis E virus recovered from humans and swine, France, 2008–2009. *Emerging Infectious Diseases*, *17*, 2018–2025.

Bouwknegt, M., Lodder-Verschoor, F., van der Poel, W. H., Rutjes, S. A., & de Roda Husman, A. M. (2007). Hepatitis E virus RNA in commercial porcine livers in The Netherlands. *Journal of Food Protection*, *70*, 2889–2895.

Brassard, J., Gagné, M. J., Généreux, M., & Côté, C. (2012). Detection of human food-borne and zoonotic viruses on irrigated, field-grown strawberries. *Applied and Environmental Microbiology*, *78*, 3763–3766.

Chandra, V., Kar-Roy, A., Kumari, S., Mayor, S., & Jameel, S. (2008). The hepatitis E virus ORF3 protein modulates epidermal growth factor receptor trafficking, STAT3 translocation, and the acute-phase response. *Journal of Virology*, *82*(14), 7100–7110. https://doi.org/10.1128/JVI.00403-08. [Epub 2008 Apr 30].

Clemente-Casares, P., Pina, S., Buti, M., Jardi, R., Martín, M., Bofill-Mas, S., et al. (2003). Hepatitis E virus epidemiology in industrialized countries. *Emerging Infectious Diseases*, *9*, 448–454.

Colson, P., Borentain, P., Motte, A., Lagrange, X., Kaba, M., Henry, M., et al. (2007). First human cases of hepatitis E infection with genotype 3c strains. *Journal of Clinical Virology*, *40*, 318–320.

Colson, P., Coze, C., Gallian, P., Henry, M., De Micco, P., & Tamalet, C. (2007). Transfusion-associated hepatitis E, France. *Emerging Infectious Diseases*, *13*, 648–649. https://doi.org/10.3201/eid1304.061387.

Colson, P., Payraudeau, E., Leonnet, C., De Montigny, S., Villeneuve, L., Motte, A., et al. (2008). Severe thrombocytopenia associated with acute hepatitis E virus infection. *Journal of Clinical Microbiology*, *46*, 2450–2452.

Colson, P., Romanet, P., Moal, V., Borentain, P., Purgus, R., Benezech, A., et al. (2012). Autochthonous infections with hepatitis E virus genotype 4, France. *Emerging Infectious Diseases*, *18*, 1361–1364.

Cook, N., D'Agostino, M., & Johne, R. (2017). Potential approaches to assess the infectivity of hepatitis E virus in pork products: A review. *Food and Environmental Virology*, *9*, 243–255.

Crossan, C., Baker, P. J., Craft, J., Takeuchi, Y., Dalton, H. R., & Scobie, L. (2012). Hepatitis E virus genotype 3 in shellfish, United Kingdom. *Emerging Infectious Diseases*, *18*, 2085–2087.

Dalton, H. R., Bendall, R., Ijaz, S., & Banks, M. (2008). Hepatitis E: An emerging infection in developed countries. *The Lancet Infectious Diseases*, *8*, 698–709.

Dalton, H. R., Fellows, H. J., Gane, E. J., Wong, P., Gerred, S., Schroeder, B., et al. (2007). Hepatitis E in New Zealand. *Journal of Gastroenterology and Hepatology*, *22*, 1236–1240.

de Deus, N., Peralta, B., Pina, S., Allepuz, A., Mateu, E., Vidal, D., et al. (2008). Epidemiological study of hepatitis E virus infection in European wild boars (*Sus scrofa*) in Spain. *Veterinary Microbiology*, *129*, 163–170.

Di Bartolo, I., Diez-Valcarce, M., Vasickova, P., Kralik, P., Hernandez, M., Angeloni, G., et al. (2012). Hepatitis E virus in pork production chain in Czech Republic, Italy, and Spain, 2010. *Emerging Infectious Diseases*, *18*, 1282–1289.

Diez-Valcarce, M., Kokkinos, P., Söderberg, K., Bouwknegt, M., Willems, K., de Roda Husman, A. M., et al. (2012). Occurrence of human enteric viruses in commercial mussels at retail level in three European countries. *Food and Environmental Virology*, *4*, 73–80.

Drexler, J. F., Seelen, A., Corman, V. M., Fumie Tateno, A., Cottontail, V., Melim Zerbinati, R., et al. (2012). Bats worldwide carry hepatitis E virus-related viruses that form a putative novel genus within the family Hepeviridae. *Journal of Virology*, *86*, 9134–9147.

Emerson, S. U., Arankalle, V. A., & Purcell, R. H. (2005). Thermal stability of hepatitis E virus. *The Journal of Infectious Diseases*, *192*, 930–933.

Emerson, S. U., & Purcell, R. H. (2003). Hepatitis E virus. *Reviews in Medical Virology*, *13*, 145–154.

Galiana, C., Fernandez-Barredo, S., Garcia, A., Gomez, M. T., & Perez-Gracia, M. T. (2008). Occupational exposure to hepatitis E virus (HEV) in swine workers. *The American Journal of Tropical Medicine and Hygiene*, *78*, 1012–1015.

Garbuglia, A. R., Scognamiglio, P., Petrosillo, N., Mastroianni, C. M., Sordillo, P., Gentile, D., et al. (2013). Hepatitis E virus genotype 4 outbreak, Italy, 2011. *Emerging Infectious Diseases*, *19*, 110–114.

Haïm-Boukobza, S., Ferey, M. P., Vétillard, A. L., Jeblaoui, A., Pélissier, E., Pelletier, G., et al. (2012). Transfusion-transmitted hepatitis E in a misleading context of autoimmunity and drug-induced toxicity. *Journal of Hepatology*, *57*, 1374–1378.

Hakze-van der Honing, R. W., van Coillie, E., Antonis, A. F., & van der Poel, W. H. (2011). First isolation of hepatitis E virus genotype 4 in Europe through swine surveillance in the Netherlands and Belgium. *PLoS One*, *6*, e22673.

Hewitt, P. E., Ijaz, S., Brailsford, S. R., Brett, R., Dicks, S., Haywood, B., et al. (2014). Hepatitis E virus in blood components: A prevalence and transmission study in southeast England. *The Lancet*, *384*, 1766–1773.

Huang, F., Li, Y., Yu, W., Jing, S., Wang, J., Long, F., et al. (2016). Excretion of infectious hepatitis E virus into milk in cows imposes high risks of zoonosis. *Hepatology*, *64*, 350–359.

Ijaz, S., Szypulska, R., Tettmar, K. I., Kitchen, A., & Tedder, R. S. (2012). Detection of hepatitis E virus RNA in plasma mini-pools from blood donors in England. *Vox Sanguinis*, *102*, 272.

Ippagunta, S. K., Naik, S., Jameel, S., Ramana, K. N., & Aggarwal, R. (2011). Viral RNA but no evidence of replication can be detected in the peripheral blood mononuclear cells of hepatitis E virus-infected patients. *Journal of Viral Hepatitis*, *18*, 668–672.

Ippagunta, S. K., Naik, S., Sharma, B., & Aggarwal, R. (2007). Presence of hepatitis E virus in sewage in northern India: Frequency and seasonal pattern. *Journal of Medical Virology*, *79*, 1827–1831.

Izopet, J., Dubois, M., Bertagnoli, S., Lhomme, S., Marchandeau, S., Boucher, S., et al. (2012). Hepatitis E virus strains in rabbits and evidence of a closely related strain in humans, France. *Emerging Infectious Diseases*, *18*, 1274–1281. https://doi.org/10.3201/eid1808.120057.

Jiménez-Clavero, M. A., Fernández, C., Ortiz, J. A., Pro, J., Carbonell, G., Tarazona, J. V., et al. (2003). Teschoviruses as indicators of fecal contamination of water. *Applied and Environmental Microbiology*, *69*, 6311–6315.

Johne, R., Plenge-Bonig, A., Hess, M., Ulrich, R. G., Reetz, J., & Schielke, A. (2010). Detection of a novel hepatitis E-like virus in faeces of wild rats using a nested broad-spectrum RT-PCR. *The Journal of General Virology*, *91*, 750–758.

Kamar, N., Weclawiack, H., Guilbeaud-Frugier, C., Legrand-Abravanel, F., Cointault, O., Ribes, D., et al. (2012). Hepatitis E virus and the kidney in solid-organ-transplant patients. *Transplantation*, *93*, 617–623.

Kasorndorkbua, C., Opriessnig, T., Huang, F. F., Guenette, D. K., Thomas, P. J., Meng, X. J., et al. (2005). Infectious swine hepatitis E virus is present in pig manure storage facilities on United States farms, but evidence of water contamination is lacking. *Applied and Environmental Microbiology*, *71*, 7831–7837.

Kokkinos, P., Kozyra, I., Lazic, S., Bouwknegt, M., Rutjes, S., Willems, K., et al. (2012). Harmonised investigation of the occurrence of human enteric viruses in the leafy green vegetable supply chain in three European countries. *Food and Environmental Virology*, *4*, 179–191.

Kumar, A., Beniwal, M., Kar, P., Sharma, J. B., & Murthy, N. S. (2004). Hepatitis E in pregnancy. *International Journal of Gynaecology and Obstetrics*, *85*, 240–244.

La Rosa, G., Pourshaban, M., Iaconelli, M., Vennarucci, V. S., & Muscillo, M. (2010). Molecular detection of hepatitis E virus in sewage samples. *Applied and Environmental Microbiology*, *76*, 5870–5873.

Legrand-Abravanel, F., Mansuy, J. M., Dubois, M., Kamar, N., Peron, J. M., Rostaing, L., et al. (2009). Hepatitis E virus genotype 3 diversity, France. *Emerging Infectious Diseases*, *15*, 110–114.

Li, X., Kamili, S., & Krawczynski, K. (2006). Quantitative detection of hepatitis E virus RNA and dynamics of viral replication in experimental infection. *Journal of Viral Hepatitis*, *13*, 835–839.

Long, F., Yu, W., Yang, C., Wang, J., Li, Y., Li, Y., et al. (2017). High prevalence of hepatitis E virus infection in goats. *Journal of Medical Virology*, *89*, 1981–1987.

Lu, L., Li, C., & Hagedorn, C. H. (2006). Phylogenetic analysis of global hepatitis E virus sequences: Genetic diversity, subtypes and zoonosis. *Reviews in Medical Virology*, *16*, 5–36.

Martin-Latil, S., Hennechart-Collette, C., Guillier, L., & Perelle, S. (2014). Method for HEV detection in raw pig liver products and its implementation for naturally contaminated food. *International Journal of Food Microbiology*, *176*, 1–8.

Matsubayashi, K., Kang, J. H., Sakata, H., Takahashi, K., Shindo, M., Kato, M., et al. (2008). A case of transfusion-transmitted hepatitis E caused by blood from a donor infected with hepatitis E virus via zoonotic food-borne route. *Transfusion*, *48*, 1368–1375.

Matsubayashi, K., Nagaoka, Y., Sakata, H., Sato, S., Fukai, K., Kato, T., et al. (2004). Transfusion-transmitted hepatitis E caused by apparently indigenous hepatitis E virus strain in Hokkaido, Japan. *Transfusion*, *44*, 934–940.

Maunula, L., Kaupke, A., Vasickova, P., Söderberg, K., Kozyra, I., Lazic, S., et al. (2013). Tracing enteric viruses in the European berry fruit supply chain. *International Journal of Food Microbiology*, *167*, 177–185.

McCreary, C., Martelli, F., Grierson, S., Ostanello, F., Nevel, A., & Banks, M. (2008). Excretion of hepatitis E virus by pigs of different ages and its presence in slurry stores in the United Kingdom. *The Veterinary Record*, *163*, 261–265.

Meng, X. J. (2013). Zoonotic and foodborne transmission of hepatitis E virus. *Seminars in Liver Disease*, *33*, 41–49.

Meng, X. J., Wiseman, B., Elvinger, F., Guenette, D. K., Toth, T. E., Engle, R. E., et al. (2002). Prevalence of antibodies to hepatitis E virus in veterinarians working with swine and in normal blood donors in the United States and other countries. *Journal of Clinical Microbiology*, *40*, 117–122.

Nakamura, M., Takahashi, K., Taira, K., Taira, M., Ohno, A., Sakugawa, H., et al. (2006). Hepatitis E virus infection in wild mongoose in Okinawa, Japan: Demonstration of anti-HEV antibodies and a full-genome nucleotide sequence. *Hepatology Research*, *34*, 137–140.

Nakano, T., Takahashi, K., Arai, M., Okano, H., Kato, H., Ayada, M., et al. (2013). Identification of European-type hepatitis E virus subtype 3e isolates in Japanese wild boars: Molecular tracing of HEV from swine to wild boars. *Infection, Genetics and Evolution*, *18*, 287–298.

Nicand, E., Armstrong, G. L., Enouf, V., Guthmann, J. P., Guerin, J. P., Caron, M., et al. (2005). Genetic heterogeneity of hepatitis E virus in Darfur, Sudan, and neighboring Chad. *Journal of Medical Virology*, *77*, 519–521.

Oliveira-Filho, E. F., Konig, M., & Thiel, H. J. (2013). Genetic variability of HEV isolates: Inconsistencies of current classification. *Veterinary Microbiology*, *165*, 148–154.

Pavio, N., et al. (2010). Zoonotic hepatitis E: Animal reservoirs and emerging risks. *Veterinary Research*, *41*, 46.

Payne, C. J., Ellis, T. M., Plant, S. L., Gregory, A. R., & Wilcox, G. E. (1999). Sequence data suggests big liver and spleen disease virus (BLSV) is genetically related to hepatitis E virus. *Veterinary Microbiology*, *68*, 119–125.

Purcell, R. H., & Emerson, S. U. (2008). Hepatitis E: An emerging awareness of an old disease. *Journal of Hepatology*, *48*, 494–503. https://doi.org/10.1016/j.jhep.2007.12.008.

Purdy, M. A., & Khudyakov, Y. E. (2011). The molecular epidemiology of hepatitis E virus infection. *Virus Research*, *161*, 31–39.

Raj, V. S., Smits, S. L., Pas, S. D., Provacia, L. B., Moorman-Roest, H., Osterhaus, A. D., et al. (2012). Novel hepatitis E virus in ferrets, the Netherlands. *Emerging Infectious Diseases*, *18*, 1369–1370.

Renou, C., Cadranel, J. F., Bourliere, M., Halfon, P., Ouzan, D., Rifflet, H., et al. (2007). Possible zoonotic transmission of hepatitis E from pet pig to its owner. *Emerging Infectious Diseases*, *13*, 1094–1096.

Rodríguez-Lázaro, D., Cook, N., Ruggeri, F. M., Sellwood, J., Nasser, A., Nascimento, M. S., et al. (2012). Virus hazards from food, water and other contaminated environments. *FEMS Microbiology Reviews*, *36*, 786–814.

Rivero-Juarez, A., Frias, M., Martinez-Peinado, A., Risalde, M. A., Rodriguez-Cano, D., Camacho, A., et al. (2017). Familial hepatitis E outbreak linked to wild boar meat consumption. *Zoonoses Public Health*, *64*, 561–565.

Rutjes, S. A., Lodder, W. J., Lodder, V. F., van den Berg, H. H., Vennema, H., Duizer, E., et al. (2009). Sources of hepatitis E virus genotype 3 in the Netherlands. *Emerging Infectious Diseases*, *15*, 381–387.

Sinha, S., Jha, R., Lakhtakia, S., & Narayan, G. (2003). Acute pancreatitis following kidney transplantation—Role of viral infections. *Clinical Transplantation*, *17*, 32–36.

Smith, D. B., Purdy, M. A., & Simmonds, P. (2013). Genetic variability and the classification of hepatitis E virus. *Journal of Virology*, *87*, 4161–4169.

Song, Y. J., Jeong, H. J., Kim, Y. J., Lee, S. W., Lee, J. B., Park, S. Y., et al. (2010). Analysis of complete genome sequences of swine hepatitis E virus and possible risk factors for transmission of HEV to humans in Korea. *Journal of Medical Virology*, *82*, 583–591.

Szabo, K., Trojnar, E., Anheyer-Behmenburg, H., Binder, A., Schotte, U., Ellerbroek, L., et al. (2015). Detection of hepatitis E virus RNA in raw sausages and liver sausages from retail in Germany using an optimized method. *International Journal of Food Microbiology*, *215*, 149–156.

Takahashi, M., Nishizawa, T., Sato, H., Sato, Y., Jirintai Nagashima, S., & Okamoto, H. (2011). Analysis of the full-length genome of a hepatitis E virus isolate obtained from a wild boar in Japan that is classifiable into a novel genotype. *The Journal of General Virology*, *92*, 902–908.

Tam, A. W., Smith, M. M., Guerra, M. E., Huang, C. C., Bradley, D. W., Fry, K. E., et al. (1991). Hepatitis E virus (HEV): Molecular cloning and sequencing of the full-length viral genome. *Virology*, *185*, 120–131.

Tei, S., Kitajima, N., Takahashi, K., & Mishiro, S. (2003). Zoonotic transmission of hepatitis E virus from deer to human beings. *The Lancet*, *362*, 371–373.

Tesse, S., Lioure, B., Fornecker, L., Wendling, M. J., Stoll-Keller, F., Bigaillon, C., et al. (2012). Circulation of genotype 4 hepatitis E virus in Europe: First autochthonous hepatitis E infection in France. *Journal of Clinical Virology*, *54*, 197–200.

Thapa, R., Biswas, B., Mallick, D., & Ghosh, A. (2009). Acute pancreatitis—Complicating hepatitis E virus infection in a 7-year-old boy with glucose 6 phosphate dehydrogenase deficiency. *Clinical Pediatrics (Phila.)*, *48*, 199–201.

van der Poel, W. H. M., Verschoor, F., van de Heide, R., Herrera, M. I., Vivo, A., Kooreman, M., et al. (2001). Hepatitis E virus sequences in swine related to sequences in humans, the Netherlands. *Emerging Infectious Diseases*, 7, 970–976.

Wenzel, J. J., Preiss, J., Schemmerer, M., Huber, B., Plentz, A., & Jilg, W. (2011). Detection of hepatitis E virus (HEV) from porcine livers in Southeastern Germany and high sequence homology to human HEV isolates. *Journal of Clinical Virology*, *52*, 50–54.

Zhao, C., Ma, Z., Harrison, T. J., Feng, R., Zhang, C., Qiao, Z., et al. (2009). A novel genotype of hepatitis E virus prevalent among farmed rabbits in China. *Journal of Medical Virology*, *81*, 1371–1379.

FURTHER READING

Feagins, A. R., Opriessnig, T., Guenette, D. K., Halbur, P. G., & Meng, X. J. (2007). Detection and characterization of infectious hepatitis E virus from commercial pig livers sold in local grocery stores in the USA. *The Journal of General Virology*, *88*, 912–917.

CHAPTER FOUR

Parasites in Food: From a Neglected Position to an Emerging Issue

Lucy J. Robertson[1]
Department of Food Safety and Infection Biology, Norwegian University of Life Sciences, Oslo, Norway
[1]Corresponding author: e-mail address: lucy.robertson@nmbu.no

Contents

Abstract

Foodborne parasites have long been a neglected group of pathogens, as they often have insidious, chronic effects, rather than being acute diseases, and they are often associated with impoverished or marginalized populations. In addition, due to the long incubation period for most foodborne parasites, source attribution is often difficult, if not

Advances in Food and Nutrition Research, Volume 86
ISSN 1043-4526
https://doi.org/10.1016/bs.afnr.2018.04.003
© 2018 Elsevier Inc.
All rights reserved.

impossible. However, global trends have enabled foodborne parasites to emerge in different populations in new locations, transmitted through different food types, and sometimes with unexpected symptoms. This emergence of foodborne parasites has brought them into focus. In this chapter, six foodborne parasites are used as examples on emergence: *Echinococcus multilocularis* is spreading to new locations; *Cryptosporidium* spp. are beginning to be associated not only with water, but also with salads; *Trypanosoma cruzi* is being manifest with acute disease due to foodborne transmission, particularly transmitted with juices; *Trichinella* spp. have become less of a burden regarding transmission via pork in many countries, but now game animals are becoming a concern; anisakiasis is becoming a global problem as the world develops a taste for sushi, and similarly for opisthorchiasis, which is increasingly being associated with cholangiocarcinoma.

However, the emergence of these foodborne parasites provides an incentive for increased efforts being made toward control. In this chapter, having described how the parasites are emerging from their neglected position, the focus turns toward control. In addition to considering control measures that may be applied to the specific parasites, an overview is provided of some of the organized collaborations, projects, and consortia, as well as some of their outputs, that have in focus the control of these emerging and important pathogens.

1. INTRODUCTION

Parasites have long been the neglected group of pathogens (compared with viruses and bacteria), and this continues to be their position today. There are several reasons that parasites are neglected, including that many, but not all, parasitic infections do not manifest as acute diseases, but rather have a chronic, more insidious impact on their hosts. Another reason that parasites are neglected is that they are often associated with poverty, with populations that are most exposed to parasitic infections being those living in areas where the basic infrastructure elements of water supply, sanitation, housing, and transport are lacking or inadequate. Such populations cannot afford costly diagnostics or treatments, and thus the financial incentive for the biomedical and pharmaceutical industries to invest in improved approaches to combating these diseases is low compared with the incentives traditionally associated with the noninfectious diseases of wealthier populations, such as obesity and cardiac diseases. Indeed, Pedrique et al. (2013) noted in a systematic assessment of drugs and vaccines for neglected diseases that only 4% (and only 1% of all approved new chemical entities) were indicated for neglected diseases, despite these diseases accounting for around 11% of the global disease burden.

As the data of Pedrique et al. (2013) demonstrate, even today, parasites are relatively neglected; on the World Health Organization (WHO) list of neglected tropical diseases (including those proposed during the 10th Meeting of the Strategic and Technical Advisory Group for Neglected Tropical Diseases in 2017, and added according to the procedures; WHO, 2017), of the 20 diseases, or groups of diseases listed, 12 (60%) are parasitic. It is also worth noting that among these parasitic diseases listed, five (42%) have the potential to be transmitted by food.

The Drugs for Neglected Diseases initiative (DNDi) has also produced a list of diseases that they believe to be neglected. In the DNDi list, among the eight diseases or groups of diseases listed, five (approximately 62%) are parasitic diseases, although the emphasis in this list is more on vectorborne parasitoses.

However, although many parasites, including foodborne parasites, remain neglected, several are also considered to be emerging threats. As there are several different types of disease emergence, for a disease to be defined as emerging is not necessarily obvious (Moutou & Pastoret, 2015). For example, an emerging disease may be one that has never been identified previously, such as Middle East respiratory syndrome (MERS) that was first identified in Saudi Arabia in 2012, and found to be due to infection with a specific novel coronavirus (MERS-CoV). However, the term "emerging disease" could also refer to the emergence of a particular disease in a geographic region where it has not previously been identified, and/or with symptoms with which the disease has not previously been associated, such as the emergence of Zika virus infections associated with microcephaly in Brazil in 2015. In addition, for diseases of animals in particular, the association of a disease with a new species, possibly in a new geographical region and/or with a new clinical spectrum, can also be considered as disease emergence; for example, the emergence of the prion disease, chronic wasting disease, in reindeer and moose in Norway in 2016. However, a disease does not necessarily have to be entirely new to a species or region in order to be considered emerging; an unexpected increase in disease incidence in an area or species where it has previously been diagnosed may also result in the disease being considered to be emerging. However, this may not necessarily indicate a real increase, but may simply reflect an improvement in our knowledge or awareness of a particular disease, and/or an increase in the sensitivity of diagnostic tools. For foodborne parasites, being considered as an emerging issue generally does not reflect new organisms being discovered (although with increasingly sophisticated tools we may now separate into individual species or subspecies parasites that were previously grouped together), but the recognition of spread and establishment of these pathogens in populations where they were previously not considered to be a problem.

As with other pathogens, the emergence of the foodborne parasites is often associated with human activity (Moutou & Pastoret, 2015), either directly or indirectly. Thus, climate change, globalization, alterations in legislation, population growth and movement, including urbanization, cultural changes, and many other factors may all result in specific pathogens, including foodborne parasites, emerging, or reemerging, in unexpected ways; it is well recognized that many current emerging infectious diseases, not just foodborne parasites, are associated with human modification of the environment (Pearce-Duvet, 2006). The commonality is that all these factors result in humans having greater exposure to a previously unfamiliar pathogen, or its natural host, or generally promote dissemination to humans from the environment or other hosts (Morse, 1995). With regard to food, the complicated trade routes, the changes in our dietary habits, healthy-eating trends, in which minimally processed, "organic" foods are considered preferable or linked to virtuosity by the consumer, and how particular sectors of the food industry may be associated with distinct population groups, are all factors that may tip a pathogen toward becoming emerging in a specific area.

In the following pages, further details are provided on six selected foodborne parasites (one cestode—*Echinococcus multilocularis*, two protozoa—*Cryptosporidium* spp. and *Trypanosoma cruzi*, two nematodes—*Trichinella* spp. and anisakids, and one trematode—*Opisthorchis* spp.), and how the factors listed above, acting in concert or alone, have moved the position of those parasites from being neglected to being recognized as emerging or reemerging issues; a summary is provided per parasite in Table 1. These selected parasites are all very different from each other not only in terms of taxonomy but also in terms of pathology, symptoms, and lifecycle. Yet there are some commonalities; the zoonotic potential (that the parasites are not only infectious to humans, but that some or all species of the group of hosts may also infect particular other animals) is also important, especially for those for which the transmission route to humans is by consumption of an animal that has already been infected itself.

The relevant factors regarding emergence or reemergence have already altered the spread and distribution of various pathogens, and will also affect their epidemiology in the future as ecosystems continue to evolve, and new technologies enable us to identify and characterize these pathogens.

Table 1 Parasites in Food: From a Neglected Position to an Emerging Issue

	Description of Emergence or Reemergence	**Relevant Factors for Emergence or Reemergence**
Cestodes		
Echinococcus multilocularis	Increasing prevalence in some areas and expansion into new areas	Definitive host populations spreading and increasing—in Europe, rabies vaccination programs have promoted the growth of the fox population, and in North America, the range of coyotes and foxes has expanded, and dogs are imported from endemic areas
Protozoa		
Cryptosporidium	Considered largely hand-to-mouth or waterborne, foodborne outbreaks are becoming increasingly recognized	Globalization of the food supply; use of organic fertilizers Improved diagnostics and detection methods
Trypanosoma cruzi	Largely considered directly vectorborne and affecting mostly impoverished rural populations, in some areas foodborne transmission has become more important and may affect all sectors of society. In addition, foodborne transmission may result in greater disease severity	Environmental changes such as urbanization, habitat fragmentation, and deforestation
Nematodes		
Trichinella spp.	Although trichinosis transmitted through infected pork has been reduced through intervention measures, transmission from game meat is becoming more important; infections may occur in countries where physicians are not familiar with trichinosis, and thus diagnosis and treatment could be delayed	Increased consumption and use of game meat, particularly associated with wild boar due to their rising populations in many countries. Illegal import of wild game/bushmeat may be a particular concern for exposing consumers in countries where physicians are not familiar with the infection

Continued

Table 1 Parasites in Food: From a Neglected Position to an Emerging Issue—cont'd

	Description of Emergence or Reemergence	Relevant Factors for Emergence or Reemergence
Anisakidae	Previously limited to countries where consumption of raw seafood is part of traditional culture, cases of anisakiasis are now increasing in other areas of the world; in addition, even if the larvae are inactivated there remains the potential for an allergenic response in some individuals and more serious effects of infection have been postulated	Increased consumption of seafood, particularly seafood consumed raw or very lightly cooked (spread of this dietary preference globally); increased prevalence of natural definitive hosts (sea mammals—partly due to protective conservation measures) may result in greater prevalence in intermediate hosts; improved diagnostics in humans, but potentially reduced skill for detection in fish and confusion over operating procedures and management plans
Trematodes		
Opisthorchis spp.	Infections have been previously limited to endemic areas where the lifecycles of the two species occur, and where consumption of raw freshwater fish are part of the culinary traditions, but cases of opisthorchiasis are now being diagnosed in other parts of the world; in addition, further research is unravelling the link between opisthorchiasis and cholangiocarcinoma (CCA)	Increased consumption of fish, and, in some areas, increased consumption of raw or inadequately cooked fish which is necessary for transmission; although establishment of the lifecycle in nonendemic areas is unlikely, human migration and tourism mean that infected people may live in places where the parasite is not endemic, and thus are less likely to be diagnosed due to lack of knowledge among diagnosticians—lack of diagnosis and treatment increases the risk of CCA developing; the increasing aquaculture market is also considered to be a probable route for the parasite to travel outside its endemic area

Change and adaptation to change are ongoing processes and mean that we should try to stay aware of the current state of the events such that we can address not only the situation today, but also the trends in the future. With this in mind, this chapter also provides a section on mitigation approaches that should be of both relevance now, and also to safeguard future public health regarding these foodborne parasites. As well as describing parasite-specific practical interventions, the chapter concludes with drawing attention to initiatives, recent, ongoing, and recently established, which indicate how foodborne parasites, both in general and the specific parasites under discussion, are being taken seriously be several groups globally. Tackling these issues from a One Health perspective, such that human infections, animal health, and the environment are all considered to have roles, should enable us to ensure that the impacts associated with foodborne parasites, as we know them now decrease and maybe disappear entirely.

2. SPECIFIC EXAMPLE PARASITES: THE TRANSITION FROM NEGLECTED POSITION TO EMERGING ISSUE

2.1 *Echinococcus multilocularis*: Becoming More Globalized

This cestode parasite does not have humans as part of its usual lifecycle, which normally involves only canids, particularly foxes, as the definitive host, and small mammals, particularly rodents, as the intermediate host. However, humans can become infected by ingesting eggs excreted in the feces of an infected canid and become an aberrant intermediate host. Although clinical signs and symptoms of alveolar echinococcosis (AE) may take decades to appear, they are severe, with proliferation of the larval stage of the parasite, particularly within the liver, resulting in a range of symptoms similar to those associated with liver cancer, possibly spreading to other organs. Without treatment, the disease is likely to be fatal within a decade. Echinococcosis is listed on the WHO list of neglected tropical diseases (WHO, 2017), due to its association with severe morbidity and mortality in the hotspot areas where human cases occur (particularly western China, Tibet, eastern Russia, and the Near East) and also because the populations affected are often poor, pastoral communities, who may be remote from the general population in the region; thus, the disease is frequently of low priority in the region's healthcare budget. Furthermore, due to the requirement for relatively expensive equipment for detecting the disease (imaging equipment such as CT scan), the infection may easily go undiagnosed in such populations; even if diagnosed, the treatment required is long-term, which is difficult to follow-up in isolated, marginalized communities (Craig et al., 2007).

Although human infection with *E. multilocularis* is rare in most European countries and definitive evidence for its foodborne transmission is lacking, due to the severity of its symptoms, this parasite has nevertheless been considered to be among the most important foodborne parasites in Europe (Bouwknegt, Devleesschauwer, Graham, Robertson, & van der Giessen, 2018). Indeed, although targeted interventions have resulted in a significant decrease in the prevalence of human infection with *Echinococcus granulosus* (causing cystic echinococcosis (CE)) in several regions that used to be highly endemic, the same has not been achieved for *E. multilocularis* (Craig, Hegglin, Lightowlers, Torgerson, & Wang, 2017). This is presumably because the domestic dog-livestock cycle associated with *E. granulosus* is relatively easier to interrupt (by worming dogs, preventing dogs from scavenging domestic animal remains at abattoirs and in the fields, and efforts at meat inspection), than the predominantly sylvatic *E. multilocularis* cycle (foxes–rodents). Not only is the prevalence of *E. multilocularis* apparently not decreasing, but the distribution of the parasite seems to be spreading in some areas of northern Europe and it seems to be emerging, becoming identified in some areas previously not considered particularly associated with the parasite, in other regions of the world (Conraths & Deplazes, 2015; Davidson, Romig, Jenkins, Tryland, & Robertson, 2012; Gottstein et al., 2015; Vuitton et al., 2015). For example, a case-finding study noted an increase in the prevalence of human AE in Switzerland over a 50-year period from 1956 to 2005, which could not be explained by improved diagnosis; the authors suggested that this change in prevalence may be associated with a rising fox population, which, in turn, is associated with a successful antirabies vaccination program (Schweiger et al., 2007). In North America, canine infections with *E. multilocularis* seem to be extending beyond their "traditional" limits of the Arctic and north-central North America, with a few cases being identified in dogs in Ontario (Trotz-Williams et al., 2017) and a relatively high prevalence being found in urban coyotes in Calgary and Edmonton (Catalano et al., 2012); this indicates the potential for an elevated threat to human health in these regions of Canada, and an unprecedented cluster of human cases was diagnosed in Alberta between 2013 and 2017. The reasons for the occurrence of *E. multilocularis* in new regions of Canada has been considered to be not only due to the range of wild hosts (coyotes, foxes) being extended, but also the import of dogs from endemic areas, including Europe, may be partly responsible for this apparent spread (Trotz-Williams et al., 2017). Indeed, the discovery of European haplotypes in Canadian wildlife does indicate the introduction of this parasite from Europe (Gesy & Jenkins, 2015).

Although there is no evidence that foodborne transmission of *E. multilocularis* is increasing, a recent meta-analysis demonstrates that transmission of AE due to the ingestion of food or water contaminated with eggs of the parasite can occur, but these risk factors appear not to elevate infection risk significantly (Conraths et al., 2017). It should be borne in mind that for an infection for which symptoms occur many years after infection, determining the vehicle of transmission is always difficult. However, it would seem probable that with increased environmental contamination, due to greater prevalence of infected definitive hosts, then the likelihood that food would be contaminated is also greater, and that other infection routes and vehicles will also be affected.

2.2 *Cryptosporidium* spp.: Transmission Emerging From Water to Salad and Other Fresh Produce

This protozoan parasite, causing diarrhea and other abdominal symptoms in the infected human host, was first described in mice over a century ago. However, its importance as a human pathogen was not recognized until around 70–80 years later when the HIV pandemic brought sharply into focus the importance of this parasite as causing severe, opportunistic infections in the immunocompromised. Almost simultaneously came the realization that the transmission stage, the oocyst, was resistant to most standard drinking water treatment technologies in use at that time, thus resulting in large waterborne outbreaks, involving hundreds, even thousands, of individuals. At this point in time, from around 1980 to 2000, *Cryptosporidium* certainly moved from being a parasite so neglected that its significance as a disease-causing agent of humans and domestic animals was unrecognized, to being an important pathogen, emerging globally, and with an impact not only in countries with poor infrastructure, but also in the wealthy countries of Europe, Australasia, and North America. The severity of the disease in some populations is exacerbated by the limitations in available treatment, a problem that continues to this day.

Although some foodborne outbreaks were identified in these earlier years of recognition of *Cryptosporidium*, these tended to be predominantly small-scale local outbreaks, frequently associated with milk and related dairy products, or with apple cider in which the apples had been contaminated prior to the drink being made. Indeed, in the 10 years from 1993 to 2003 just 10 foodborne outbreaks were recorded, with fewer than 450 cases in total (see table 1 in Robertson & Chalmers, 2013). However, in the 10 years from 2005 to 2015 the number of foodborne outbreaks recorded has increased by 50% (15 outbreaks listed; see table 2 in Ryan, Hijjawi, & Xiao, 2018), with over 1800 cases recorded, an increase of over 400% (Ryan et al., 2018). Thus, although *Cryptosporidium* had already become an emerging issue 20 years ago, more recently it seems to be reemerging as a foodborne pathogen. Interestingly, also, the predominant food transmission vehicles recorded seem to have changed, shifting from dairy products and apple cider, which were the main transmission vehicles during the first decade (1993–2003), to over 45% of the outbreaks and more than 90% of the cases being associated with salad ingredients or garnish in more recent times. These later outbreaks also seem to affect larger numbers of people; of the nonsalad/garnish-associated outbreaks the mean number of people affected per outbreak was around 30 (ranging from 4 with raw meat to 74 with the vehicle of infection not identified), whereas for those outbreaks associated with salad ingredients, the mean number of people infected was around 200 (ranging from 18 to 648). The reason for this reemergence of *Cryptosporidium* as a foodborne pathogen, particularly associated with salad vegetables, has not been closely investigated but potential factors could include a general rise in the per capita consumption of salad, the increase in popularity of prewashed read-to-eat (RTE) salad vegetables, the rise in international trade in salad ingredients, particularly with transport from warmer countries to colder countries during the winter months, more intensive farming decreasing the gap between fresh produce and animals, and improved awareness, diagnostics, and trace back during outbreaks, enabling not only cryptosporidiosis cases and outbreaks to be identified, but the implicated product also. Although greater awareness of cryptosporidiosis and improvements in diagnostic sensitivity undoubtedly play a role in more outbreaks being detected, for the particular transmission vehicle, the second factor listed here may be of particular relevance. Bagged, prewashed RTE salad vegetables were introduced in the United States in the mid-1990s, and soon became a popular consumer choice, with the number of consumers continuing to rise steadily (in United States 223.95 million in 2011, 232.91 million in 2015; https://www.statista.com). Similar trends are occurring elsewhere in the world. Although surveys of RTE salads in UK indicate that the majority are of acceptable microbiological quality (Little & Gillespie, 2008), and similar data have been obtained in Italy (De Giusti et al., 2010), such studies tend not to consider parasites. One problem with the bulk washing of salad prior to bagging is that point-source contamination can be spread throughout a large batch, and the sanitizers used for salad washwater are usually aimed at reducing bacterial contamination (on the produce itself, but, more importantly, within the washwater; Gil, Selma, López-Gálvez, & Allende, 2009) and are not necessarily effective at killing hardy *Cryptosporidium* oocysts. Thus, in this way, given the distribution of RTE salad, there is the potential for many people to become exposed to a contamination that, initially at least, may have been limited in spread. Indeed, the largest foodborne outbreak of cryptosporidiosis is associated with precut mixed salad leaves obtained from a particular supermarket chain, with leaves from growers in UK, Spain, Italy, and France (Ryan et al., 2018). This indicates also the complexity in traceback when an outbreak occurs, and is probably particularly difficult for products with a short-shelf life (such that the food is rapidly consumed or discarded) and an infectious agent, such as *Cryptosporidium*, with an incubation period that exceeds or matches the shelf-life of the implicated product.

2.3 *Trypanosoma cruzi*: Foodborne Transmission Becoming More Common Than Vectorborne and Results in More Severe Symptoms

Chagas disease, caused by infection with the protozoan parasite *T. cruzi*, is listed by the World Health Organization as a neglected tropical disease (WHO, 2017) and has also been described as one of the "social diseases" of poverty, along with malnutrition, diarrhea, tuberculosis, and other parasitic diseases (Storino, 2000). Chagas disease may be fatal, and around 12,000 people die annually from this infection (de Noya, Gonzalez, & Robertson, 2015). The disease develops in two distinct stages, in which an acute stage, which occurs shortly after infection, is followed by a chronic stage that usually takes several years to develop; the latter stage is most commonly associated with the clinical pathology. Cell death in the target tissues results in clinical manifestations due to the damage to the affected organs, often the digestive system, nervous system, or the heart. The disease has long been associated with less affluent socioeconomic groups in specific rural areas of South America as the usual vectors, triatomines, which thrive in ecotopes such as palm trees, piles of rocks, hollow trees, and mammal burrows, are also well adapted to living in the sort of human homes that are particularly associated with rural poverty, being poorly constructed or made of adobe (mud) bricks, not plastered internally, and with thatched roofs. In such locations, the triatomines can shelter and reproduce, emerging at night to feed on human hosts, and, if infected with trypanosomes, may then infect the host by defecating into the bite wound (de Noya et al., 2015). Although initiatives directed against vectors and improvements in housing have decreased vectorborne transmission through the skin in recent years, oral (foodborne) transmission appears to be on the rise (de Noya et al., 2015). Of the many foodborne cases reported in the literature, a high proportion are associated with fruit juice, with contamination via triatomines (either being ground up in the juice preparation, or defecating into the juice). There are several important differences between the two transmission routes, including foodborne infection more often occurring as an outbreak, that not only triatomines with fast reflex defecation are involved in the lifecycle for foodborne transmission, that the parasite load can be very high (if one or more whole insects are ground into the vehicle of infection), and, importantly in the context of the current discussion, rather than being particularly associated with poor people living in rural areas in nonimproved housing, that large numbers of people of any social status may be exposed (de Noya et al., 2015). This latter point may be particularly exemplified by the outbreak in Caracas in 2007, in which infection was confirmed in 103 people, of whom 75% were symptomatic and over 20% required hospitalization, and one child died (Alarcón de Noya et al., 2010). What was particularly noticeable about this outbreak was not only more obvious and severe clinical signs than expected in the exposed people, but that the population affected was predominantly urban and middleclass, a demographic group not normally associated with Chagas disease. The authors suggested that environmental changes had altered the behavior and ecology of the infection reservoirs, resulting in the urbanization and domiciliation of lifecycle. Indeed, oral transmission is now considered to be the most important route of infection for Chagas disease in Venezuela and the Brazilian Amazon (Silva-Dos-Santos et al., 2017), and environmental changes such as deforestation, habitat fragmentation, urbanization, etc., are again considered to be the reason for the emergence of this infection (Nava, Shimabukuro, Chmura, & Luz, 2017).

Although Chagas disease is generally considered a serious disease, regardless of transmission route, a further concern with foodborne transmission is that disease severity seems to be greater, particularly with prolonged fever in the initial phases of infection (de Noya et al., 2015). The reasons for the greater disease severity with oral transmission have not been fully elucidated, but experiments comparing oral and intraperitoneal (i.p.) infection in mice, using the same strain and dose of parasite have shown that with oral transmission, as well as transmission being more successful, there is also a higher maximum peak of parasitemia and parasite loads in different tissues are greater during acute infection than in mice infected via the i.p. route (Margioto Teston, de Abreu, Abegg, Gomes, & de Ornelas Toledo, 2017).

The various foodborne outbreaks recorded, along with the higher clinical burden of disease (de Noya et al., 2015), have brought further attention to this parasite, with calls to policy makers and stakeholders to focus attention on control of transmission of this parasite via the foodborne route (Robertson, Devleesschauwer, Alarcón de Noya, Noya González, & Torgerson, 2016), and to use integrated surveillance systems and effective outreach programs to mitigate or control transmission of this parasite (Nava et al., 2017). Indeed, with this background, Chagas disease is now sometimes considered a worldwide problem, and to address source tracking for foodborne transmission, qPCR has been recently evaluated as a methodology for confirming implicated food commodities in outbreaks (de Souza Godoi et al., 2017; Mattos et al., 2017).

2.4 *Trichinella* spp.: Game Animals Replace Undercooked Pork as the Major Vehicle of Infection in Some Countries

Human trichinosis, in which people are infected by consumption of larvae of the nematode *Trichinella* in the undercooked meat of an infected animal, has long been recognized as an important foodborne parasitosis. In many countries of the world, including throughout Europe, testing of pork at the slaughterhouse level, using a recommended methodology or equivalent, is compulsory unless the pig production system has been certified as *Trichinella*-free due to meeting a particular standard of controlled housing (European Commission, 2015). The symptoms of trichinosis depend on the stage of infection, with abdominal symptoms (diarrhea, vomiting, abdominal pain) associated with invasion of the intestine, followed by fever, inflammation, swelling, being associated with migration of the new larvae about a week after initial infection, and then rash and myalgia, possibly with heart, lung, or CNS involvement, associated with the subsequent encystation of these larvae into the tissue. Meat control and enclosed pig farming mean that in Europe, human infections with *Trichinella spiralis*, the species closely associated with domestic pork, occur relatively infrequently apart from in locations where infrastructure insufficiencies, including socioeconomic problems, lack of veterinary controls, and inadequate education, may result in infected pork being included in traditional cured, dried, or smoked products (see, for example, Cacciò, Chalmers, Dorny, & Robertson, 2018). Thus, although considerable budget is spent on control of this parasite in many countries, the global burden of disease (measured in disability adjusted life years, DALYs) is, compared to that of many of other foodborne parasitic diseases, relatively how (Devleesschauwer et al., 2015). However, although pork may no longer present the biggest risk for trichinosis, other animal species may act as hosts for *Trichinella* spp., and nonpork meat sources may represent the emergence or reemergence of this infection and human outbreaks of trichinosis (Rostami, Gamble, Khazan, & Bruschi, 2017). As these outbreaks are most likely to be small, family-size outbreaks, they are unlikely to receive as much media attention, or even scientific interest as those associated with pork. Although the European legislation does, indeed, address testing for *Trichinella* in animals other than pigs (listed are horses, wild boar, bears, walruses, crocodiles, and birds, and other carnivorous mammals (including marine mammals) are also mentioned in general; European Commission, 2015), the fact that many of these animals, probably with the exception of horses, are often not slaughtered through a legislated system, but maybe hunted by individuals, means that meat from these animals is more likely to evade being tested, although this is not always the case. Testing of meat for *Trichinella* larvae is particularly likely to be ignored if the animals have been hunted illegally. Furthermore, some countries outside Europe do not necessarily legislate for testing such animals. For example, it has been noted that in China there is currently no mandatory testing for *Trichinella* larvae in meats other than pork, despite a range of less usual animal meats (wild animals, raw meat, and under-cooked foods such as dumplings or scalded dog meat) being considered as delicacies by some consumers, and, indeed, may be consumed quite widely (Bai, Hu, Liu, Tang, & Liu, 2017). Indeed, review papers from China indicate that dog and game meat may be of increasing significance as sources of trichinosis infections in people, although pork still remains the most usual infection vehicle at present (Cui, Wang, & Xu, 2011; Wang, Cui, & Xu, 2006). Dogs, which are known scavengers, are particularly likely to be infected with *Trichinella*, and outbreaks of trichinosis associated with consumption of dog meat have been reported, particularly in China (Rostami et al., 2017). It is worth noting that over 10% of outbreaks of trichinosis reported from China in the period 2000–03 were associated with consumption of infected dog meat (Wang et al., 2006).

Nevertheless, in general, wild boar, horse, and bear are relatively common nonpork meat sources of trichinosis, whereas although infections from consumption of meat from dog, turtle, jackal, cougar, and walrus have occurred, they are more unusual, presumably because these are less usual meat sources (Rostami et al., 2017). An overview comparison of sources of meat types associated with trichinosis cases and outbreaks divided by region or country (Murrell & Pozio, 2011) indicated that of 27 geographic areas listed, domestic pigs were most associated with trichinosis for 11 of them, but for 13 of these regions wild game was the equivalent or predominant source, with all cases associated with wild game in seven of these regions (Ethiopia, Canada, Iran, Lebanon, Greece, Israel, South Korea).

From the available data, it is clear that the wild boar populations globally are experiencing an unprecedented demographic explosion that has been documented in a range of countries including in Europe, USA, and Australia (Ruiz-Fons, 2017). The expanding populations of wild boar may increase the likelihood of meat from these animals being consumed, either as a part of hunting bags at the individual level or supplied to shops and other establishments. It is perhaps worth noting that a major outbreak of trichinosis in Belgium in November 2014 was associated with consumption of wild boar imported into Belgium from Spain and used at three different restaurants (Messiaen et al., 2016). The reason for how this heavily infected wild boar meat evaded detection in the import and supply chain is not clear.

Hunters may also be particularly exposed to *Trichinella* if, rather than bringing the meat home for preparation, they attempt to cook it while out in the field; one example of this was a small outbreak that occurred in Alaska in 2014, when a group of hunters attempted to cook bear meat from the bear they had killed over an open fire (reported in Rostami et al., 2017). As previously mentioned, when animals are hunted illegally then it is highly unlikely that the meat will undergo the relevant veterinary controls. For example, a small outbreak occurred in southern Italy in 2016 that was associated with illegally hunted wild boars in a national park (Turiac et al., 2017), and another larger outbreak occurred in Serbia during winter 2016–17, with 114 people diagnosed with trichinosis (*T. britovi*), associated with consumption of wild boar that had not been through veterinary controls, although it was not noted whether the hunting was legal or not (Cacciò et al., 2018).

Tourists traveling to exotic destinations and participating in safari-type experiences are a further group that are more often associated with trichinosis associated with unusual meat, that has frequently been prepared by smoking or barbecuing or grilling on an open fire (e.g., Dupouy-Camet, Lecam, Talabani, & Ancelle, 2009). Indeed, it has been speculated (Robertson, Sprong, Ortega, van der Giessen, & Fayer, 2014) that in such situations, local people may be less likely to expose themselves to infected meat as their culture is not to eat meat "rare," but that tourists may be unaware of the potential dangers of meat in a different setting than their own home countries and cultures, and thus do not alter their preferences accordingly. An example provided in the review paper of Robertson et al. (2014) is an outbreak of trichinosis, acquired in the Arctic (Nunavut, Canada) but diagnosed in France, which was associated with consumption of grizzly bear meat by five travelers. The meat not consumed by the travelers was consumed locally, but well cooked, and resulted in no suspected cases, but the travelers consumed the meat either raw or pan-fried (Houzé et al., 2009).

Thus, whereas postmortem control of meat and controlled swine rearing has been effective in interrupting the domestic cycle of trichinosis in many countries, the disease is nevertheless reemerging in specific demographic groups, with game meat of different sorts now becoming the predominant source of infection, at least in Europe and North America. In a review from 2015 of *Trichinella* imported with live animals and meat (Pozio, 2015), it was noted that at that time point there was not a large problem with cases of trichinosis due to imported wild animal meat. However, that wild boar and bear meat have been introduced illegally to Europe with personal baggage, and that tons of bushmeat from Africa are also apparently imported illegally, clearly suggests that a risk of imported parasites exists; one specific concern with cases of trichinosis derived from such imported meat is that if cases of infection occur in countries where physicians are not familiar with the disease, then diagnosis, and thus treatment, may be delayed (Pozio, 2015).

2.5 Anisakiasis—And the Global Spread of Sushi

Consumption of raw or undercooked marine fish has long been known to be associated with infection by various nematodes in the family Anisakidae, the causative agents of anisakiasis, in which humans are aberrant hosts. The species of particular importance to human health are those in the genera, *Anisakis* and *Pseudoterranova*, although not limited to these genera, with the species *Anisakis simplex* and *Pseudoterranova decipiens* of greatest relevance.

In the regular lifecycle of species in this family, marine mammals are the definitive hosts and the intermediate hosts include marine crustaceans followed by various species of marine fish or cephalopods. When humans become infected, by consuming undercooked seafood containing the infective larvae, the immune response to the larvae burrowing into the wall of the digestive tract is usually the main cause of the pathology, for which severe abdominal pain is the most obvious manifestation. Two forms of anisakiasis are recognized depending on where larval invasion occurs, intestinal, which is more common in Europe, and gastric, which predominates in Japan. Intestinal anisakiasis, in particular, is often misdiagnosed, and many patients require surgery due to perforation or occlusion of the bowel.

In addition, some people may be allergic to antigens associated with the larvae, which may also be in the surrounding flesh of the fish, and acute allergic manifestations may occur in the consumer, even if the larvae are dead. Furthermore, some work has indicated that *Anisakis* infection could be a risk factor for the development of some cancers associated with the gastrointestinal tract (Garcia-Perez et al., 2015), due not only to the inflammatory reaction elicited during infection, but also neoplastic alterations (Speciale et al., 2017).

Anisakiasis was previously considered to be restricted only to those cultures or areas where consumption of raw fish was considered to be a regular part of the diet; namely, coastal areas of South America where ceviche is consumed, the Netherlands where raw herring are eaten, Spain where raw anchovies are consumed, and Japan, the land of sushi and sashimi, from where most cases have been diagnosed. Due to the restricted geographical locations, global awareness of this foodborne parasitosis has previously been likewise limited. However, a review from 2005 describes the reported increase in prevalence of anisakiasis in the previous two decades as "dramatic" (Chai, Murrell, & Lymbery, 2005), and a recent case report describes anisakiasis as "a growing disease in Western countries" (Carmo, Marques, Bispo, & Serra, 2017). Furthermore, another case report, from Portugal, where although seafood is part of the traditional diet, raw seafood is not, describes anisakiasis as "an emerging cosmopolitan zoonosis" (Baptista-Fernandes et al., 2017).

Although this increase, which is considered to be still continuing, probably partially reflects improvements in diagnostic techniques, particularly endoscopy, another very relevant parameter is alteration in dietary preferences. Although meat consumption per capita is greater than that of seafood and is increasing, between 1961 and 2013, the rise in consumption was almost twice that for aquatic animals than for meat (FAOSTAT, http://www.fao.org/faostat/en/#compare). The various meat-related food scares and scandals in recent decades, such as mad cow disease in the 1990s and horsemeat food fraud in 2013, may be partially responsible for pushing consumers to explore alternative protein sources than meat. The consumer demand is not only rising or seafood, but, in particular, the demand for raw or lightly cooked fish is also increasing. As explained in the prize-winning documentary from 2011, *Sushi: The Global Catch* (Director, Mark Hall), within a relatively short period of time, sushi has expanded being from a particularly Japanese dish for special occasions, to a global phenomenon that can be found for sale in supermarkets, restaurants—in petrol stations and at football games—all over Europe, North America, and Australasia; and not only through Europe and North America, but also wider afield in Africa and Asia—during filming of *Sushi: The Global Catch* the first sushi restaurant in Rwanda opened. But consumption of raw fish involves not only sushi and sashimi; several other raw fish dishes are also increasing in popularity, including, but not limited to, carpaccio, ceviche, crudo, gravlax, koi pla, poke, and tartare. With such dishes becoming more common worldwide, the potential for exposure to Anisakid larvae is also becoming a more global phenomenon, representing an emerging parasitic disease in regions where consumption of raw fish was previously unknown or unusual, although it is also considered to be an emerging disease in countries where raw fish are a traditional dish (for example, "boquerones en vinagre" (anchovies in vinegar) in some regions of Spain; Bao et al., 2017). Given that some surveys have indicated that the prevalence of infection in anchovies is affected by where they are caught, and that the likelihood of fish being infected in a particular region is also closely affected by the presence of the parasite definitive host in that region, there is certainly a strong possibility for human exposure to vary with time, not only according to human consumption of raw fish, but also associated to where fish are caught, and the presence of marine mammals in that area (Rello, Adroher, Benítez, & Valero, 2009). Although the relationship between the population size of the definitive hosts of a parasite, and the parasite population size in intermediate hosts is complex, it has been speculated that as coastal marine cetacean populations have recovered in size due to implementation of protective conservation strategies (Magera, Mills Flemming, Kaschner, Christensen, & Lotze, 2013), so has the likelihood that fish will be infected with anisakid larvae (Chai et al., 2005). Indeed, in addition, in the Baltic sea an increased occurrence of the anisakid worms *P. decipiens* and *Contracaecum osculatum* has been associated with a rising gray seal population in the area (Zuo, Kania, Mehrdana, Marana, & Buchmann, 2018). Finally, alterations in the fishery supply chain, with control today no longer being the task of veterinary inspectors, but maybe more likely to be the job of the food business operator, has also been suggested to be a reason why infected fish may not be removed from the chain due to training in the detection of the larvae in fish being insufficient (D'amico et al., 2014). Indeed, the same authors suggest that concerns about transmission of this foodborne pathogen in raw fish have resulted in a complex legal framework regarding management of the product chain that, rather than protecting the consumer, has given rise to confusion and a wide range of differences in operating procedures and management plans (D'amico et al., 2014).

2.6 *Opisthorchis* spp.: Tourism, Travel, and More Raw Fish

Members of the Opisthorchiidae family are considered to be neglected tropical diseases by WHO, being within the category of foodborne trematodiases (WHO, 2017). As with all trematodes, these parasites have indirect lifecycles, with mollusks acting as one of the intermediate hosts. Among the Opisthorchiidae family are three important genera with respect to public health, *Opisthorchis, Clonorchis*, and *Metorchis*, although information about the third of these, *Metorchis*, is very limited. Although the lifecycles of all three of these genera of parasites are very similar, for the purposes of this chapter the focus is on *Opisthorchis*. Within this genus, two species are of relevance, *Opisthorchis viverreni* and *Opisthorchis felineus*. The definitive hosts of these parasites are fish-eating mammals including humans; the main reservoir hosts for *O. viverreni* are pigs, rodents, dogs, and cats, and for *O. felineus* are cats, canids, mustelids. In humans, after consumption of the metacercariae (encysted in the skin or flesh of the second intermediate host, various freshwater fish in the cyprinid family), the excysted juveniles move from the duodenum to the biliary ducts and take up residence there (also in the liver, gall bladder, and, for *O. felineus*, pancreatic ducts). Eggs are passed in the feces, and if they are ingested by the first intermediate host, an appropriate freshwater snail, particularly those in the family Bithyniidae, they hatch and then undergo several stages of asexual reproduction, resulting ultimately in the release of free-swimming cercariae. These actively seek their second intermediate host, which they penetrate, encysting to form the metacercariae, either in the muscles or below the scales. It is this stage that is infective to the definitive hosts, including humans. That other fish-eating mammals also act as definitive hosts means that control of the lifecycle is complicated, as the lifecycle can be maintained even when steps are taken to prevent human feces contaminating freshwater where the fish and snails reside.

Although many infections with either species of *Opisthorchis* can be asymptomatic or presenting as only mild symptoms, such as dyspepsia, abdominal discomfort, malaise, indigestion, diarrhea, they can also have more serious clinical presentation, such as hepatomegaly and liver cirrhosis, cholecystitis, and malnutrition. However, the most serious outcome of infection, and which is associated with chronic high worm burdens, is bile duct cancer (cholangiocarcinoma; CCA). The etiology behind the development of CCA in infected people is likely to be multifactorial, being associated with chronic inflammation resulting from a combination of mechanical damage, parasite secretions, and immunopathology (Sripa et al., 2007). It should be noted that although reports of associations between CCA tend to be more concerned with *O. viverrini* infection than *O. felineus*, investigations using an experimental hamster model indicate that actually *O. felineus* is likely to produce greater pathogenesis than *O. viverrini* (Lvova et al., 2012), and that in this model *O. felineus* has carcinogenic potential in terms of development of bile duct cancer (Maksimova et al., 2017), and development of precancerous lesions (Gouveia et al., 2017). Nevertheless, although some studies also clearly indicate an epidemiological association (Pakharukova & Mordvinov, 2016), a study investigating associations between *O. felineus* infection and CCA in the Russian Federation does not provide an unequivocal answer (Fedorova et al., 2017); although the incidence of liver and intrahepatic bile duct cancers (code C22 in ICD-10) was significantly higher in regions with high *O. felineus* infection, compared with low incidence regions, in another region with high C22 cancer incidence, new cases of the infection had not been reported. As the authors point out, however, CCA usually develops a decade or more after *Opisthorchis* infection, and the study is also limited by the lack of distinction between liver and bile duct cancers (Fedorova et al., 2017).

An important difference between the two parasites is their geographical distribution. Whereas, *O. viverrini* is mainly found in South East Asia (Cambodia, Lao PDR, Thailand, Vietnam) where over 10 million people are considered to be harboring the infection, *O. felineus* has a more northern and western distribution, occurring in Belorussia, Kazakhstan, Russia, Ukraine, and various foci in Europe, with between 1 and 2 million people considered to be infected (Keiser & Utzinger, 2009); for both species together, the median number of DALYs in 2010 was around 200,000 (Torgerson et al., 2015).

The reasons for both these species of parasites being generally considered neglected are various, but among them is their association often with conditions of poverty and that the symptoms are often not obvious, and morbidity may be subtle (Fürst, Keiser, & Utzinger, 2012). In addition, the most serious public health consequence of infection, CCA, may take years to develop; although infection can be relatively readily diagnosed (standard formal-ether sedimentation and microscopy or ELISA either for coproantigens or antibodies) and cheaply treated with prazinquantel, the lack of pathognomic symptoms means that CCA-affected people may not be detected until the end stages of the disease; the prognosis without early diagnosis and intervention is very poor (Hughes et al., 2017).

As with anisakiasis, transmission of the *Opisthorchis* spp. is dependent on consumption of inadequately cooked fish, although in this case freshwater fish rather than marine. Thus, the regions with which opistorchiasis cases are originally associated, are those with a particular tradition for raw freshwater fish dishes. However, for the reasons previously outlined regarding dietary habits for anisakiasis (increased consumption of fish in general, and particularly a rising increase in lightly cooked or raw fish), opistorchiasis has moved from becoming a wide-spread, but neglected, foodborne parasitic disease to an emerging issue. Tourists to Southeast Asia and Thai laborers have apparently been regularly reported to carry *O. viverrini* beyond the normal distribution of infection (Andrews, Sithithaworn, & Petney, 2008), and it has also been noted that, due to the lack of diagnostic symptoms and the prolonged duration of infection, infected persons may remain undiagnosed for a long time. Indeed, as tourism to SE Asia has risen markedly (for example, the number of tourists to Thailand has risen from 11.6 million in 2004 to 24.81 million tourists in 2014, to over 32 million in 2016), the likelihood of visitors to the area becoming infected and bringing their infections back to their own country with them has also risen. The increasing movement of people from endemic countries, for employment reasons as well as tourism or visiting family who have already moved abroad, means that patients with *Opisthorchis* infections will be living far beyond the endemic regions, and this infection is becoming a global problem, far exceeding being a medical problem associated only with limited regions (Maksimova et al., 2017). Although this transport is unlikely to result in establishment of the lifecycle elsewhere (as both intermediate hosts would be required, along with contamination of the aquatic environment with the trematode eggs from the feces of the infected person), it may well be very detrimental to the health of the infected person, due to lack of diagnosis or treatment. However, as also pointed out by Andrews et al. (2008), the potential for spread of *O. viverrini* beyond SE Asia is even greater when considering the fish export/import market. Asia is the world's largest producer of freshwater aquaculture products, with production of finfish in inland aquaculture well over 40 million tonnes in 2014, compared with under 0.5 million tonnes in Europe (FAO, 2016). Indeed, carp, which are cyprinids, produced by aquaculture in Asia, are responsible for over 50% of the global finfish aquaculture production (Penman, Gupta, & Dey, 2005) and are also used in sushi and thus eaten raw.

Although SE Asia, the endemic area for *O. viverrini,* has the most sizeable inland aquaculture, one case reported in the literature regarding acquisition of opisthorchiasis from imported fish is concerned with *O. felineus* that was transmitted to a family after eating illegally imported smoked carp, imported from Siberia (Yossepowitch et al., 2004). In addition to this outbreak, several outbreaks of opisthorchiasis have been reported from Italy in more recent years; of eight outbreaks reported between 2003 and 2011, together resulting in over 200 confirmed infections, all involved consumption of raw tench (*Tinca tinca*) that had been caught in lakes in central Italy (Pozio, Armignacco, Ferri, & Gomez Morales, 2013). It has been noted that the occurrence of these outbreaks in Italy since 2003 may reflect changes in fish consumption habits (Armignacco et al., 2008); in particular, the authors noted that tench has previously not been used much, due to low commercial value, and also that in Italy it is traditional that fish are well cooked, with raw fish only becoming popular in recent years. In addition, some of the outbreaks demonstrated particular features of importance. For example, in the outbreak from 2007 that resulted in infection in 20 individuals, the fish had been frozen for 3 days at −10°C, before being cut into fillets and marinated in vinegar and wine for 24 h before consumption (Armignacco et al., 2008). Thus, it is clear that the metacercariae of *O. felineus* not only survive smoking (Yossepowitch et al., 2004), but also freezing and marinating. A larger outbreak that occurred during 2011 and involved around 80 infected individuals was partially due to the restaurant using tench rather than whitefish due to cost and availability factors, thus food fraud issues may be of relevance (Cacciò et al., 2018). In addition, it seems likely that among the people exposed were several tourists (of the infected people traced in this outbreak two were from Austria and seven from the Netherlands); not only might tourists be more likely to be unable to recognize the taste of different locally caught fish, but also (especially for asymptomatic infections) it is possible that the people infected may not be diagnosed, particularly if they do not become linked to an outbreak. Living with chronic or cryptic infections may mean that they are at risk of later development of CCA (Cacciò et al., 2018).

3. INTERVENTIONS

3.1 General Comments

For each of the parasites, improvements in diagnostics and treatment are likely to improve the clinical situation at the individual patient level, and this is particularly so for those parasites for which lack of identification may result in devastating long-term or chronic diseases, such as AE due to infection with *E. multilocularis*, Chagas disease for *T. cruzi*, various prolonged gastrointestinal problems with anisakiasis, or CCA for *Opisthorchis* spp. Indeed, even for cryptosporidiosis, the potential for long-term sequelae has been reported (Osman et al., 2017; Rehn et al., 2015; Stiff, Davies, Mason, Hutchings, & Chalmers, 2017); although for most people infected it is more likely to manifest as an acute, but short-lived, self-limiting episode of diarrhea. However, for most of the parasites described here, such improvements are unlikely to have a significant direct impact on transmission at the community or population level, particularly for *E. multilocularis* and *Anisakis* spp., for which humans are a dead-end host, and therefore further transmission will not occur.

Among the other interventions that could be considered, some are parasite-specific, whereas some are more general and can be broadly divided into two groups: interrupting the lifecycle, and preventing foodborne transmission. Both these groups include interventions that are focused upon specific measures and more general, often educational, efforts.

Interventions that may reduce foodborne transmission are considered according to the specific selected parasites under consideration are raised and discussed in the following sections. However, it should be noted that in order to determine whether the interventions suggested are worthwhile implementing, a cost-benefit analysis (or, if possible, a social cost-benefit analysis) should be conducted to determine whether the "cost" involved in the intervention provides an acceptable saving in DALYs and/or economically. It should also be noted that not all the parasites listed here are solely foodborne (other transmission routes exist for some parasites, notably, *E. multilocularis, Cryptosporidium* spp., and *T. cruzi*) thus interventions that may reduce foodborne transmission need not necessarily completely prevent the transmission cycle.

3.2 Parasite-Specific Interventions: *E. multilocularis*

As already described, foodborne transmission of *E. multilocularis* results from contamination of food that is eaten without heat treatment, usually fresh produce, with *Echinococcus* eggs. Thus, any intervention that reduces environmental contamination with *E. multilocularis* eggs will reduce the likelihood of contamination of food. Canids are the definitive hosts of this parasite, so regular worming of dogs and keeping the stray dog population under control are important strategies. In areas that are endemic for the parasite and where dogs are an important definitive host, such strategies of limiting dog populations and the prevalence of *Echinococcus* infection in dogs are likely to reduce environmental contamination from these definitive hosts (Hegglin & Deplazes, 2013; Ito, Romig, & Takahashi, 2003). In countries where the parasite currently is not found, mandatory worming of dogs at the border may protect not only potential contamination of food (such as berries) from the particular infected dog but also introduction and establishment of the parasite; however, it is important to note that compulsory dog treatment may not keep an area free of this parasite, even with 100% treatment compliance, due to the sylvatic lifecycle. In areas where the lifecycle is established, then control of the parasite by eliminating wildlife hosts entirely (foxes, voles) is not feasible or appropriate, and treating foxes by setting out bait that includes suitable antihelminthic treatment (praziquantel) has been discussed vigorously. Indeed, König et al. (2008) demonstrated that in less than a year of intensive baiting, the prevalence of *E. multilocularis* in foxes in some regions could be reduced to close to zero. However, even after such a significant decrease, to ensure that elimination is achieved, this intensive baiting needs to be continued (Hegglin & Deplazes, 2008). Furthermore, it is important to be aware that not only foxes will be enticed by bait, and thus if this strategy is to be pursued then it is important that the removal of bait by other animals is considered; removal of bait by wild boars has been suggested to have a significant impact on whether this strategy is effective or not (Antolova, Miterpakova, Reiterova, & Dubinsky, 2006). Cost-effectiveness or cost-benefit studies, which also take into account ecological parameters, are of clear importance here (Janko & König, 2011), and factors such as available financial resources, priority setting of political decision-makers, and public attitudes are also of relevance (Hegglin & Deplazes, 2013).

3.3 Parasite-Specific Interventions: *Cryptosporidium* spp.

Any interventions that reduce the potential for contamination of food with matter derived from feces, particularly human feces or feces of young ruminants such as calves and lambs, are likely to be effective at reducing the risk of contamination of food with oocysts of *Cryptosporidium*. However, with such a generalized pathway, with many different host species, it is difficult to select parasite-specific interventions to reduce foodborne cryptosporidiosis. Use of a HACCP approach in any food industry that may be relevant for transmission of this parasite may assist in pinpointing where contamination could occur and places where interventions may be of most value. Relevant interventions are thus based around general hygiene principles, ensuring that irrigation water is free from contamination with animal feces or sewage effluent, and ensuring proper hygiene among food handlers, including that persons who have diarrheal disease, or have recently suffered from diarrheal disease, do not handle foods. Pasteurization of milk is a good control measure for dairy products, not just for *Cryptosporidium*, and may also be relevant for fruit juices. Given the potential for spread of *Cryptosporidium* oocysts throughout a batch during commercial washing of fresh produce in the production of RTE salads, specific attention should be focused upon the washwater; given the high biological oxygen demand of this water, disinfection is not easy. Indeed, the washing process, that is intended to make the produce cleaner and safer, may, in fact, do the opposite.

3.4 Parasite-Specific Interventions: *T. cruzi*

As already described, foodborne transmission of *T. cruzi* results from contamination of food, or more frequently beverages (fruit juice), with trypomastigotes from the triatomine vectors, or, less commonly, from reservoir hosts such as opossums. Reducing the likelihood that triatomines and reservoir hosts can gain access to food such as fruit juices, such as by storing food and beverages covered, or keeping them in a refrigerator in endemic areas are obvious approaches to reducing the likelihood of contamination. In consideration of prophylactic and control measures for foodborne Chagas diseases (Robertson and Noya 2015), the authors not only consider prevention of how food can become contaminated, using a HACCP approach to consider the weakest points in the food chain, from production to consumption, but, due to the inextricable link of this illness with both poverty and the vector reduviid bug, also discuss vector control in general. Within buildings where high-risk food products may be prepared, stored, or served, two approaches are both worthy of consideration; these are residual spraying of insecticides and also improving housing infrastructure, including plastering of walls, use of concrete flooring and roofs of suitable materials, and also using screens on windows and doors.

Educational tools are also considered of importance, and the use of mandatory rules to prevent food contamination, particularly in places such as canteens and restaurants, is also recommended. The authors also note how blenders, used in the preparation of fruit juices, should be considered as high-risk equipment regarding the potential for contamination, particularly by nymph stages of the triatomines. These stages, which are very small, may fall into the blender, but, due to the smooth sides, be unable to climb out again, and, as nymph stages do not possess wings, are also unable to fly out (Robertson & Noya, 2015). Thus, keeping blenders in a sealed unit, such as a cupboard, when not in use, and rinsing them before use in the preparation of juices or other blended products are simple approaches toward limiting contamination.

3.5 Parasite-specific interventions: *Trichinella* spp. in game animals

In western Europe, at least, the transmission of *Trichinella spiralis* in the domestic pork industry is negligible. This is largely due to strict controls and biosafety in pork husbandry, and thus the majority of pigs raised for slaughter do not have the opportunity to ingest any meat containing viable *Trichinella* larvae. These controls are backed up by the mandatory testing of slaughter pigs for *Trichinella* larvae by an approved method. It is clear that in order to control *Trichinella* transmission on the basis of the sylvatic cycle, that is not via pork but through consumption of game animals, education of hunters and game meat consumers is key. It has been noted that investment of funds into relevant stakeholders, such as hunters, should be a priority for public health services concerned with control of this foodborne parasite (Pozio, 2014). Although hunters should also have the opportunity to have their "bag" tested, how this would be paid for is unclear, and hunters themselves may be unwilling to take on this additional expense. Given that such testing may be difficult to implement, the importance of adequate cooking should be emphasized. In addition, and as noted by Turiac et al. (2017), it is necessary continually raising the awareness on the epidemiological and clinical features of this zoonosis among healthcare personnel for an immediately suspicion of the disease.

3.6 Parasite-Specific Interventions: Anisakidae

Despite the various reasons for anisakiasis being considered an emerging/reemerging parasitic disease (e.g., Zanelli et al., 2017), it is clear that proactive risk management and consumer protection are on the agenda.

In Europe, the European Food Safety Authority (EFSA) conducted a risk assessment regarding parasites in fishery products, with particular emphasis on *Anisakis* (EFSA, 2010). In particular, EFSA considered the potential for allergic reactions, evaluated alternative treatments for killing viable parasites in fishery products and assessed their effectiveness in comparison with freezing, and discussed whether criteria could be set regarding fish that may not present a health hazard regarding the presence of parasites when eaten raw or cold smoked (EFSA, 2010). EFSA concluded that freezing or heat treatments were the most effective methods for killing the larvae, with heating at >60°C for at least 1 min, and freezing either at −35°C for at least 15 h, at −20°C for not less than 24 h, or at −15°C for at least 96 h. As noted by Bao et al. (2017), their QRA simulation clearly shows that should an education campaign results in an *X*% increase in the number of anchovy meals that are frozen, then the incidence of anisakiasis in the population will also reduce by *X*%. However, Bao et al. (2017) also note that although consumers may be aware that freezing prevents transmission of this parasite, most do not actually do so—indicating the need to target this consumer group, and to determine why they do not do this, particularly in those regions where the disease incidence is highest.

Marinating and cold smoking were acknowledged as not providing a sufficient level of safety, with no sea fishing grounds considered to be known to be free of *A. simplex*. However, the risk from aquaculture salmon, farmed in floating cages or onshore tanks, and fed on compound feed, was considered to be negligible (EFSA, 2010) and has been latterly supported by a large-scale study of farmed Norwegian salmon (Levsen & Maage, 2016). A risk assessment focusing specifically on the likelihood of farmed salmon being sold containing viable anisakid larvae also supports this finding (Crotta, Ferrari, & Guitian, 2016).

A further consideration regarding management of anisakiasis has been delivered through considering "horizon scanning," which resulted in a proposal for collaborative software to provide multilevel management of parasites (not limited to anisakids) in seafood (Llarena-Reino, Abollo, Regueira, Rodríguez, & Pascual, 2015). Professional training was considered to be a key driver. It should also be noted that the presence of anisakid larvae in imported fish has resulted in several notifications to the European Rapid Alert System for Food and Feed (RASFF), with over 91% of parasitic infestations in the RASFF database from 2012 due to import of fish in which anisakid larvae were detected (Robertson et al., 2014). More recently, data from 2017 (1st January until 31st December) show a similar awareness of this parasite, as from 41 parasite infestation reports in RASFF, 35 (ca. 85%)

mention *Anisakis* specifically, whereas others not included among the 35 could be anisakid larvae (e.g., parasitic infestation of fish mentioned, but the parasite not specified).

3.7 Parasite-Specific Interventions: *Opisthorchis* spp.

A cross-sectional study in Thailand found that prioritization of the parasite *Opisthorchis viverrini* by village-level health centers had an impact on risk of infection (Ong et al., 2016). Although, interestingly, behavior regarding consumption of raw fish did not have a significant impact on risk of infection, the authors emphasize the need for a holistic approach in considering control measures for this pathogen, particularly consideration of those factors that constitute the broader pathogenic landscape (Ong et al., 2016). At the same time, other authors seem to consider that interventions directed toward lifecycle interruption for this parasite are destined to fail, citing failure to alter eating practices and the relatively high prevalence of infection in reservoir hosts, such as dogs and cats (Hughes et al., 2017). These authors instead suggest that identification of biomarkers that can be used as indicators of the carcinogenic pathway being activated may be more relevant, enabling detection of the most serious sequelae of this infection, CCA, and thus enabling medical interventions to have a higher likelihood of being successful (Hughes et al., 2017). Various biomarkers have already been suggested, including overexpression of proteins orosmucoid 2 and kinesin 18A (Rucksaken et al., 2012), annexin A1 (Hongsrichan et al., 2014), and various other dysregulated proteins (Khoontawad et al., 2017). Other suggested markers, include, for example, a carbohydrate antigen associated with CCA, on which particular epitopes may be recognized using monoclonal antibody-based techniques (Sawanyawisuth et al., 2012). With regards to *O. felineus*, which has a different geographical distribution, the emphasis remains predominantly on control at the fish level; a landmark paper following the outbreaks in Italy summarized the treatments that could be used to inactivate the metacercariae in fish, with particular reference to the fact that one outbreak had occurred despite the fish being frozen at −10°C (Pozio et al., 2013). Other control mechanisms suggested at the local level are to try to reduce infection of dogs and cats that are otherwise maintaining the lifecycle, by educating fishermen not to discard unwanted catch on the lakeshore where they can be eaten by these animals, and for restaurants also to ensure disposal of fish leftovers or waste such that they are not accessible to dogs and cats (Pozio et al., 2013).

3.8 Current and New Efforts Toward Research and Control

For all foodborne parasites, realization of the problem associated with them is probably the fundamental initial step that enables the implementation of other preventative initiatives. In this respect, the transition from being a neglected subject to an emerging or reemerging problem is actually of assistance, as people are more engaged when they realize that a particular issue is of direct concern to themselves, rather than merely to a group of people who may live very far away and whose problems may seem to be of little global or wider relevance. Although foodborne parasites have previously been a focus of only a very limited group of research scientists, doctors, and veterinarians, various broader interest networks indicate that foodborne parasites are climbing up the agenda and capturing attention from a wider audience. Below an overview is provided of both some general foodborne parasite initiatives and also some parasite-specific initiatives; key points are summarized in Table 2.

For example, WHO and FAO have made some concerted efforts in recent years to compare different foodborne parasites with risk-ranking exercises and also establishing the actual burden due to foodborne parasites (see, for example, FAO/WHO, 2014; Hald et al., 2016; Havelaar et al., 2015; Kirk et al., 2015; Robertson et al., 2014; Torgerson et al., 2015). Although the information published from the work by the WHO Foodborne Disease Burden Epidemiology Reference Group (FERG) did not focus on foodborne parasites alone, their inclusion at all, and the accompanying recognition of the relevance of foodborne parasites (e.g., *Taenia solium* being one of the major causes of deaths due to foodborne diseases) brought this pathogen group into greater focus. Some selectivity of the parasites included was, however, noticed—for example, the exclusion of *T. cruzi* on the basis of its regional occurrence (Robertson et al., 2016).

The increased focus on foodborne parasites in general in more recent times is also reflected in specific actions like the establishment of the Food and Environmental Parasitology Network (FEPN) in Canada in 2009 (see http://www.fepn.net/), with the intention of identifying and communicating risks and research, facilitating discussion and collaboration, developing and validating methods, generating data, and providing advice, the International Association for Food and Waterborne Parasitology (IAFWP) in 2015 (see https://www.iafwp.org/), with the mission to promote and facilitate research and collaboration on this subject with the overall intention of reducing the global burden of parasites transmitted by food or water, along with the companion journal (Food and Waterborne Parasitology Journal,

Table 2 Parasites in Food: From a Neglected Position to an Emerging Issue

	Initiatives Established	Relevant Links or References
Foodborne parasites in general	Food and Environmental Parasitology network (FEPN) in Canada; International Association for Food and Waterborne Parasitology (IAFWP), with associated journal; COST Action, FA1408, A European Network for Foodborne Parasites (Euro-FBP); OIE (World Organization for Animal Health) Collaborating Centers for foodborne parasites: Food-Borne Parasites from the Asia-Pacific Region, Food-Borne Zoonotic Parasites, and Food-Borne Zoonotic Parasites from the European Region; European Food Safety Authority (EFSA) Opinion on Foodborne Parasites	http://www.fepn.net; https://www.iafwp.org/; https://www.journals.elsevier.com/food-and-waterborne-parasitology; https://www.euro-fbp.org/; http://www.cost.eu/COST_Actions/fa/FA1408; http://www.oie.int/en/our-scientific-expertise/collaborating-centres/annual-reports; http://www.efsa.europa.eu/en/events/event/171206
Specific foodborne parasites		
Cestodes		
Echinococcus multilocularis	EFSA Opinion on *Echinococcus multilocularis*; EMIA consortium project (*Echinococcus multilocularis* infection in animals)	European Food Safety Authority (2015) and Oksanen et al., 2016
Protozoa		
Cryptosporidium	ACCORD (ACcelerator for CryptOsporidium Research & Drug Development to Reduce Child Mortality); US CDC CryptoNet	Shoultz, de Hostos, & Choy, 2016; https://www.cdc.gov/parasites/crypto/pdf/cryptonet_fact_sheet508c.pdf

Trypanosoma cruzi	WHO Program on Control of Chagas Disease; The International Federation of Associations of People Affected by Chagas Disease (FINDECHAGAS)	http://www.who.int/chagas/en/; http://www.findechagas.com
Nematodes		
Trichinella spp.	CDC Trichinellosis Information for Hunters; U.K. Food Standards Agency *Trichinella* testing of wild boar carcasses; testing of hunting dog sera	https://www.cdc.gov/parasites/trichinellosis/hunters.html; https://www.food.gov.uk/sites/default/files/multimedia/pdfs/trichinellatestingwildboar.pdf; Gómez-Morales et al. (2016)
Anisakidae	EFSA Opinion on parasites in fishery products; Parasite risk assessment with integrated tools in EU fish production value chains (PARASITE); Scanisakis, for UV-based detection of Anisakids	European Food Safety Authority (2010); http://parasite-project.eu/project; Levsen et al., 2018; https://cordis.europa.eu/result/rcn/189395_en.html
Trematodes		
Opisthorchis spp.	Lawa Model, uses an EcoHealth/One Health tactic; Cholangiocarcinoma Screening and Care Program (CASCAP); Tomsk OPIsthorchiasis Consortium (TOPIC)	Sripa et al., 2015; http://www.who.int/neglected_diseases/news/fbti_thailand_uses_integrated_ecosystems_health_approach/en/; Khuntikeo, Loilome, Thinkhamrop, Chamadol, & Yongvanit, 2016; Ogorodova et al., 2015

published by Elsevier; see https://www.journals.elsevier.com/food-and-waterborne-parasitology), and, in Europe, the COST Action, FA1408, A European Network for Foodborne Parasites (Euro-FBP), an EU-funded networking project running between 2015 and 2019 (see https://www.euro-fbp.org/ and http://www.cost.eu/COST_Actions/fa/FA1408), with the ultimate goal of decreasing the impact on human health from foodborne parasites through establishing a risk-based control program containing robust and appropriate protective strategies. In addition, there are three OIE (World Organization for Animal Health) Collaborating Centers for foodborne parasites: Food-Borne Parasites from the Asia-Pacific Region (based in Changchun, China), Food-Borne Zoonotic Parasites (based in Saskatchewan, Canada), and Food-Borne Zoonotic Parasites from the European Region (based in Maisons-Alfort Cedex, France). The remits of these three centers are similar, although within a regional focus; in their annual reports from 2016 (http://www.oie.int/en/our-scientific-expertise/collaborating-centres/annual-reports/) all three Centers mention in particular *Trichinella* and *Toxoplasma* activities, the Canadian Center also mentions *Taenia saginata* in cattle (Cysticercus bovis), *Cyclospora*, and *Giardia*, the Chinese Center also mentions *T. solium* (Cysticercus) in pigs, *Clonorchis sinensis*, and *Cryptosporidium*, and the European Center also mentions *Cryptosporidium* and *Alaria alata* (which is not currently considered to be zoonotic). Thus, of the six foodborne parasites in focus in this chapter, only two (*Trichinella* and *Cryptosporidium*) were of focus for the OIE Foodborne Parasite Collaborating Centers in 2016, indicating, perhaps, that even these Centers need to expand their considerations.

Also within Europe, the EFSA has taken on the task of considering and evaluating the public health risks associated with three specific foodborne parasites (*Cryptosporidium*, *Echinococcus*, and *Toxoplasma*), with the opinion document due in October 2018 (see http://www.efsa.europa.eu/en/events/event/171206).

As noted, in addition to these parasite-wide initiatives, there have also been some more parasite-specific initiatives. With regard to the six parasites considered here and their foodborne transmission, *E. multilocularis* is part of the ongoing EFSA opinion, but it is a measure perhaps of the potential severity of this infection that EFSA already published an opinion on this parasite in 2015 (European Food Safety Authority, 2015) and, in addition, funded a consortium project between 2012 and 2015 known as EMIA (*E. multilocularis* infection in animals), which included six European consortium partners, and five external experts.

Cryptosporidium is also part of the ongoing EFSA opinion, but also has been very much in focus with respect to the Euro-FBP COST Action (e.g., Cacciò et al., 2018; Chalmers & Cacciò, 2016). As *Cryptosporidium* is largely considered to be a waterborne, rather than foodborne, pathogen, much of the emphasis still remains on the water mode of transmission, or, more particularly directed toward effective drug development, with initiatives such as ACCORD (ACcelerator for CryptOsporidium Research & Drug Development to Reduce Child Mortality) that are intended to develop effective treatments for cryptosporidiosis (Shoultz et al., 2016), and is now associated with PATH—Program for Appropriate Technology in Health (http://sites.path.org/drugdevelopment/projects/edd/accord/). Furthermore, the US Center for Disease Control and Prevention (CDC) has launched an initiative called CryptoNet (https://www.cdc.gov/parasites/crypto/pdf/cryptonet_fact_sheet508c.pdf), the purpose of which is to facilitate systematic collection and molecular characterization of *Cryptosporidium* isolates, thereby providing better understanding of cryptosporidiosis epidemiology in United States, which, among other objectives, intends to improve detection and investigation of foodborne outbreaks.

For *T. cruzi*, the WHO Programme on Control of Chagas Disease (http://www.who.int/chagas/en/) has enabled various subregional initiatives through the Pan American Health Organization (PAHO), which, although not specifically concerned with foodborne transmission, as vector control and development of treatment has been in focus for many years, has enabled strong collaboration to develop. This was exemplified using a Partnership Assessment Tool (Salerno, Salvatella, Issa, & Anzola, 2015). The International Federation of Associations of People Affected by Chagas Disease (FINDECHAGAS) is another patient-centric, multicountry group that was created in Brazil in 2009 with the main goal being to improve social policies, especially in health, with actions that are targeted toward prevention, diagnosis, treatment, and social and psychological protection for carriers and their families (http://www.findechagas.com). Thus, although the main focus is not foodborne transmission, this is obviously also a relevant element.

With education considered a key intervention to reduce transmission of *Trichinella* via game animals, targeted initiatives have been developed. For example, the U.S. Center for Disease Control and Prevention has a web page specifically aimed at hunters (Trichinellosis Information for Hunters; https://www.cdc.gov/parasites/trichinellosis/hunters.html) that explains not only why hunters should be aware of this infection, but also how animals with trichinellosis may appear and how to prevent infection. Similarly, the

U.K. Food Standards Agency has published a leaflet to provide guidance to hunters regarding *Trichinella* testing of wild boar carcasses, including information on the infection itself, samples that should be taken for testing, and a form to accompany samples sent in for analysis (Food Standards Agency, 2010; see https://www.food.gov.uk/sites/default/files/multimedia/pdfs/trichinellatestingwildboar.pdf). Various other countries have similar information for hunters, usually in national languages. Obviously, it would be useful for hunters to know the likelihood of animals that they hunt being infected, and, given that testing of wildlife is impractical, work by Gómez-Morales et al. (2016) has suggested that one approach to obtain such data would be by testing the sera of hunting dogs in defined locations, such that they act as sentinels for circulation of this infection among the wildlife. As a test, Gómez-Morales et al. (2016) analyzed sera in hunting dogs from hunting dogs from 23 districts in a particular region of Italy where there is extensive hunting of wild boar, and an outbreak due to consumption of wild boar meat has been recorded; results indicated that serological testing of hunting dogs could provide an indication on the circulation of *Trichinella* spp. in the wildlife in a specific region during a particular timeframe. As the authors note, however, as both hunters and their dogs may travel between districts, this information must also be taken into account.

In addition to the EFSA opinion on parasites in fishery products (EFSA, 2010), that had a particular emphasis on anisakiasis, an EU-funded project "Parasite risk assessment with integrated tools in EU fish production value chains (PARASITE), Grant Agreement (GA) no. 312068; http://parasite-project.eu/project" which ended in 2016 had particular focus on Anisakids, with objectives (in work packages) focusing on exposure assessment, DNA bar-coding, determination of allergenic capacity, improved detection, investigation of interventions that could inactivate the parasites and reduce allergenic capacity, and quantitative risk analysis. The project has resulted in the development of a graphical exposure risk profile, which includes those fish species or their products, which are considered to be of greatest risk as a source of anisakiasis within Europe (Levsen et al., 2018). As well as other outcomes of this project (see https://cordis.europa.eu/result/rcn/189395_en.html), the project resulted in the development of an automatic device, Scanisakis, for UV-based detection of the zoonotic species within the genera *Anisakis*, *Pseudoterranova*, and *Contracaecum*. In addition, the project developed a device for determining the viability of anisakid larvae, being able to distinguish between live and dead larvae on the basis of various selected viability features and was tested for use on frozen, marinated, and salted products.

Of the six parasites considered in this chapter, *Opistorchis* spp. is, perhaps, the one that remains more neglected than emerging, despite perhaps being the one that currently exerts the greatest public health burden, in terms of the severity and prevalence of infection on a global scale. Nevertheless, there are initiatives in place that seek to tackle this parasite. One approach, now known as the Lawa Model, uses an EcoHealth/One Health tactic; first introduced into the Lawa Lake area in Khon Kaen province, Thailand, where *O. viverrini* is endemic, the program used a combination of anthelminthic treatment, intensive health education, and ecosystem monitoring, all with community participation (Sripa et al., 2015). The results were so positive that the Lawa Model has been hailed as a flagship approach by the World Health Organization (see http://www.who.int/neglected_diseases/news/fbti_thailand_uses_integrated_ecosystems_health_approach/en/) and has been recommended by WHO as an approach worth implementing in other areas and countries. Another approach that has also been initiated in Thailand is the Cholangiocarcinoma Screening and Care Program (CASCAP), which is primarily to instigate long-term screening of population at risk of *O. viverrini* infection and CCA (of whom approximately 20 million are in Thailand, where this initiative is located) such that precancerous changes to the biliary tract and liver are identified in addition to early stage CCA that can be successfully treated (Khuntikeo et al., 2016). Despite being targeted at the clinical level, CASCAP also seeks to address research needs (particularly regarding diagnostics and treatment), to address the socioeconomic aspects of CCA at the community level with the intention of developing policies to address the impact, and to review the efficacy of current control and prevention programs, including education, in order to develop measures for control of *O. viverrini* infections and CCA. Hughes et al. (2017) note that longer-term public education schemes, such as that organized by CASCAP, should be commenced and enlarged such that communities are provided with education about the dangers associated with raw, partially cooked, or fermented fish. The hope is that, over time, attitudes toward consumption of raw fish will modify, even in communities where it is an important part of the local culture. Another initiative concerned with control of opisthorchiasis includes both species (and *C. sinensis*) and is based around a group of professionals who have formed a consortium called TOPIC (Tomsk OPIsthorchiasis Consortium) who wish to raise awareness, strengthen integrated control, and conduct research in order to combat these parasites; the Lawa Model is proposed to be followed by TOPIC also (Ogorodova et al., 2015).

4. CONCLUSION

Pathogens that are neglected because their effects are limited to particular populations or particular locations are, in our increasingly mobile and globalized world, ripe to emerge—they will evolve to adopt new transmission routes, invade new hosts, use new vehicles of infection, and produce new pathologies. As many parasitic infections have been neglected, it is no surprise to see that many are now emerging, appearing in unexpected hosts, in new locations, using different transmission vehicles, or resulting in a different spectrum of symptoms. In this chapter, just six foodborne parasites are used as examples, but others could also have been selected. In recognizing these emerging foodborne parasites and rising to combat them in their new situations, we do ourselves the additional favor of also having the opportunity of addressing pathogens that, although neglected, have been a significant burden, both in terms of health and socioeconomy, often in impoverished or otherwise marginalized communities.

REFERENCES

Alarcón de Noya, B., Díaz-Bello, Z., Colmenares, C., Ruiz-Guevara, R., Mauriello, L., Zavala-Jaspe, R., et al. (2010). Large urban outbreak of orally acquired acute Chagas disease at a school in Caracas, Venezuela. *The Journal of Infectious Diseases*, *201*(9), 1308–1315. https://doi.org/10.1086/651608.

Andrews, R. H., Sithithaworn, P., & Petney, T. N. (2008). *Opisthorchis viverrini*: An underestimated parasite in world health. *Trends in Parasitology*, *24*(11), 497–501. https://doi.org/10.1016/j.pt.2008.08.011.

Antolova, D., Miterpakova, M., Reiterova, K., & Dubinsky, P. (2006). Influence of anthelmintic baits on the occurrence of causative agents of helminthozoonoses in red foxes (*Vulpes vulpes*). *Helminthologia*, *43*, 226–231.

Armignacco, O., Caterini, L., Marucci, G., Ferri, F., Bernardini, G., Natalini Raponi, G., et al. (2008). Human illnesses caused by Opisthorchis felineus flukes, Italy. *Emerging Infectious Diseases*, *14*(12), 1902–19025. https://doi.org/10.3201/eid1412.080782.

Bai, X., Hu, X., Liu, X., Tang, B., & Liu, M. (2017). Current research of Trichinellosis in China. *Frontiers in Microbiology* *8*, 1472. https://doi.org/10.3389/fmicb.2017.01472.

Bao, M., Pierce, G. J., Pascual, S., González-Muñoz, M., Mattiucci, S., Mladineo, I., et al. (2017). Assessing the risk of an emerging zoonosis of worldwide concern: Anisakiasis. *Scientific Reports* 7, 43699. https://doi.org/10.1038/srep43699.

Baptista-Fernandes, T., Rodrigues, M., Castro, I., Paixão, P., Pinto-Marques, P., Roque, L., et al. (2017). Human gastric hyperinfection by *Anisakis simplex*: A severe and unusual presentation and a brief review. *International Journal of Infectious Diseases*, *64*, 38–41. https://doi.org/10.1016/j.ijid.2017.08.012.

Bouwknegt, M., Devleesschauwer, B., Graham, H., Robertson, L. J., & van der Giessen, J. (2018). Prioritization of foodborne parasites in Europe. *Eurosurveillance*, *23*(9) pii: 17-00161.

Cacciò, S. M., Chalmers, R. M., Dorny, P., & Robertson, L. J. (2018). Foodborne parasites: Outbreaks and outbreak investigations. A meeting report from the European Network for Foodborne Parasites (Euro-FBP). *Food and Waterborne Parasitology, 10.* https://doi.org/10.1016/j.fawpar.2018.01.001. in press.

Carmo, J., Marques, S., Bispo, M., & Serra, D. (2017). Anisakiasis: A growing cause of abdominal pain!. *BMJ Case Reports.* https://doi.org/10.1136/bcr-2016-218857.

Catalano, S., Lejeune, M., Liccioli, S., Verocai, G. G., Gesy, K. M., Jenkins, E. J., et al. (2012). *Echinococcus multilocularis* in urban coyotes, Alberta, Canada. *Emerging Infectious Diseases, 18*(10), 1625–1628. https://doi.org/10.3201/eid.1810.120119.

Chai, J. Y., Murrell, K. D., & Lymbery, A. J. (2005). Fish-borne parasitic zoonoses: Status and issues. *International Journal for Parasitology, 35*(11 – 12), 1233–1254.

Chalmers, R. M., & Cacciò, S. M. (2016). Towards a consensus on genotyping schemes for surveillance and outbreak investigations of *Cryptosporidium*; Berlin, June 2016. *Euro Surveillance, 21*(37). https://doi.org/10.2807/1560-7917.ES.2016.21.37.30338.

Conraths, F. J., & Deplazes, P. (2015). *Echinococcus multilocularis*: Epidemiology, surveillance and state-of-the-art diagnostics from a veterinary public health perspective. *Veterinary Parasitology, 213*(3–4), 149–161. https://doi.org/10.1016/j.vetpar.2015.07.027.

Conraths, F. J., Probst, C., Possenti, A., Boufana, B., Saulle, R., La Torre, G., et al. (2017). Potential risk factors associated with human alveolar echinococcosis: Systematic review and meta-analysis. *PLoS Neglected Tropical Diseases, 11*(7), e0005801. https://doi.org/10.1371/journal.pntd.0005801.

Craig, P. S., Budke, C. M., Schantz, P. M., Li, T., Qiu, J., Yang, Y., et al. (2007). Human echinococcosis: A neglected disease? *Tropical Medicine and Health, 35*(4), 283–292.

Craig, P. S., Hegglin, D., Lightowlers, M. W., Torgerson, P. R., & Wang, Q. (2017). Echinococcosis: Control and prevention. *Advances in Parasitology, 96*, 55–158. https://doi.org/10.1016/bs.apar.2016.09.002.

Crotta, M., Ferrari, N., & Guitian, J. (2016). Qualitative risk assessment of introduction of anisakid larvae in Atlantic salmon (*Salmo salar*) farms and commercialization of products infected with viable nematodes. *Food Control, 69*, 275–284.

Cui, J., Wang, Z. Q., & Xu, B. L. (2011). The epidemiology of human trichinellosis in China during 2004-2009. *Acta Tropica, 118*(1), 1–5. https://doi.org/10.1016/j.actatropica.2011.02.00.

D'amico, P., Malandra, R., Costanzo, F., Castigliego, L., Guidi, A., Gianfaldoni, D., et al. (2014). Evolution of the *Anisakis* risk management in the European and Italian context. *Food Research International, 64*, 348–362.

Davidson, R. K., Romig, T., Jenkins, E., Tryland, M., & Robertson, L. J. (2012). The impact of globalisation on the distribution of *Echinococcus multilocularis*. *Trends in Parasitology, 28*(6), 239–247. https://doi.org/10.1016/j.pt.2012.03.004.

De Giusti, M., Aurigemma, C., Marinelli, L., Tufi, D., De Medici, D., Di Pasquale, S., et al. (2010). The evaluation of the microbial safety of fresh ready-to-eat vegetables produced by different technologies in Italy. *Journal of Applied Microbiology, 109*(3), 996–1006. https://doi.org/10.1111/j.1365-2672.2010.04727.x.

de Noya, B. A., Gonzalez, O. N., & Robertson, L. J. (2015). Trypanosoma cruzi as a Foodborne Pathogen. In *Springer briefs in food, health and nutrition.* New York, Heidelberg, Dordrecht, London: Springer, ISBN: 978-3-319-23409-0.

de Souza Godoi, P. A., Piechnik, C. A., de Oliveira, A. C., Sfeir, M. Z., de Souza, E. M., Rogez, H., et al. (2017). qPCR for the detection of foodborne *Trypanosoma cruzi*. *Parasitology International, 66*(5), 563–566. https://doi.org/10.1016/j.parint.2017.06.001.

Devleesschauwer, B., Praet, N., Speybroeck, N., Torgerson, P. R., Haagsma, J. A., De Smet, K., et al. (2015). The low global burden of trichinellosis: Evidence and implications. *International Journal for Parasitology, 45*(2–3), 95–99. https://doi.org/10.1016/j.ijpara.2014.05.006.

Dupouy-Camet, J., Lecam, S., Talabani, H., & Ancelle, T. (2009). Trichinellosis acquired in Senegal from warthog ham. *Euro Surveillance, 14*, 1–2.

European Commission. (2015). Commission implementing regulation (Eu) 2015/1375 of 10 August 2015 laying down specific rules on official controls for *Trichinella* in meat. *Official Journal of the European Union*. 11.8.2015. L212/7–L212/34.

European Food Safety Authority. (2010). EFSA panel on biological hazards (BIOHAZ); scientific opinion on risk assessment of parasites in fishery products. *EFSA Journal*, *8*(4), 1543. 91 pp. https://doi.org/10.2903/j.efsa.2010.1543.

European Food Safety Authority. (2015). EFSA panel on animal health and welfare (AHAW); scientific opinion on *Echinococcus multilocularis* infection in animals. *EFSA Journal*, *13*(12), 4373. 129 pp. https://doi.org/10.2903/j.efsa.2015.4373.

FAO. (2016). The state of world fisheries and aquaculture 2016. In *Contributing to food security and nutrition for all* (p. 200). Rome: Food and Agriculture Organization of the United Nations.

FAO/WHO. (2014). Multicriteria-based ranking for risk management of foodborne parasites. In *Microbiological Risk Assessment Series: Vol. 23. Report of a Joint FAO/WHO Expert Meeting, 3–7 September 2012*. Rome, Italy: FAO Headquarters. ISBN 978 92 4 156470 0 (WHO); ISBN 978-92-5-108199-0 (print) (FAO); E-ISBN 978-92-5-108200-3(PDF) (FAO); ISSN 1726-5274.

Fedorova, O. S., Kovshirina, Y. V., Kovshirina, A. E., Fedotova, M. M., Deev, I. A., Petrovskiy, F. I., et al. (2017). *Opisthorchis felineus* infection and cholangiocarcinoma in the Russian federation: A review of medical statistics. *Parasitology International*, *66*(4), 365–371. https://doi.org/10.1016/j.parint.2016.07.010.

Food Standards Agency. (2010). *Guidance for Trichinella testing in feral wild boar*. Available from, https://www.food.gov.uk/sites/default/files/multimedia/pdfs/trichinellatestingwildboar.pdf.

Fürst, T., Keiser, J., & Utzinger, J. (2012). Global burden of human food-borne trematodiasis: A systematic review and meta-analysis. *The Lancet. Infectious Diseases*, *12*(3), 210–221. https://doi.org/10.1016/S1473-3099(11)70294-8.

Garcia-Perez, J. C., Rodríguez-Perez, R., Ballestero, A., Zuloaga, J., Fernandez-Puntero, B., Arias-Díaz, J., et al. (2015). Previous exposure to the fish parasite *Anisakis* as a potential risk factor for gastric or colon adenocarcinoma. *Medicine (Baltimore)*, *94*(40), e1699. https://doi.org/10.1097/MD.0000000000001699.

Gesy, K. M., & Jenkins, E. J. (2015). Introduced and native haplotypes of *Echinococcus multilocularis* in wildlife in Saskatchewan, Canada. *Journal of Wildlife Diseases*, *51*(3), 743–748. https://doi.org/10.7589/2014-08-214.

Gil, M. I., Selma, M. V., López-Gálvez, F., & Allende, A. (2009). Fresh-cut product sanitation and wash water disinfection: Problems and solutions. *International Journal of Food Microbiology*, *134*(1–2), 37–45. https://doi.org/10.1016/j.ijfoodmicro.2009.05.021.

Gómez-Morales, M. A., Selmi, M., Ludovisi, A., Amati, M., Fiorentino, E., Breviglieri, L., et al. (2016). Hunting dogs as sentinel animals for monitoring infections with *Trichinella* spp. in wildlife. *Parasites & Vectors 9*, 154. https://doi.org/10.1186/s13071-016-1437-1.

Gottstein, B., Stojkovic, M., Vuitton, D. A., Millon, L., Marcinkute, A., & Deplazes, P. (2015). Threat of alveolar echinococcosis to public health—A challenge for Europe. *Trends in Parasitology*, *31*(9), 407–412. https://doi.org/10.1016/j.pt.2015.06.001.

Gouveia, M. J., Pakharukova, M. Y., Laha, T., Sripa, B., Maksimova, G. A., Rinaldi, G., et al. (2017). Infection with *Opisthorchis felineus* induces intraepithelial neoplasia of the biliary tract in a rodent model. *Carcinogenesis*, *38*(9), 929–937. https://doi.org/10.1093/carcin/bgx042.

Hald, T., Aspinall, W., Devleesschauwer, B., Cooke, R., Corrigan, T., Havelaar, A. H., et al. (2016). World Health Organization estimates of the relative contributions of food to the burden of disease due to selected foodborne hazards: A structured expert elicitation. *PLoS One*, *11*(1), e0145839. https://doi.org/10.1371/journal.pone.0145839.

Havelaar, A. H., Kirk, M. D., Torgerson, P. R., Gibb, H. J., Hald, T., Lake, R. J., et al. (2015). World Health Organization global estimates and regional comparisons of the burden of foodborne disease in 2010. *PLoS Medicine*, 12(*12*), e1001923. https://doi.org/10.1371/journal.pmed.1001923.

Hegglin, D., & Deplazes, P. (2008). Control strategy for *Echinococcus multilocularis*. *Emerging Infectious Diseases*, *14*, 1626–1628.

Hegglin, D., & Deplazes, P. (2013). Control of *Echinococcus multilocularis*: Strategies, feasibility and cost-benefit analyses. *International Journal for Parasitology*, *43*(5), 327–337. https://doi.org/10.1016/j.ijpara.2012.11.013. [Epub 2013 Feb 4].

Hongsrichan, N., Intuyod, K., Pinlaor, P., Khoontawad, J., Yongvanit, P., Wongkham, C., et al. (2014). Cytokine/chemokine secretion and proteomic identification of upregulated annexin A1 from peripheral blood mononuclear cells cocultured with the liver fluke *Opisthorchis viverrini*. *Infection and Immunity*, *82*(5), 2135–2147. https://doi.org/10.1128/IAI.00901-13.

Houzé, S., Ancelle, T., Matra, R., Boceno, C., Carlier, Y., Gajadhar, A. A., et al. (2009). Trichinellosis acquired in Nunavut, Canada in September 2009: Meat from grizzly bear suspected. *Euro Surveillance*, *14*(44) pii: 19383.

Hughes, T., O'Connor, T., Techasen, A., Namwat, N., Loilome, W., Andrews, R. H., et al. (2017). Opisthorchiasis and cholangiocarcinoma in Southeast Asia: An unresolved problem. *International Journal of General Medicine*, *10*, 227–237. https://doi.org/10.2147/IJGM.S133292.

Ito, A., Romig, T., & Takahashi, K. (2003). Perspective on control options for Echinococcus multilocularis with particular reference to Japan. *Parasitology*, *127*(Suppl), S159–72.

Janko, C., & König, A. (2011). Disappearance rate of praziquantel-containing bait around villages and small towns in Southern Bavaria, Germany. *Journal of Wildlife Diseases*, *47*, 373–380.

Keiser, J., & Utzinger, J. (2009). Food-borne trematodiases. *Clinical Microbiology Reviews*, *22*(3), 466–483. https://doi.org/10.1128/CMR.00012-0.

Khoontawad, J., Pairojkul, C., Rucksaken, R., Pinlaor, P., Wongkham, C., Yongvanit, P., et al. (2017). Differential protein expression marks the transition from infection with *Opisthorchis viverrini* to cholangiocarcinoma. *Molecular & Cellular Proteomics*, *16*(5), 911–923. https://doi.org/10.1074/mcp.M116.064576.

Khuntikeo, N., Loilome, W., Thinkhamrop, B., Chamadol, N., & Yongvanit, P. (2016). A comprehensive public health conceptual framework and strategy to effectively combat cholangiocarcinoma in Thailand. *PLoS Neglected Tropical Diseases*, *10*(1), e0004293. https://doi.org/10.1371/journal.pntd.0004293.

Kirk, M. D., Pires, S. M., Black, R. E., Caipo, M., Crump, J. A., Devleesschauwer, B., et al. (2015). World Health Organization estimates of the global and regional disease burden of 22 foodborne bacterial, protozoal, and viral diseases, 2010: A data synthesis. *PLoS Medicine*, *12*(12), e1001921. https://doi.org/10.1371/journal.pmed.1001921.

König, A., Romig, T., Janko, C., Hildenbrand, R., Holzhofer, E., Kotulski, Y., et al. (2008). Integrated-baiting concept against *Echinococcus multilocularis* in foxes is successful in southern Bavaria Germany. *European Journal of Wildlife Research*, *54*, 439–447.

Levsen, A., & Maage, A. (2016). Absence of parasitic nematodes in farmed, harvest quality Atlantic salmon (*Salmo salar*) in Norway—Results from a large scale survey. *Food Control*, *68*, 25–29.

Levsen, A., Svanevika, C. S., Cipriani, P., Mattiucci, S., Gayd, M., Hastie, L. C., et al. (2018). A survey of zoonotic nematodes of commercial keyfish species from major European fishing grounds—Introducing the FP7 PARASITE exposure assessment study. *Fisheries Research*, *202*, 4–21. https://doi.org/10.1016/j.fishres.2017.09.009.

Little, C. L., & Gillespie, I. A. (2008). Prepared salads and public health. *Journal of Applied Microbiology*, *105*(6), 1729–1743. https://doi.org/10.1111/j.1365-2672.2008.03801.x.

Llarena-Reino, M., Abollo, E., Regueira, M., Rodríguez, H., & Pascual, S. (2015). Horizon scanning for management of emerging parasitic infections in fishery products. *Food Control, 49*, 49–58.

Lvova, M. N., Tangkawattana, S., Balthaisong, S., Katokhin, A. V., Mordvinov, V. A., & Sripa, B. (2012). Comparative histopathology of *Opisthorchis felineus* and *Opisthorchis viverrini* in a hamster model: An implication of high pathogenicity of the European liver fluke. *Parasitology International, 61*(1), 167–172. https://doi.org/10.1016/j.parint.2011.08.005.

Magera, A. M., Mills Flemming, J. E., Kaschner, K., Christensen, L. B., & Lotze, H. K. (2013). Recovery trends in marine mammal populations. *PLoS One, 8*(10), e77908. https://doi.org/10.1371/journal.pone.0077908.

Maksimova, G. A., Pakharukova, M. Y., Kashina, E. V., Zhukova, N. A., Kovner, A. V., Lvova, M. N., et al. (2017). Effect of *Opisthorchis felineus* infection and dimethylnitrosamine administration on the induction of cholangiocarcinoma in Syrian hamsters. *Parasitology International, 66*(4), 458–463. https://doi.org/10.1016/j.parint.2015.10.002.

Margioto Teston, A. P., de Abreu, A. P., Abegg, C. P., Gomes, M. L., & de Ornelas Toledo, M. J. (2017). Outcome of oral infection in mice inoculated with *Trypanosoma cruzi* IV of the Western Brazilian Amazon. *Acta Tropica, 166*, 212–217. https://doi.org/10.1016/j.actatropica.2016.11.019.

Mattos, E. C., Meira-Strejevitch, C. D. S., Marciano, M. A. M., Faccini, C. C., Lourenço, A. M., & Pereira-Chioccola, V. L. (2017). Molecular detection of *Trypanosoma cruzi* in acai pulp and sugarcane juice. *Acta Tropica, 176*, 311–315. https://doi.org/10.1016/j.actatropica.2017.08.025.

Messiaen, P., Forier, A., Vanderschueren, S., Theunissen, C., Nijs, J., Van Esbroeck, M., et al. (2016). Outbreak of trichinellosis related to eating imported wild boar meat, Belgium, 2014. *Euro Surveillance 21*, https://doi.org/10.2807/1560-7917.ES.2016.21.37.30341.

Morse, S. S. (1995). Factors in the emergence of infectious diseases. *Emerging Infectious Diseases, 1*(1), 7–15.

Moutou, F., & Pastoret, P. P. (2015). Defining an emerging disease. *Revue Scientifique et Technique, 34*(1), 41–52.

Murrell, K. D., & Pozio, E. (2011). Worldwide occurrence and impact of human trichinellosis, 1986-2009. *Emerging Infectious Diseases, 17*(12), 2194–2202. https://doi.org/10.3201/eid1712.110896.

Nava, A., Shimabukuro, J. S., Chmura, A. A., & Luz, S. L. B. (2017). The impact of global environmental changes on infectious disease emergence with a focus on risks for Brazil. *ILAR Journal*. https://doi.org/10.1093/ilar/ilx034.

Ogorodova, L. M., Fedorova, O. S., Sripa, B., Mordvinov, V. A., Katokhin, A. V., Keiser, J., et al. (2015). Opisthorchiasis: An overlooked danger. *PLoS Neglected Tropical Diseases, 9*(4), e0003563. https://doi.org/10.1371/journal.pntd.0003563.

Oksanen, A., Siles-Lucas, M., Karamon, J., Possenti, A., Conraths, F. J., Romig, T., et al. (2016). The geographical distribution and prevalence of *Echinococcus multilocularis* in animals in the European Union and adjacent countries: A systematic review and meta-analysis. *Parasites & Vectors, 9*(1), 519.

Ong, X., Wang, Y. C., Sithithaworn, P., Namsanor, J., Taylor, D., & Laithavewat, L. (2016). Uncovering the pathogenic landscape of helminth (*Opisthorchis viverrini*) infections: A cross-sectional study on contributions of physical and social environment and healthcare interventions. *PLoS Neglected Tropical Diseases, 10*(12), e0005175. https://doi.org/10.1371/journal.pntd.0005175.

Osman, M., Benamrouz, S., Guyot, K., Baydoun, M., Frealle, E., Chabe, M., et al. (2017). High association of *Cryptosporidium* spp. infection with colon adenocarcinoma in Lebanese patients. *PLoS One, 12*(12), e0189422. https://doi.org/10.1371/journal.pone.0189422.

Pakharukova, M. Y., & Mordvinov, V. A. (2016). The liver fluke *Opisthorchis felineus*: Biology, epidemiology and carcinogenic potential. *Transactions of the Royal Society of Tropical Medicine and Hygiene, 110*(1), 28–36. https://doi.org/10.1093/trstmh/trv085.

Pearce-Duvet, J. M. (2006). The origin of human pathogens: Evaluating the role of agriculture and domestic animals in the evolution of human disease. *Biological Reviews of the Cambridge Philosophical Society, 81*(3), 369–382.

Pedrique, B., Strub-Wourgaft, N., Some, C., Olliaro, P., Trouiller, P., Ford, N., et al. (2013). The drug and vaccine landscape for neglected diseases (2000 – 11): A systematic assessment. *The Lancet, Global Health, 1*(6), e371–9. https://doi.org/10.1016/S2214-109X(13)70078-0.

Penman, D. J., Gupta, M. V., & Dey, M. M. (2005). Carp genetic resources for aquaculture in Asia. *WorldFish Center Technical Report, 65*, 152.

Pozio, E. (2014). Searching for *Trichinella*: Not all pigs are created equal. *Trends in Parasitology, 30*(1), 4–11.

Pozio, E. (2015). *Trichinella* spp. imported with live animals and meat. *Veterinary Parasitology, 213*(1–2), 46–55. https://doi.org/10.1016/j.vetpar.2015.02.017.016/j.pt.2013.11.001.

Pozio, E., Armignacco, O., Ferri, F., & Gomez Morales, M. A. (2013). *Opisthorchis felineus*, an emerging infection in Italy and its implication for the European Union. *Acta Tropica, 126*(1), 54–62. https://doi.org/10.1016/j.actatropica.2013.01.005.

Rehn, M., Wallensten, A., Widerström, M., Lilja, M., Grunewald, M., Stenmark, S., et al. (2015). Post-infection symptoms following two large waterborne outbreaks of *Cryptosporidium hominis* in Northern Sweden, 2010-2011. *BMC Public Health, 15*, 529. https://doi.org/10.1186/s12889-015-1871-6.

Rello, F. J., Adroher, F. J., Benítez, R., & Valero, A. (2009). The fishing area as a possible indicator of the infection by anisakids in anchovies (*Engraulis encrasicolus*) from southwestern Europe. *International Journal of Food Microbiology, 129*(3), 277–281. https://doi.org/10.1016/j.ijfoodmicro.2008.12.009.

Robertson, L. J., & Chalmers, R. M. (2013). Foodborne cryptosporidiosis: Is there really more in Nordic countries? *Trends in Parasitology, 29*(1), 3–9. https://doi.org/10.1016/j.pt.2012.10.003.

Robertson, L. J., Devleesschauwer, B., Alarcón de Noya, B., Noya González, O., & Torgerson, P. R. (2016). *Trypanosoma cruzi*: Time for international recognition as a foodborne parasite. *PLoS Neglected Tropical Diseases, 10*(6), e0004656. https://doi.org/10.1371/journal.pntd.0004656.

Robertson, L. J., & Noya, O. (2015). Prophylactic measures and implementation of control measures in foodborne Chagas Disease. In B. A. de Noya, O. N. Gonzalez, & L. J. Robertson (Eds.), *Trypanosoma cruzi as a Foodborne Pathogen*. Springer Briefs in Food, Health and Nutrition. New York, Heidelberg, Dordrecht, London: Springer. ISBN: 978-3-319-23409-0.

Robertson, L. J., Sprong, H., Ortega, Y. R., van der Giessen, J. W., & Fayer, R. (2014). Impacts of globalisation on foodborne parasites. *Trends in Parasitology, 30*(1), 37–52. https://doi.org/10.1016/j.pt.2013.09.005.

Rostami, A., Gamble, H. R., Dupouy-Camet, J., Khazan, H., & Bruschi, F. (2017). Meat sources of infection for outbreaks of human trichinellosis. *Food Microbiology, 64*, 65–71. https://doi.org/10.1016/j.fm.2016.12.012.

Rucksaken, R., Khoontawad, J., Roytrakul, S., Pinlaor, P., Hiraku, Y., Wongkham, C., et al. (2012). Proteomic analysis to identify plasma orosomucoid 2 and kinesin 18A as potential biomarkers of cholangiocarcinoma. *Cancer Biomarkers: Section A of Disease Markers, 12*(2), 81–95. https://doi.org/10.3233/CBM-130296.

Ruiz-Fons, F. (2017). A review of the current status of relevant zoonotic pathogens in wild swine (*Sus scrofa*) populations: Changes modulating the risk of transmission to humans. *Transboundary and Emerging Diseases*, *64*(1), 68–88. https://doi.org/10.1111/tbed.12369.

Ryan, U., Hijjawi, N., & Xiao, L. (2018). Foodborne cryptosporidiosis. *International Journal for Parasitology*, *48*(1), 1–12. https://doi.org/10.1016/j.ijpara.2017.09.004.

Salerno, R., Salvatella, R., Issa, J., & Anzola, M. C. (2015). A regional fight against Chagas disease: Lessons learned from a successful collaborative partnership. *Revista Panamericana de Salud Pública*, *37*(1), 38–43.

Sawanyawisuth, K., Silsirivanit, A., Kunlabut, K., Tantapotinan, N., Vaeteewoottacharn, K., & Wongkham, S. (2012). A novel carbohydrate antigen expression during development of Opisthorchis viverrini-associated cholangiocarcinoma in golden hamster: A potential marker for early diagnosis. *Parasitology International*, *61*(1), 151–154. https://doi.org/10.1016/j.parint.2011.07.013.

Schweiger, A., Ammann, R. W., Candinas, D., Clavien, P. A., Eckert, J., Gottstein, B., et al. (2007). Human alveolar echinococcosis after fox population increase, Switzerland. *Emerging Infectious Diseases*, *13*(6), 878–882.

Shoultz, D. A., de Hostos, E. L., & Choy, R. K. (2016). Addressing *Cryptosporidium* infection among young children in low-income settings: The crucial role of new and existing drugs for reducing morbidity and mortality. *PLoS Neglected Tropical Diseases*, *10*(1), e0004242. https://doi.org/10.1371/journal.pntd.0004242.

Silva-Dos-Santos, D., Barreto-de-Albuquerque, J., Guerra, B., Moreira, O. C., Berbert, L. R., Ramos, M. T., et al. (2017). Unraveling Chagas disease transmission through the oral route: Gateways to *Trypanosoma cruzi* infection and target tissues. *PLoS Neglected Tropical Diseases*, *11*(4), e0005507. https://doi.org/10.1371/journal.pntd.0005507.

Speciale, A., Trombetta, D., Saija, A., Panebianco, A., Giarratana, F., Ziino, G., et al. (2017). Exposure to *Anisakis* extracts can induce inflammation on in vitro cultured human colonic cells. *Parasitology Research*. https://doi.org/10.1007/s00436-017-5551-6.

Sripa, B., Kaewkes, S., Sithithaworn, P., Mairiang, E., Laha, T., Smout, M., et al. (2007). Liver fluke induces cholangiocarcinoma. *PLoS Medicine*, *4*(7), e201.

Sripa, B., Tangkawattana, S., Laha, T., Kaewkes, S., Mallory, F. F., Smith, J. F., et al. (2015). Toward integrated opisthorchiasis control in northeast Thailand: The Lawa project. *Acta Tropica*, *141*(Pt. B), 361–367. https://doi.org/10.1016/j.actatropica.2014.07.017.

Stiff, R. E., Davies, A. P., Mason, B. W., Hutchings, H. A., & Chalmers, R. M. (2017). Long-term health effects after resolution of acute *Cryptosporidium parvum* infection: A 1-year follow-up of outbreak-associated cases. *Journal of Medical Microbiology*, *66*(11), 1607–1611. https://doi.org/10.1099/jmm.0.000609.

Storino, R. (2000). La cara oculta de la enfermedad de chagas. *Revista de la Federación Argentina de Cardiología*, *29*, 31–44.

Torgerson, P. R., Devleesschauwer, B., Praet, N., Speybroeck, N., Willingham, A. L., Kasuga, F., et al. (2015). World Health Organization estimates of the global and regional disease burden of 11 foodborne parasitic diseases, 2010: A data synthesis. *PLoS Medicine*, *12*(12), e1001920. https://doi.org/10.1371/journal.pmed.1001920.

Trotz-Williams, L. A., Mercer, N. J., Walters, J. M., Wallace, D., Gottstein, B., Osterman-Lind, E., et al. (2017). Public health follow-up of suspected exposure to *Echinococcus multilocularis* in Southwestern Ontario. *Zoonoses and Public Health*, *64*(6), 460–467. https://doi.org/10.1111/zph.12326.

Turiac, I. A., Cappelli, M. G., Olivieri, R., Angelillis, R., Martinelli, D., Prato, R., et al. (2017). Trichinellosis outbreak due to wild boar meat consumption in southern Italy. *Parasites & Vectors*, *10*(1), 107. https://doi.org/10.1186/s13071-017-2052-5.

Vuitton, D. A., Demonmerot, F., Knapp, J., Richou, C., Grenouillet, F., Chauchet, A., et al. (2015). Clinical epidemiology of human AE in Europe. *Veterinary Parasitology*, *213*(3–4), 110–120. https://doi.org/10.1016/j.vetpar.2015.07.036.

Wang, Z. Q., Cui, J., & Xu, B. L. (2006). The epidemiology of human trichinellosis in China during 2000-2003. *Acta Tropica*, *97*(3), 247–251.

World Health Organization. (2017). *Neglected tropical diseases.* The World Health Organization. http://www.who.int/neglected_diseases/diseases/en/.

Yossepowitch, O., Gotesman, T., Assous, M., Marva, E., Zimlichman, R., & Dan, M. (2004). Opisthorchiasis from imported raw fish. *Emerging Infectious Diseases*, *10*(12), 2122–2126.

Zanelli, M., Ragazzi, M., Fiorino, S., Foroni, M., Cecinato, P., Del Mar Jordana Sanchez, M., et al. (2017). An Italian case of intestinal anisakiasis with a presurgical diagnosis: Could this parasite represent an emerging disease? *Pathology, Research and Practice*, *213*(5), 558–564. https://doi.org/10.1016/j.prp.2017.01.027.

Zuo, S., Kania, P. W., Mehrdana, F., Marana, M. H., & Buchmann, K. (2018). *Contracaecum osculatum* and other anisakid nematodes in grey seals and cod in the Baltic Sea: Molecular and ecological links. *Journal of Helminthology*, *92*(1), 81–89. https://doi.org/10.1017/S0022149X17000025.

CHAPTER FIVE

Antimicrobial Resistance in the Food Chain in the European Union

Diego Florez-Cuadrado*[,1], Miguel A. Moreno*[,†], María Ugarte-Ruíz*, Lucas Domínguez*[,†]

*Foodborne Zoonoses and Antimicrobial Resistance Unit, VISAVET Health Surveillance Center, Complutense University, Madrid, Spain
[†]Department of Animal Health, Veterinary Faculty, Complutense University, Madrid, Spain
[1]Corresponding author: e-mail address: diflorez@ucm.es

Contents

Abstract

Consumers require safety foods but without losing enough supply and low prices. Food concerns about antimicrobial residues and antimicrobial-resistant (AMR) bacteria are not usually appropriately separated and could be perceived as the same problem. The monitoring of residues of antimicrobials in animal food is well established at different levels (farm, slaughterhouse, and industry), and it is preceded by the legislation of veterinary medicines where maximum residues limits are required for medicines to be used in food animal. Following the strategy of the World Health Organization, one of the proposed measures consists in controlling the use of critical antibiotics. The European Union surveillance program currently includes the animal species with the highest meat production (pigs, chickens, turkeys, and cattle) and the food derived from them, investigating antimicrobial resistance of zoonotic (*Salmonella* and *Campylobacter*) and indicator (*Escherichia coli* and enterococci) bacteria. AMR mechanisms encoded by genes have a greater impact on transfer than mutations. Sometimes these genes are found in mobile genetic elements such as plasmids, transposons, or integrons, capable of

Advances in Food and Nutrition Research, Volume 86
ISSN 1043-4526
https://doi.org/10.1016/bs.afnr.2018.04.004
© 2018 Elsevier Inc.
All rights reserved.

passing from one bacterium to another by horizontal transfer. It is important to know that depending on how the resistance mechanism is transferred, the power of dissemination is different. By vertical transfer of the resistance gene, whatever its origin, will be transmitted to the following generations. In the case of horizontal transfer, the resistance gene moves to neighboring bacteria and therefore the range of resistance can be much greater.

1. INTRODUCTION

Until the discovery of antimicrobials, there were no effective treatments against bacterial infectious diseases. The fact that bacterial infections were clinically uncontrollable led to epidemics, such as the plague of Athens (431 BC) (Littman, 2009) or the Black Death (XIV century) (Bos et al., 2011), the most devastating pandemic of plague in the history of mankind. Prior to the discovery of antimicrobials, many attempts were made to identify effective treatments against bacterial infections (Aminov, 2010). One of the objectives of the scientific community at the beginning of the 20th century was to identify chemical compounds capable of acting exclusively on the microorganism without affecting the infected person. This is how drugs, such as arsphenamine, also known as Salvarsan or compound 606 (Zaffiri, Gardner, & Toledo-Pereyra, 2012), and the sulfonamide Prontosil emerge (Jacob, 1938), treatments that were used until they were unmarked by penicillin in 1928.

Since the discovery of penicillin by Alexander Fleming (Bornstein, 1940), antimicrobials have meant, together with anesthesia and sanitary hygienic practices, a real revolution in health. Antimicrobials are substances that kill microorganisms or inhibit their growth and are used to treat and control bacterial infections (Martinez, 2009). Antimicrobials began to be used in human medicine as well as in animal health and production. In the absence of diseases, antimicrobials were sometimes used as prophylaxis or as growth promoters in animals (Castanon, 2007). Antimicrobials can cause changes in the digestive and metabolic processes of animals, which translate into increases in the efficiency of food use and significant improvements in weight gain, although the mechanisms are still not exactly known (Feighner & Dashkevicz, 1987). The first experiences (in chickens) that showed their beneficial effects date from the late 1940s, and in the 1960s, their commercial employment was widespread in Europe (Castanon, 2007; Feighner & Dashkevicz, 1987). Owing to the public health risk, the

European Union (EU) has been established in 2006 the total ban on the use in animal feed of antimicrobials as growth promoters. The use of antimicrobials in animals could cause the selection and propagation of antimicrobial-resistant (AMR) bacteria, and AMR traits that could reach to humans through the consumption of animal-derived foods.

For all this it is important to control the use of antimicrobials in animals and monitor resistance to antimicrobials that have zoonotic bacteria. It has been seen that interventions that restrict the use of antimicrobials in animals destined for food production reduce antimicrobials resistant bacteria in these animals by up to 39% (Postma, Vanderhaeghen, Sarrazin, Maes, & Dewulf, 2017). The selective pressure of antimicrobials has selected bacteria such as *Campylobacter* resistant to quinolones (Diarrassouba et al., 2007; Kwon et al., 2017; Pedersen & Wedderkopp, 2003) that would have emerged, at least in part from farms and pose a great public health risk. The World Health Organization (WHO) places the problem of AMR as one of the main health challenges of the 21st century.

Food chain is an ecosystem where numerous bacteria coexist, sometimes at the selective pressure exerted by antimicrobials. Food can be contaminated with AMR bacteria and/or AMR genes in many ways. Animal products may contain AMR bacteria as a result of fecal contamination during slaughter. The environment, including humans, can also contaminate food. Such contamination can occur after the processing of food and then it is called later contamination.

2. SELECTION AND TRANSMISSION OF RESISTANCE

The resistance of bacteria to antimicrobials can be natural or acquired (Martinez, Coque, & Baquero, 2015). Natural resistance means that all isolates belonging to the same species are resistant to an antimicrobial (Munita & Arias, 2016). This can be caused by peculiarities of the bacterial cell wall that prevents access to the antimicrobial to its target, as is the case of gram-negative bacteria that are impervious to penicillin G (Sutherland, 1964), or mycoplasmas that lack a typical cell wall are resistant to penicillin (Taylor-Robinson & Bebear, 1997). Acquired resistance refers to a loss of susceptibility to an antimicrobial by some isolates of a species, which is the most common form of its presentation. The AMR mechanisms can be grouped into three categories: (I) antimicrobial reduction inside the bacteria, (II) antimicrobial inactivation, and (III) modification of the target on which the antimicrobial acts (Blair, Webber, Baylay, Ogbolu, & Piddock, 2015).

In the first case, the bacterium controls the amount of antimicrobial that is inside preventing their entry (porins) or expelling it outdoors (efflux pumps) (Maria-Neto, de Almeida, Macedo, & Franco, 2015). The second category of resistance mechanisms is based on the presence of genes capable of expressing enzymes that degrade or modify the antimicrobial (van Hoek et al., 2011). Finally, there is the strategy of modifying the molecular target of antimicrobial action, by mutations or methylation, thus preventing it from acting on the bacterium (Munita & Arias, 2016). In short, all these mechanisms are determined by specific mutations or by the expression of AMR genes.

2.1 Vertical Transfer: Specific Mutations

A spontaneous mutation is a genetic change that arises naturally and not as a result of exposure to mutagens but as consequence of error in the DNA proofreading after its replication. These types of mutations can affect any gene and occur with a frequency between 10^{-5} and 10^{-10} per cell and division, depending on the type of bacteria and environmental characteristics (O'Brien, Rodrigues, & Buckling, 2013). A bacterium that possesses an AMR gene due to a mutation will transmit that resistance mechanism to its daughter cells by vertical transfer (Lawrence, 2005). The use of an antimicrobial is able to select resistant isolates, allowing the propagation of these clones by natural selection.

Resistance to quinolones is a classic example of resistance mediated by mutations, although in some cases there may be mutations that confer simultaneous resistance to several antimicrobial from different families (Gomez et al., 2017). Much of this resistance is related to the use of fluoroquinolones in food-producing animals, and resistance to this antimicrobial in Campylobacter is frequently observed in both animal and human isolates (Pugajeva et al., 2018). The recent emergence of resistance to antimicrobials in foodborne pathogens is a matter of concern. These resistances include the following: (i) transferable low-level resistance to fluoroquinolones in Enterobacteriaceae, (ii) presence of methicillin-resistant *Staphylococcus aureus* (MRSA) in animals, and (iii) worldwide occurrence of human and animal isolates of *Escherichia coli* and *Salmonella* with extended-spectrum beta-lactamases (Infosan, 2008). There may also be mutations that modify a known resistance gene, broadening its effects. This is the case of the genes that encode some beta-lactamases that inactivate the cephalosporin derived by mutation of a gene that codes for an enzyme whose specificity was restricted to penicillin. As a result of this mutation, the enzyme produced now has a double activity that affects both penicillin and cephalosporin (Shaikh, Fatima, Shakil, Rizvi, & Kamal, 2015). Resistance to quinolones typically arises as a result of specific mutations and of changes in drug entry and efflux (Jacoby, 2005). Quinolones are a group of synthetic chemotherapeutic agents, which mean that they are not produced by microorganisms, unlike classical antimicrobials. These antimicrobials are bactericidal substances used throughout the world but the increase in resistance in different bacterial species makes their use is threatened. Quinolones cause the lysis and death of the bacterium, while bacteriostatic antimicrobials are those that inhibit bacterial growth (Emmerson & Jones, 2003).

Resistance to macrolides is other example of bacterial resistance mediated by mutations. Mutations that produce resistance to macrolides are located in the 23S ribosomal gene mainly and prevent the correct binding of the antimicrobial to the ribosome (Fyfe, Grossman, Kerstein, & Sutcliffe, 2016). It is important to highlight this mechanism of resistance in a zoonotic bacterium such as *Campylobacter* since the macrolides, specifically erythromycin, are the treatment of choice against campylobacteriosis. The main mechanism of resistance to erythromycin in *Campylobacter* is the A2075G mutation of the 23S gene (Gibreel et al., 2005). Also mutations A2074C, A2074G, and A2074T produce high levels of resistance to erythromycin but their frequency of detection is much lower because they affect the fitness of the bacteria (Gibreel et al., 2005; Mamelli, Prouzet-Mauleon, Pages, Megraud, & Bolla, 2005).

2.2 Horizontal Transfer: AMR Genes

The issue of horizontal transfer of AMR genes is considered a direct and indirect risk in the food industry. The direct risk is related to the presence in the food of AMR pathogenic bacteria resistant to antimicrobials, which can be transmitted to the consumer by ingestion or contact and cause disease (Hald, Lo Fo Wong, & Aarestrup, 2007). The indirect risk to human health consists in the horizontal transfer of mobile genetic elements containing AMR genes from nonpathogenic bacteria to pathogenic bacteria. This horizontal transfer can occur at different points in the food chain: environment, facilities, and equipment of the food industry, in food or in people or in animals (Lester, Frimodt-Moller, Sorensen, Monnet, & Hammerum, 2006).

Currently there is several horizontal transfer vehicles described as plasmids (intercellular), transposons, or integrons (both intracellular). The plasmids are circular sequences of extrachromosomal DNA that generally confer advantages to the host, the most characteristic being those that carry

AMR genes. The transfer of plasmids can occur between bacteria of the same or of different genera, however, the maintenance of the plasmid supposes an energetic cost for the bacterium (Bennett, 2008). The presence of an antimicrobial in the medium allows the selective survival of the AMR isolates and the transfer of the mechanism of resistance to other neighboring bacteria. The use of antimicrobials coupled with the ease of genetic mobilization of transposons, facilitates the selection of bacterial isolates that carry AMR genes to different classes of antimicrobials (Davies & Davies, 2010). This is how multiresistant genomic islands can be generated, which can be found both in plasmids and in the bacterial chromosome (Wang et al., 2014). The integrons are the main system of capture of genes of resistance on the part of the plasmids thanks to the fact that they have a specific site of recombination that captures them (Lee et al., 2002).

The mechanisms that allow horizontal transfer are transduction, transformation, and conjugation (Kurland, Canback, & Berg, 2003). In transduction, the vector is a bacteriophage that transfers a DNA fragment from one bacterium to another. It is well known that bacteriophages contribute to the spread of AMR genes among foodborne pathogens as *Salmonella* or *E. coli* (Colavecchio, Cadieux, Lo, & Goodridge, 2017). The transformation allows the acquisition and incorporation of naked exogenous DNA. When bacteria die and their membrane has been more or less destroyed they release DNA fragments that can be picked up by other bacteria. This mode of transfer is very widespread and has been described in zoonotic bacteria such as *Campylobacter*. Conjugation is a process during which DNA is transferred from a donor bacterium to a receptor bacterium through a mechanism that involves close cell contact.

3. EUROPEAN SURVEILLANCE OF AMR

At European level, AMR monitoring in the food chain has been established by a stepwise coordinated approach involving the scientific advice provided by the European Food Safety Agency (EFSA) and the legislative authority of the European Commission. The Directive 2003/99/EC "on the monitoring of zoonoses and zoonotic agents" (2003/99/EC, 2003) comprised also the monitoring of the AMR associated to bacterial zoonotic agents at the level of the primary production (preharvest), but also at other stages of the food chain, including in food (postharvest) and feed (Article 4.2), and the specific requirements for this monitoring described in annex II state that "Member States must ensure that the monitoring system provides relevant information at least with regard to a representative number of isolates of *Salmonella* spp., *Campylobacter jejuni* and *Campylobacter coli* from cattle, pigs and poultry and food of animal origin derived from those species." Nevertheless, the details of each national monitoring system had to be established by the member states (MS).

The first report about "Trends and sources of zoonoses, zoonotic agents and AMR in the EU" (EFSA, 2005) published by EFSA covered data from 2004. Concerning the food chain, this report summarized information at both, pre- and postharvest. At the primary production level, the report summarized data of AMR in cattle (*Salmonella typhimurium*, 17 MS; *C. jejuni*, 5 MS; *E. coli* indicator, 12 MS), pigs (*S. typhimurium*, 19 MS; *C. coli* 6 MS; *E. coli* indicator, 16 MS), and *Gallus gallus*/poultry (*S. typhimurium* 14 MS, *S. enteritidis*, 18 MS; *C. coli*, 6 MS, *C. jejuni*, 9 MS; *E. coli* indicator, 16 MS). At the postharvest level, the report included AMR data in bovine meat (*Salmonella*, 7 MS; *E. coli* indicator, 3 MS), pig meat (*Salmonella*, 11 MS; *Campylobacter*, 1 MS; *E. coli* indicator, 4 MS), and broiler meat (*Salmonella*, 14 MS; *Campylobacter*, 5 MS; *E. coli* indicator, 4 MS). However, these data come from different and nonharmonized sources (national monitoring programs or others), and, although the main objective was to collect information, comparison between data should be carefully considered. As a proof, the only paragraph about AMR on the executive summary state "the submitted information indicated that animals and food of animal origin might serve as reservoirs for resistant bacteria with the risk of direct or indirect transfer of resistance bacteria to humans."

The Commission Decision 2007/407/EC (2007/407/EC, 2007) on "a harmonized monitoring of AMR in *Salmonella* in poultry and pigs" laid down the first detailed rules for AMR using the combinations salmonella-pigs and salmonella-poultry as the starting point. The main achievements of this decision were the sequential sampling calendar, the sampling size (fixed as 170 isolates/animal species/year), and the list of antimicrobial substances and cut-off values. The Commission Decision 2007/516/EC also established sampling size (170 isolates) and the list of antimicrobial substances and cut-off values (2007/516/EC, 2007) for AMR monitoring in campylobacter. Both decisions were based on the scientific reports previously published by EFSA regarding these topics (EFSA, 2008). Equally, EFSA published another scientific report for AMR monitoring of indicator bacteria, specifically *E. coli* and enterococci (EFSA, 2017a).

Finally, on 2012, EFSA published two reports: a scientific report on technical specifications on the harmonized monitoring and reporting of

AMR in *Salmonella*, and indicator commensal *E. coli* and *Enterococcus* spp. bacteria transmitted through food (EFSA, 2010) and a scientific report on technical specifications on the harmonized monitoring and reporting of AMR in MRSA in food-producing animals and food (EFSA, 2012).

The Commission implementing Decision 2013/652/EU (2013/652/EU, 2013) laid down the rules for the harmonized monitoring and reporting of AMR by MS. This decision strengthen the previous legislative work on AMR in terms of bacterial species and food animals covered, and updated the critical points for proper monitoring like the panel of antimicrobial substances per bacterial species (including interpretative thresholds and range of concentrations) and the sampling sizes. The combinations of animal populations/food categories and bacteria that must be included are summarized on Tables 1 (food categories) and 2 (animal populations). Voluntary monitoring is summarized in Table 3. The decision established a biennial sampling frequency in a rotary system whit poultry and poultry meat on even years (from 2014 to 2020) and pigs, bovines, and their meats on odds years (from 2015 to 2019).

Having in mind that National Control Programs for *Samonella* in laying hens, broilers, and turkeys are mandatory for MS and that these programs establish the collection and storage of the isolates, these isolates must be used for the AMR monitoring. This is also valid for isolates collected according to Regulation 2073/2005 about microbiological criteria for foodstuffs (2005/2073/EC, 2005). Accordingly, AMR monitoring of *Salmonella* is mainly based on a retrospective sampling (preexisting isolates), whereas the remaining bacterial species/phenotypes must be isolated through prospective samplings designed specifically for this purpose.

Table 1 Mandatory Combination of Bacterial Species/Phenotypes and Foods Where Antimicrobial Resistance Must be Monitored According to Commission Implementing Decision 2013/652/EU (2013)

Bacterial Species/ Phenotypes	Foods	Sample Size
ESBL- or ampC- or carbapenemase-producing *E. coli*	Fresh meat of broilers, pig meat, and bovine meat gathered at retail	300 samples of each food category (150 if production is less than 100,000 ton of poultry or pig meat, or less than 50,000 ton of bovine meat)

Table 2 Mandatory Combination of Bacterial Species/Phenotypes and Animal Populations Where Antimicrobial Resistance Must be Monitored According to Commission Implementing Decision 2013/652/EU (2013)

Bacterial Species/Phenotypes	Animal Populations	Sample Size
Salmonella spp.	(i) Each population of laying hens, broilers, and fattening turkeys sampled in the framework of the national control programs (ii) Carcases of both broilers and fattening turkeys sampled for testing and verification of compliance, in accordance with Regulation (EC) No. 2073/2005 (iii) Carcases of fattening pigs sampled for testing and verification of compliance, in accordance with to Regulation (EC) No. 2073/2005 Carcases of bovines under 1 year of age where the production of meat of those bovines in the Member State is more than 10,000 ton slaughtered per year sampled for testing and verification of compliance, in accordance with Regulation (EC) No. 2073/2005	170 (85[a])
C. jejuni	Cecal samples gathered at slaughter from broilers and from fattening turkeys where the production of turkey meat in the Member State is more than 10,000 ton slaughtered per year	170 (85[a])
Indicator commensal *E. coli*	(i) Cecal samples gathered at slaughter from broilers and from fattening turkeys where the production of turkey meat in the Member State is more than 10,000 ton slaughtered per year (ii) Cecal samples gathered at slaughter from fattening pigs and bovines under 1 year of age where the production of meat of those bovines in the Member State is more than 10,000 ton slaughtered per year	170 (85[a])
ESBL- or AmpC- or carbapenemase-producing *E. coli*	(i) Cecal samples gathered at slaughter from broilers and from fattening turkeys where the production of turkey meat in the Member State is more than 10,000 ton slaughtered per year (ii) Cecal samples gathered at slaughter from fattening pigs and bovines under 1 year of age where the production	300 (150[b])

[a]Member States with a production of less than 100,000 ton of poultry meat slaughtered per year and less than 100,000 ton of pig meat slaughtered per year.
[b]Member States with a production of less than 100,000 ton of poultry meat slaughtered per year, less than 100,000 ton of pig meat slaughtered per year and less than 50,000 ton bovine meat slaughtered per year.

Table 3 Voluntary Combination of Bacterial Species/Phenotypes and Foods Where Antimicrobial Resistance Must be Monitored According to Commission Implementing Decision 2013/652/EU (2013)

Bacterial Species/ Phenotypes	Animal Populations	Sample Size
C. coli	(i) Cecal samples gathered at slaughter from broilers (ii) Cecal samples gathered at slaughter from fattening pigs	170 (85[a])
E. faecalis/E. faecium	(i) Cecal samples gathered at slaughter from broilers and from fattening turkeys where the production of turkey meat in the Member State is more than 10,000 ton slaughtered per year (ii) cecal samples gathered at slaughter from fattening pigs and bovines under 1 year of age where the production of meat of those bovines in the Member State is more than 10,000 ton slaughtered per year	170 (85[a])

[a]Member States with a production of less than 100,000 ton of poultry meat slaughtered per year and less than 100,000 ton of pig meat slaughtered per year.

4. AMR BACTERIA IN THE FOOD CHAIN

Currently, surveillance programs are being carried out on the levels of resistance found in food animals, animals, and people in the EU, and these data are published annually in the EU summary report on antimicrobial resistance in zoonotic and indicator bacteria from humans (EFSA and the European Centre for Disease Prevention and Control (ECDC)) (EFSA, 2017a). These surveillance programs allow comparing the evolution of AMR resistance levels and profiles over time.

4.1 Campylobacter

The genus *Campylobacter* is the zoonotic agent that produces the largest number of gastroenteritis of food transmission in humans annually in the EU (EFSA, 2017b). The infection caused by bacteria of the genus *Campylobacter* is called campylobacteriosis and is mainly due to the species *C. jejuni* (approximately 90%) and *C. coli* (around 10%) (Sheppard, Jolley, & Maiden, 2012). During 2016, a total of 246,307 people infected with *Campylobacter* were reported in the EU, placing this bacterium in the first position of bacterial infections caused by food consumption and far surpassing others such as *Salmonella* or verotoxin-producing *E. coli* (EFSA, 2017b). The clinical symptoms in people infected with *C. jejuni* or *C. coli* are diarrhea, fever, abdominal pain, and weight loss (Man, 2011). It is a self-limiting disease and the symptoms usually last for 5–6 days (Peterson, 1994). Although gastroenteritis is the main symptom of the infection, these microorganisms have been associated with other pathologies such as Guillain Barré syndrome or Miller Fisher syndrome (Baker et al., 2012; Koga et al., 2005). Generally, the treatment of infections caused by thermophilic *Campylobacter* is based on the application of antimicrobials only in specific cases. Currently, in cases where this treatment is necessary, quinolones and especially macrolides are the drug of choice (Allos, 2001), although in cases of bacteremia or systemic infection, the use of intravenous aminoglycosides is common (Alfredson & Korolik, 2007).

With respect to quinolones, in the last 2 decades, there has been a rapid increase in the percentage of resistance to ciprofloxacin in strains of *Campylobacter* throughout the world. According to EFSA data, 60.8% of strains of *C. jejuni* and 70.6% of *C. coli* from clinical cases in humans in the EU were resistant to ciprofloxacin (EFSA, 2017a). Some studies have linked this increase in resistance with the use of these antimicrobials in food animals, especially in the poultry industry (McDermott et al., 2002; Smith et al., 1999). In the EU, the high levels of resistance to ciprofloxacin in *Campylobacter* from samples of broilers and, especially meat (65.6% *C. jejuni* and 85.8% *C. coli*), have become a serious problem of public health, since it is estimated that up to 30% of *Campylobacter* infections in humans are attributed to the handling and/or consumption of this type of samples/food (EFSA, 2017a).

Regarding resistance to erythromycin, the percentages detected in clinical isolates in the EU are low for *C. jejuni* (1.5%) and moderately high for *C. coli* (14.4%) (EFSA, 2017a). In recent years, an increase in erythromycin resistance has been described, especially in animal isolates of *C. coli*, in some regions of the world. For example, percentages of erythromycin resistance greater than 40% in strains of *C. coli* from turkeys and pigs have been reported in the United States (Luangtongkum et al., 2009). In *Campylobacter* isolates from broilers in the EU, the percentage of resistance to erythromycin is also higher in *C. coli* (14.5%) than in *C. jejuni* (5.9%). This trend is maintained in isolates of turkeys for fattening (43.3% *C. coli* and 2.5% in *C. jejuni*) while in isolates of fattening pigs only *C. coli* data are available where the percentage is 21.6%, due to the fact that practically no *C. jejuni* is isolated from this host (Thakur & Gebreyes, 2005). The percentage of multiresistant isolates, those that show resistance to three or more classes of antimicrobials, are higher also in *C. coli* than in *C. jejuni* and usually correspond to ciprofloxacin, erythromycin, and tetracycline (EFSA, 2017a).

Campylobacter has mechanisms of resistance against antimicrobials that are inherent to the bacteria, while others have been acquired through mutations or horizontal gene transfer (Aarestrup, McDermott, & Wegener, 2008). Some of the most frequent mechanisms described in this microorganism are the synthesis of modifying or inactivating enzymes, the alteration or protection of the antimicrobial binding site, the expulsion of the antimicrobial agent outside the cell by means of efflux pumps or the reduction of the permeability of the bacterium (Tang, Fang, Xu, & Zhang, 2017). Resistance to erythromycin in *Campylobacter* is related to mutations in ribosomal genes, efflux pumps, and the presence of the *erm*(B) gene (Florez-Cuadrado et al., 2016). This gene is located in genomic islands of multiresistance, along with other AMR genes, to aminoglycosides mainly (Florez-Cuadrado et al., 2017; Wang et al., 2011).

4.2 Salmonella

Nontyphoidal *Salmonella* enterica is a leading cause of foodborne disease in both developing and developed countries and characterized by presenting febrile syndromes associated with gastrointestinal or systemic manifestations, often severe (Coburn, Grassl, & Finlay, 2007). According to WHO is estimated that annually affects tens of millions of people around the world and causes more than 100,000 deaths. Serotypes or serovars of *Salmonella* can be classified into groups from an epidemiological point of view as they are more or less adapted to a host species (Kingsley & Baumler, 2000). Thus, there are serovars strictly adapted to a specific host (e.g., *S. typhi* only associated with infections in humans or *S. gallinarum* in birds), serovars adapted to a specific host but which in some cases can be isolated in other hosts (e.g., *S. cholerasuis* that has been associated with severe systemic processes in pigs and humans) and serovars not adapted to specific hosts (e.g., *S. typhimurium* that is isolated from a wide variety of animals and the environment) (Uzzau et al., 2000). The latter are the ones that most frequently cause outbreaks of salmonellosis in humans, associated with the consumption of contaminated products, mainly eggs and meat.

The growing evolution of *Salmonella* isolates resistant to multiple antimicrobials is a problem over the control of this bacterium. Resistance to conventional antimicrobials such as ampicillin, chloramphenicol, or sulfonamides has become relatively frequent in clinical isolates since the 1990s. The presence of multiresistant isolates is associated with increased mortality, risk of infection, and hospitalization rates in infected humans (Varma et al., 2005). The clinical isolates of *Salmonella* show high rates of resistance to sulfonamides, tetracyclines, and ampicillin. On the other hand, ESBL-producing *Salmonellas* were identified in 0.5% of the isolates of human origin in the EU, with more than 10 different serovars being represented (EFSA, 2017a). Regarding multiresistance data in the EU, the highest rates correspond to *S. typhimurium* monophasic. The monophasic *S. typhimurium* is currently the third most frequent serovar that causes human infection in Europe, with 5770 cases in 2015, besides being the second most represented in pigs and the first in terms of multiresistance (EFSA, 2017a).

According to EFSA data, among *Salmonella* isolated from pig meat, the highest levels of resistance corresponded to antimicrobials ampicillin, sulfamethoxazole, and tetracyclines (EFSA, 2017a), in line with the data from human isolates. In the case of bovine meat, *Salmonella* shows lower resistance rates than pig meat, except for the antimicrobials tetracycline and tigecycline (EFSA, 2017a).

4.3 Indicator E. coli

According to its pathogenesis and epidemiological characteristics, this bacterium is divided into several pathotypes: Shiga toxin-producing *E. coli* (STEC), enterotoxigenic *E. coli* (ETEC), enteropathogenic *E. coli* (EPEC), enteroaggregative *E. coli* (EAEC), enteroinvasive *E. coli* (EIEC), and diffusely adherent *E. coli* (DAEC) (Jafari, Aslani, & Bouzari, 2012). STEC is undoubtedly the most important pathogen from the point of view of animal health as it is the only one so far considered to cause zoonosis or foodborne disease (EFSA, 2017b). The clinical picture of infections caused by STEC in humans includes diarrhea, which can sometimes progress to hemorrhagic colitis, abdominal pain, fever, and vomiting (Caprioli, Morabito, Brugere, & Oswald, 2005). The pathogenicity of STEC is attributed mainly to the production of virulence factors known as Shiga toxins. The main reservoirs of STEC are ruminants, especially cattle (Diaz-Sanchez et al., 2013). The transmission of STEC occurs generally through the consumption of contaminated meat that has been undercooked. Hamburgers made with beef are the meat derivative most involved in outbreaks in man (Bell et al., 1994). However, the intake of contaminated water, unpasteurized food, and vegetables are also frequent transmission routes (Cody et al., 1999; Karmali, 2004; Taormina, Beuchat, & Slutsker, 1999). The treatment should focus on a liquid therapy, dialysis, and appropriate antimicrobials depending on the strain. However, the use of antimicrobials sometimes aggravates the disease depending on the causative strain. In the case of infections caused by *E. coli* strain O104:H4, the use of carbapenems was recommended because this strain was resistant to penicillins and cephalosporins (Goldwater & Bettelheim, 2012; Muniesa, Hammerl, Hertwig, Appel, & Brussow, 2012).

Resistance to antimicrobials found in *E. coli*, both of human origin and isolated from animal and environmental reservoirs, is a cause of growing global concern. The *E. coli* indicators show resistance to various antimicrobials, susceptible to being transferred to other strains naturally, which can reach humans through the food chain (EFSA, 2017a). Isolates of *E. coli* from meat show a higher percentage of resistance to tetracycline, ampicillin, and streptomycin, being higher in broiler, swine, and cattle in decreasing order (EFSA, 2014). In recent years, resistance to antimicrobials found in strains isolated from humans has increased in number, especially new β-lactams such as third-generation cephalosporins (ceftazidime and cefotaxime) used as the treatment of choice in infections caused by *E. coli* and among others (Manninen, Auvinen, Huovinen, & The Finnish Study Group for Antimicrobial, 1997). In these cases, the mechanism of resistance is based on the production of extended-release β-lactamases (ESBLs) and other enzymes such as AmpC. This phenomenon has great relevance since the group of β-lactams is the most widely used in the treatment of bacterial infections (French, 2010). Both the commensal and the pathogen *C. coli* can transfer the genes of both types of enzymes to other bacteria and even to other bacterial species. EU data for 2015 showed that 7.9% of pork samples produced *E. coli* with an ESBL phenotype and 1.1% with an AmpC phenotype. In bovine meat, the total prevalence found was 5% of *E. coli* isolates with an ESBL phenotype and 0.3% with an AmpC phenotype (EFSA, 2017a).

5. ANTIMICROBIALS OF LAST RESORT

The presence of bacteria resistant to antimicrobials of last resort isolated from food makes the writing of this paragraph necessary (Garcia-Graells et al., 2017). Since 1983, a large number of beta-lactamases have been emerging that are capable of conferring resistance to beta-lactam antimicrobials. Thus, infections caused by ESBL-producing gram-negative bacilli are extremely serious and can be fatal (Paterson & Bonomo, 2005). In these cases, the antimicrobials of choice are carbapenems (imipenem, meropnem, etc.), since they resist the hydrolysis of ESBL-type enzymes (Zhanel et al., 2007). For this reason, carbapenems are an example of antimicrobials qualified as a "last resort" against infections caused by multiresistant bacteria, since it is a family classified as broad spectrum that are not hydrolyzed by the majority of beta-lactamases described. Unfortunately, there are already known cases of infections caused by bacteria resistant to these antimicrobials (Meletis, 2016). As a consequence of the appearance of strains resistant to carbapenems, it is necessary to use the few antimicrobials against which these bacteria are still sensitive, as is the case of colistin, despite its known adverse effects of nephrotoxicity and neurotoxicity (Wolinsky & Hines, 1962). Colistin (polymyxin E) is one of the few antimicrobials that can still be used to fight infections caused by microorganisms resistant to carbapenems in humans. It had been described that the ability of the bacteria to develop resistance to colistin was reduced due to the physiological cost causing the poor viability of this phenotype, together with the absence of horizontal transmission processes of resistance (Beceiro et al., 2014). In this way, this antimicrobial has been used on a daily basis in the metaphylactic treatment in slaughter animals, especially in pigs and poultry. In 2016, the first mechanism of plasmid-mediated colistin resistance was identified, the *mcr-1* gene in *E. coli* and *K. pneumonia* isolated from humans in China (Liu et al., 2016). In the same year, a second resistance gene, *mcr-2*, was identified in *E. coli* isolated from porcine and bovine cattle in Belgium (Xavier et al., 2016), and a year later, the gene *mcr-3* was identified in *E. coli* isolated from pigs from Malaysia, *K. pneumonia* from Thailand, and *S. enterica* serovar *typhimurium* from the United States (Yin et al., 2017).

Regarding surveillance, 2014 was the first year in which the monitoring of colistin resistance in *E. coli* isolated from animals was mandatory. The 0.9% and 7.4% of *E. coli* isolated from broiler chickens and turkeys, respectively, were resistant to this antimicrobial (EFSA, 2016). Next year, indicator *E. coli* resistant to colistin were found by several isolates from pigs and calves (0.4% and 0.9%, respectively), similar to the figure observed in broilers in 2014 (EFSA, 2015). Many countries around the world have reported the presence of *mcr-1* gene in Enterobacteriaceae recovered from humans, food, or animals (Skov & Monnet, 2016). These studies also showed that the plasmids carrying *mcr-1* had been transferred between different bacteria, because unrelated *E. coli* strains carried *mcr-1* (Haenni, Metayer, Gay, & Madec, 2016). *E. coli* isolates from pigs in Germany and calves in France also produced extended-spectrum beta-lactamases (Falgenhauer et al., 2016; Haenni et al., 2016). Colistin resistance was reported in 1.3% isolates of *Salmonella* spp. from pork meat, 1.3% of bovine meat, 0% of fattening pigs, and 2.2% of *Salmonella* spp. of calves (EFSA, 2017a). In the meat of fattening pigs, a variety of serovars with colistin resistance was detected. Only one of these serovars (*S. Dublin*) belonged to serogroup D, a serogroup that shows a lower level of intrinsic susceptibility to colistin compared to other serovars. The monophasic *S. typhimurium* was the serovar most commonly detected (EFSA, 2017a).

6. CONCLUSIONS

AMR bacteria in animal foods are a new topic that must be adequately communicated to consumers. This is a particular piece of a well-known food hazard that are zoonotic bacteria transmitted to humans by animal food, but adding a new aspect related to AMR genes that could also be harbored by commensal bacteria of food and move to pathogenic bacteria, especially on the human gut. EU legislation paid attention to this new hazard adding AMR testing of zoonotic bacteria (*Salmonella* and *Campylobacter*), as well as in fecal indicator bacteria, especially *E. coli*. In addition, different measures taken at farm level will decrease the load of AMR bacteria by healthy animals at the slaughterhouse level, that remain a critical control point of the food chain for public health.

REFERENCES

2003/99/EC. (2003). *Directive of the European Parliament and of the council of 17 November 2003 on the monitoring of zoonoses and zoonotic agents, amending council decision 90/424/EEC and repealing council directive 92/117/EEC*. The Commission of the European Communities.

2005/2073/EC. (2005). *Commission regulation (EC) no 2073/2005 of 15 November 2005 on microbiological criteria for foodstuffs*. The Commission of the European Communities.

2007/407/EC. (2007). *Commission decision of 12 June 2007 concerning a financial contribution from the community towards a survey on the prevalence and antimicrobial resistance of* Campylobacter *spp. in broiler flocks and on the prevalence of* Campylobacter *spp. and* Salmonella *spp. in broiler carcasses to be carried out in the member states*. The Commission of the European Communities.

2007/516/EC. (2007). *Commission decision of 19 July 2007 concerning a financial contribution from the community towards a survey on the prevalence and antimicrobial resistance of* Campylobacter *spp. in broiler flocks and on the prevalence of* Campylobacter *spp. and* Salmonella *spp. in broiler carcasses to be carried out in the member states*. The Commission of the European Communities.

2013/652/EU. (2013). *Commission Implementing Decision of 12 November 2013 on the monitoring and reporting of antimicrobial resistance in zoonotic and commensal bacteria*. The Commission of the European Communities.

Aarestrup, F. M., McDermott, P. F., & Wegener, H. C. (2008). Transmission of antibiotic resistance from food animals to humans. *2008* (pp. 645–665). ASM Press.

Alfredson, D. A., & Korolik, V. (2007). Antibiotic resistance and resistance mechanisms in Campylobacter jejuni and Campylobacter coli. *FEMS Microbiology Letters*, *277*(2), 123–132. https://doi.org/10.1111/j.1574-6968.2007.00935.x.

Allos, B. M. (2001). Campylobacter jejuni infections: Update on emerging issues and trends. *Clinical Infectious Diseases*, *32*(8), 1201–1206. https://doi.org/10.1086/319760.

Aminov, R. I. (2010). A brief history of the antibiotic era: Lessons learned and challenges for the future. *Frontiers in Microbiology*, *1*, 134. https://doi.org/10.3389/fmicb.2010.00134.

Baker, M. G., Kvalsvig, A., Zhang, J., Lake, R., Sears, A., & Wilson, N. (2012). Declining Guillain–Barre syndrome after campylobacteriosis control, New Zealand, 1988–2010. *Emerging Infectious Diseases*, *18*(2), 226–233. https://doi.org/10.3201/eid1802.111126.

Beceiro, A., Moreno, A., Fernandez, N., Vallejo, J. A., Aranda, J., Adler, B., et al. (2014). Biological cost of different mechanisms of colistin resistance and their impact on virulence in Acinetobacter baumannii. *Antimicrobial Agents and Chemotherapy*, *58*(1), 518–526. https://doi.org/10.1128/AAC.01597-13.

Bell, B. P., Goldoft, M., Griffin, P. M., Davis, M. A., Gordon, D. C., Tarr, P. I., et al. (1994). A multistate outbreak of Escherichia coli O157:H7-associated bloody diarrhea and hemolytic uremic syndrome from hamburgers. The Washington experience. *JAMA*, *272*(17), 1349–1353.

Bennett, P. M. (2008). Plasmid encoded antibiotic resistance: Acquisition and transfer of antibiotic resistance genes in bacteria. *British Journal of Pharmacology*, *153*(Suppl. 1), S347–357. https://doi.org/10.1038/sj.bjp.0707607.

Blair, J. M., Webber, M. A., Baylay, A. J., Ogbolu, D. O., & Piddock, L. J. (2015). Molecular mechanisms of antibiotic resistance. *Nature Reviews. Microbiology*, *13*(1), 42–51. https://doi.org/10.1038/nrmicro3380.

Bornstein, S. (1940). Action of penicillin on enterococci and other streptococci. *Journal of Bacteriology*, *39*(4), 383–387.

Bos, K. I., Schuenemann, V. J., Golding, G. B., Burbano, H. A., Waglechner, N., Coombes, B. K., et al. (2011). A draft genome of Yersinia pestis from victims of the black death. *Nature*, *478*(7370), 506–510. https://doi.org/10.1038/nature10549.

Caprioli, A., Morabito, S., Brugere, H., & Oswald, E. (2005). Enterohaemorrhagic Escherichia coli: Emerging issues on virulence and modes of transmission. *Veterinary Research*, *36*(3), 289–311. https://doi.org/10.1051/vetres:2005002.

Castanon, J. I. (2007). History of the use of antibiotic as growth promoters in European poultry feeds. *Poultry Science*, *86*(11), 2466–2471. https://doi.org/10.3382/ps.2007-00249.

Coburn, B., Grassl, G. A., & Finlay, B. B. (2007). Salmonella, the host and disease: A brief review. *Immunology and Cell Biology*, *85*(2), 112–118. https://doi.org/10.1038/sj.icb.7100007.

Cody, S. H., Glynn, M. K., Farrar, J. A., Cairns, K. L., Griffin, P. M., Kobayashi, J., et al. (1999). An outbreak of Escherichia coli O157:H7 infection from unpasteurized commercial apple juice. *Annals of Internal Medicine*, *130*(3), 202–209.

Colavecchio, A., Cadieux, B., Lo, A., & Goodridge, L. D. (2017). Bacteriophages contribute to the spread of antibiotic resistance genes among foodborne pathogens of the enterobacteriaceae family—A review. *Frontiers in Microbiology*, *8*, 1108. https://doi.org/10.3389/fmicb.2017.01108.

Davies, J., & Davies, D. (2010). Origins and evolution of antibiotic resistance. *Microbiology and Molecular Biology Reviews*, *74*(3), 417–433. https://doi.org/10.1128/MMBR.00016-10.

Diarrassouba, F., Diarra, M. S., Bach, S., Delaquis, P., Pritchard, J., Topp, E., et al. (2007). Antibiotic resistance and virulence genes in commensal Escherichia coli and Salmonella isolates from commercial broiler chicken farms. *Journal of Food Protection*, *70*(6), 1316–1327.

Diaz-Sanchez, S., Sanchez, S., Herrera-Leon, S., Porrero, C., Blanco, J., Dahbi, G., et al. (2013). Prevalence of Shiga toxin-producing *Escherichia coli*, Salmonella spp. and Campylobacter spp. in large game animals intended for consumption: Relationship with management practices and livestock influence. *Veterinary Microbiology*, *163*(3–4), 274–281. https://doi.org/10.1016/j.vetmic.2012.12.026.

EFSA, EFSA (European Food Safety Authority). Trends and source of zoonoses, zoonotic agents and antimicrobial resistance in the European Union. The EFSA Journal, 2005. ISBN: 92-9199-016-7.

EFSA, EFSA (European Food Safety Authority). (2008). Report of the task force on zoonoses data collection including guidance for harmonized monitoring and reporting of antimicrobial resistance in commensal *Escherichia coli* and Enterococcus spp. from food animals. *The EFSA Journal*. https://doi.org/10.2903/j.efsa.2008.141r.

EFSA, EFSA (European Food Safety Authority). (2010). The community summary report on antimicrobial resistance in zoonotic and indicator bacteria from animals and food in the European Union in 2004–2007. *The EFSA Journal*. https://doi.org/10.2903/j.efsa.2010.1309.

EFSA, EFSA (European Food Safety Authority). (2012). Technical specifications on harmonised monitoring and reporting of MRSA. *The EFSA Journal*. https://doi.org/10.2903/j.efsa.2012.2897.

EFSA, EFSA (European Food Safety Authority) and ECDC (European Centre for Disease Prevention and Control). (2014). The European Union summary report on antimicrobial resistance in zoonotic and indicator bacteria from humans, animals and food in 2012. *The EFSA Journal*. https://doi.org/10.2903/j.efsa.2014.3590.

EFSA, EFSA (European Food Safety Authority) and ECDC (European Centre for Disease Prevention and Control). (2015). The European Union summary report on antimicrobial resistance in zoonotic and indicator bacteria from humans, animals and food in 2013. *The EFSA Journal*, *13*(2), 4036.

EFSA, EFSA (European Food Safety Authority) and ECDC (European Centre for Disease Prevention and Control). (2016). The European Union summary report on antimicrobial resistance in zoonotic and indicator bacteria from humans, animals and food in 2014. *The EFSA Journal*. https://doi.org/10.2903/j.efsa.2016.4380.

EFSA. (2017a). The European Union summary report on antimicrobial resistance in zoonotic and indicator bacteria from humans, animals and food in 2015. *The EFSA Journal*, *15*(2), 212. https://doi.org/10.2903/j.efsa.2017.4694.

EFSA, EFSA (European Food Safety Authority) and ECDC (European Centre for Disease Prevention and Control). (2017b). The European Union summary report on trends and sources of Zoonoses, zoonotic agents and food-borne outbreaks in 2016. *The EFSA Journal*. https://doi.org/10.2903/j.efsa.2017.5077.

Emmerson, A. M., & Jones, A. M. (2003). The quinolones: Decades of development and use. *The Journal of Antimicrobial Chemotherapy*, *51*(Suppl. 1), 13–20. https://doi.org/10.1093/jac/dkg208.

Falgenhauer, L., Waezsada, S. E., Yao, Y., Imirzalioglu, C., Kasbohrer, A., Roesler, U., et al. (2016). Colistin resistance gene mcr-1 in extended-spectrum beta-lactamase-producing and carbapenemase-producing gram-negative bacteria in Germany. *The Lancet Infectious Diseases*, *16*(3), 282–283. https://doi.org/10.1016/S1473-3099(16)00009-8.

Feighner, S. D., & Dashkevicz, M. P. (1987). Subtherapeutic levels of antibiotics in poultry feeds and their effects on weight gain, feed efficiency, and bacterial cholyltaurine hydrolase activity. *Applied and Environmental Microbiology*, *53*(2), 331–336.

Florez-Cuadrado, D., Ugarte-Ruiz, M., Meric, G., Quesada, A., Porrero, M. C., Pascoe, B., et al. (2017). Genome comparison of erythromycin resistant Campylobacter from turkeys identifies hosts and pathways for horizontal spread of erm(B) genes. *Frontiers in Microbiology*, *8*, 2240. https://doi.org/10.3389/fmicb.2017.02240.

Florez-Cuadrado, D., Ugarte-Ruiz, M., Quesada, A., Palomo, G., Dominguez, L., & Porrero, M. C. (2016). Description of an erm(B)-carrying Campylobacter coli isolate in Europe. *The Journal of Antimicrobial Chemotherapy*, *71*(3), 841–843. https://doi.org/10.1093/jac/dkv383.

French, G. L. (2010). The continuing crisis in antibiotic resistance. *International Journal of Antimicrobial Agents*, *36*(Suppl. 3), S3–7. https://doi.org/10.1016/S0924-8579(10)70003-0.

Fyfe, C., Grossman, T. H., Kerstein, K., & Sutcliffe, J. (2016). Resistance to macrolide antibiotics in public health pathogens. *Cold Spring Harbor Perspectives in Medicine, 6*(10). https://doi.org/10.1101/cshperspect.a025395.

Garcia-Graells, C., De Keersmaecker, S. C. J., Vanneste, K., Pochet, B., Vermeersch, K., Roosens, N., et al. (2017). Detection of plasmid-mediated colistin resistance, mcr-1 and mcr-2 genes, in Salmonella spp. isolated from food at retail in Belgium from 2012 to 2015. *Foodborne Pathogens and Disease*. https://doi.org/10.1089/fpd.2017.2329.

Gibreel, A., Kos, V. N., Keelan, M., Trieber, C. A., Levesque, S., Michaud, S., et al. (2005). Macrolide resistance in Campylobacter jejuni and Campylobacter coli: Molecular mechanism and stability of the resistance phenotype. *Antimicrobial Agents and Chemotherapy, 49*(7), 2753–2759. https://doi.org/10.1128/AAC.49.7.2753-2759.2005.

Goldwater, P. N., & Bettelheim, K. A. (2012). Treatment of enterohemorrhagic Escherichia coli (EHEC) infection and hemolytic uremic syndrome (HUS). *BMC Medicine, 10*, 12. https://doi.org/10.1186/1741-7015-10-12.

Gomez, J. E., Kaufmann-Malaga, B. B., Wivagg, C. N., Kim, P. B., Silvis, M. R., Renedo, N., et al. (2017). Ribosomal mutations promote the evolution of antibiotic resistance in a multidrug environment. *eLife, 6*, e20420, 1–25. https://doi.org/10.7554/eLife.20420.

Haenni, M., Metayer, V., Gay, E., & Madec, J. Y. (2016). Increasing trends in mcr-1 prevalence among extended-spectrum-beta-lactamase-producing Escherichia coli isolates from French calves despite decreasing exposure to colistin. *Antimicrobial Agents and Chemotherapy, 60*(10), 6433–6434. https://doi.org/10.1128/AAC.01147-16.

Hald, T., Lo Fo Wong, D. M., & Aarestrup, F. M. (2007). The attribution of human infections with antimicrobial resistant Salmonella bacteria in Denmark to sources of animal origin. *Foodborne Pathogens and Disease, 4*(3), 313–326. https://doi.org/10.1089/fpd.2007.0002.

Infosan. (2008). *Red Internacional de Autoridades en materia de Inocuidad de los Alimentos (INFOSAN). INFOSAN Nota informativa No 2/2008—Resistencia a los antimicrobianos.* 7 de marzo de.

Jacob, F. H. (1938). Prontosil for meningitis. *British Medical Journal, 1*(4033), 887–888.

Jacoby, G. A. (2005). Mechanisms of resistance to quinolones. *Clinical Infectious Diseases, 41*(Suppl. 2), S120–126. https://doi.org/10.1086/428052.

Jafari, A., Aslani, M. M., & Bouzari, S. (2012). Escherichia coli: A brief review of diarrheagenic pathotypes and their role in diarrheal diseases in Iran. *Iranian Journal of Microbiology, 4*(3), 102–117.

Karmali, M. A. (2004). Infection by Shiga toxin-producing Escherichia coli: An overview. *Molecular Biotechnology, 26*(2), 117–122. https://doi.org/10.1385/MB:26:2:117.

Kingsley, R. A., & Baumler, A. J. (2000). Host adaptation and the emergence of infectious disease: The Salmonella paradigm. *Molecular Microbiology, 36*(5), 1006–1014.

Koga, M., Gilbert, M., Li, J., Koike, S., Takahashi, M., Furukawa, K., et al. (2005). Antecedent infections in fisher syndrome: A common pathogenesis of molecular mimicry. *Neurology, 64*(9), 1605–1611. https://doi.org/10.1212/01.WNL.0000160399.08456.7C.

Kurland, C. G., Canback, B., & Berg, O. G. (2003). Horizontal gene transfer: A critical view. *Proceedings of the National Academy of Sciences of the United States of America, 100*(17), 9658–9662. https://doi.org/10.1073/pnas.1632870100.

Kwon, J. H., Reske, K. A., Hink, T., Seiler, S. M., Wallace, M. A., Bommarito, K. M., et al. (2017). An evaluation of the prevalence of vancomycin-resistant enterococci (VRE) and methicillin-resistant Staphylococcus aureus (MRSA) in hospital food. *Infection Control and Hospital Epidemiology, 38*(11), 1373–1375. https://doi.org/10.1017/ice.2017.207.

Lawrence, J. G. (2005). Horizontal and vertical gene transfer: The life history of pathogens. *Contributions to Microbiology, 12*, 255–271. https://doi.org/10.1159/000081699.

Lee, M. D., Sanchez, S., Zimmer, M., Idris, U., Berrang, M. E., & McDermott, P. F. (2002). Class 1 integron-associated tobramycin-gentamicin resistance in Campylobacter jejuni isolated from the broiler chicken house environment. *Antimicrobial Agents and Chemotherapy, 46*(11), 3660–3664.

Lester, C. H., Frimodt-Moller, N., Sorensen, T. L., Monnet, D. L., & Hammerum, A. M. (2006). In vivo transfer of the vanA resistance gene from an enterococcus faecium isolate of animal origin to an E. faecium isolate of human origin in the intestines of human volunteers. *Antimicrobial Agents and Chemotherapy*, *50*(2), 596–599. https://doi.org/10.1128/AAC.50.2.596-599.2006.

Littman, R. J. (2009). The plague of Athens: Epidemiology and paleopathology. *Mount Sinai Journal of Medicine*, *76*(5), 456–467. https://doi.org/10.1002/msj.20137.

Liu, Y. Y., Wang, Y., Walsh, T. R., Yi, L. X., Zhang, R., Spencer, J., et al. (2016). Emergence of plasmid-mediated colistin resistance mechanism MCR-1 in animals and human beings in China: A microbiological and molecular biological study. *The Lancet Infectious Diseases*, *16*(2), 161–168. https://doi.org/10.1016/S1473-3099(15)00424-7.

Luangtongkum, T., Jeon, B., Han, J., Plummer, P., Logue, C. M., & Zhang, Q. (2009). Antibiotic resistance in Campylobacter: Emergence, transmission and persistence. *Future Microbiology*, *4*(2), 189–200. https://doi.org/10.2217/17460913.4.2.189.

Mamelli, L., Prouzet-Mauleon, V., Pages, J. M., Megraud, F., & Bolla, J. M. (2005). Molecular basis of macrolide resistance in Campylobacter: Role of efflux pumps and target mutations. *The Journal of Antimicrobial Chemotherapy*, *56*(3), 491–497. https://doi.org/10.1093/jac/dki253.

Man, S. M. (2011). The clinical importance of emerging Campylobacter species. *Nature Reviews. Gastroenterology & Hepatology*, *8*(12), 669–685. https://doi.org/10.1038/nrgastro.2011.191.

Manninen, R., Auvinen, H., Huovinen, P., & The Finnish Study Group for Antimicrobial Resistance. (1997). Resistance to second- and third-generation cephalosporins among Escherichia coli and Klebsiella species is rare in Finland. *Clinical Microbiology and Infection*, *3*(4), 408–413.

Maria-Neto, S., de Almeida, K. C., Macedo, M. L., & Franco, O. L. (2015). Understanding bacterial resistance to antimicrobial peptides: From the surface to deep inside. *Biochimica et Biophysica Acta*, *1848*(11 Pt. B), 3078–3088. https://doi.org/10.1016/j.bbamem.2015.02.017.

Martinez, J. L. (2009). The role of natural environments in the evolution of resistance traits in pathogenic bacteria. *Proceedings of the Biological Sciences*, *276*(1667), 2521–2530. https://doi.org/10.1098/rspb.2009.0320.

Martinez, J. L., Coque, T. M., & Baquero, F. (2015). What is a resistance gene? Ranking risk in resistomes. *Nature Reviews Microbiology*, *13*(2), 116–123. https://doi.org/10.1038/nrmicro3399.

McDermott, P. F., Bodeis, S. M., English, L. L., White, D. G., Walker, R. D., Zhao, S., et al. (2002). Ciprofloxacin resistance in Campylobacter jejuni evolves rapidly in chickens treated with fluoroquinolones. *The Journal of Infectious Diseases*, *185*(6), 837–840. https://doi.org/10.1086/339195.

Meletis, G. (2016). Carbapenem resistance: Overview of the problem and future perspectives. *Therapeutic Advances in Infectious Disease*, *3*(1), 15–21. https://doi.org/10.1177/2049936115621709.

Muniesa, M., Hammerl, J. A., Hertwig, S., Appel, B., & Brussow, H. (2012). Shiga toxin-producing Escherichia coli O104:H4: A new challenge for microbiology. *Applied and Environmental Microbiology*, *78*(12), 4065–4073. https://doi.org/10.1128/AEM.00217-12.

Munita, J. M., & Arias, C. A. (2016). Mechanisms of antibiotic resistance. *Microbiology Spectrum*, *4*(2), 481–511. https://doi.org/10.1128/microbiolspec.VMBF-0016-2015.

O'Brien, S., Rodrigues, A. M., & Buckling, A. (2013). The evolution of bacterial mutation rates under simultaneous selection by interspecific and social parasitism. *Proceedings of the Biological Sciences*, *280*(1773), 20131913. https://doi.org/10.1098/rspb.2013.1913.

Paterson, D. L., & Bonomo, R. A. (2005). Extended-spectrum beta-lactamases: A clinical update. *Clinical Microbiology Reviews*, *18*(4), 657–686. https://doi.org/10.1128/CMR.18.4.657-686.2005.

Pedersen, K., & Wedderkopp, A. (2003). Resistance to quinolones in Campylobacter jejuni and Campylobacter coli from Danish broilers at farm level. *Journal of Applied Microbiology*, *94*(1), 111–119.

Peterson, M. C. (1994). Clinical aspects of Campylobacter jejuni infections in adults. *The Western Journal of Medicine*, *161*(2), 148–152.

Postma, M., Vanderhaeghen, W., Sarrazin, S., Maes, D., & Dewulf, J. (2017). Reducing antimicrobial usage in pig production without jeopardizing production parameters. *Zoonoses and Public Health*, *64*(1), 63–74. https://doi.org/10.1111/zph.12283.

Pugajeva, I., Avsejenko, J., Judjallo, E., Berzins, A., Bartkiene, E., & Bartkevics, V. (2018). High occurrence rates of enrofloxacin and ciprofloxacin residues in retail poultry meat revealed by an ultra-sensitive mass-spectrometric method, and antimicrobial resistance to fluoroquinolones in Campylobacter spp. *Food Additives & Contaminants. Part A, Chemistry, Analysis, Control, Exposure & Risk Assessment*. https://doi.org/10.1080/19440049.2018.1432900.

Shaikh, S., Fatima, J., Shakil, S., Rizvi, S. M., & Kamal, M. A. (2015). Antibiotic resistance and extended spectrum beta-lactamases: Types, epidemiology and treatment. *Saudi Journal of Biological Sciences*, *22*(1), 90–101. https://doi.org/10.1016/j.sjbs.2014.08.002.

Sheppard, S. K., Jolley, K. A., & Maiden, M. C. (2012). A gene-by-gene approach to bacterial population genomics: Whole genome MLST of Campylobacter. *Genes (Basel)*, *3*(2), 261–277. https://doi.org/10.3390/genes3020261.

Skov, R. L., & Monnet, D. L. (2016). Plasmid-mediated colistin resistance (mcr-1 gene): Three months later, the story unfolds. *Euro Surveillance*, *21*(9), 30155. https://doi.org/10.2807/1560-7917.ES.2016.21.9.30155.

Smith, K. E., Besser, J. M., Hedberg, C. W., Leano, F. T., Bender, J. B., Wicklund, J. H., et al. (1999). Quinolone-resistant Campylobacter jejuni infections in Minnesota, 1992–1998. Investigation team. *The New England Journal of Medicine*, *340*(20), 1525–1532. https://doi.org/10.1056/NEJM199905203402001.

Sutherland, R. (1964). The nature of the insensitivity of gram-negative bacteria towards Penicillins. *Journal of General Microbiology*, *34*, 85–98. https://doi.org/10.1099/00221287-34-1-85.

Tang, Y., Fang, L., Xu, C., & Zhang, Q. (2017). Antibiotic resistance trends and mechanisms in the foodborne pathogen, Campylobacter. *Animal Health Research Reviews*, *2*, 1–12. https://doi.org/10.1017/S1466252317000135.

Taormina, P. J., Beuchat, L. R., & Slutsker, L. (1999). Infections associated with eating seed sprouts: An international concern. *Emerging Infectious Diseases*, *5*(5), 626–634. https://doi.org/10.3201/eid0505.990503.

Taylor-Robinson, D., & Bebear, C. (1997). Antibiotic susceptibilities of mycoplasmas and treatment of mycoplasmal infections. *The Journal of Antimicrobial Chemotherapy*, *40*(5), 622–630.

Thakur, S., & Gebreyes, W. A. (2005). Campylobacter coli in swine production: Antimicrobial resistance mechanisms and molecular epidemiology. *Journal of Clinical Microbiology*, *43*(11), 5705–5714. https://doi.org/10.1128/JCM.43.11.5705-5714.2005.

Uzzau, S., Brown, D. J., Wallis, T., Rubino, S., Leori, G., Bernard, S., et al. (2000). Host adapted serotypes of Salmonella enterica. *Epidemiology and Infection*, *125*(2), 229–255.

van Hoek, A. H., Mevius, D., Guerra, B., Mullany, P., Roberts, A. P., & Aarts, H. J. (2011). Acquired antibiotic resistance genes: An overview. *Frontiers in Microbiology*, *2*, 203. https://doi.org/10.3389/fmicb.2011.00203.

Varma, J. K., Molbak, K., Barrett, T. J., Beebe, J. L., Jones, T. F., Rabatsky-Ehr, T., et al. (2005). Antimicrobial-resistant nontyphoidal Salmonella is associated with excess bloodstream infections and hospitalizations. *The Journal of Infectious Diseases*, *191*(4), 554–561. https://doi.org/10.1086/427263.

Wang, Y., Zhang, M., Deng, F., Shen, Z., Wu, C., Zhang, J., et al. (2014). Emergence of multidrug-resistant Campylobacter species isolates with a horizontally acquired rRNA methylase. *Antimicrobial Agents and Chemotherapy*, *58*(9), 5405–5412. https://doi.org/10.1128/AAC.03039-14.

Wang, X., Zhao, S., Harbottle, H., Tran, T., Blickenstaff, K., Abbott, J., et al. (2011). Antimicrobial resistance and molecular subtyping of Campylobacter jejuni and Campylobacter coli from retail meats. *Journal of Food Protection*, *74*(4), 616–621. https://doi.org/10.4315/0362-028X.JFP-10-432.

Wolinsky, E., & Hines, J. D. (1962). Neurotoxic and nephrotoxic effects of colistin in patients with renal disease. *The New England Journal of Medicine*, *266*, 759–762. https://doi.org/10.1056/NEJM196204122661505.

Xavier, B. B., Lammens, C., Ruhal, R., Kumar-Singh, S., Butaye, P., Goossens, H., et al. (2016). Identification of a novel plasmid-mediated colistin-resistance gene, mcr-2, in Escherichia coli, Belgium, June 2016. *Euro Surveillance*, *21*(27). https://doi.org/10.2807/1560-7917.ES.2016.21.27.30280.

Yin, W., Li, H., Shen, Y., Liu, Z., Wang, S., Shen, Z., et al. (2017). Novel plasmid-mediated colistin resistance gene mcr-3 in Escherichia coli. *mBio*, *8*(3). https://doi.org/10.1128/mBio.00543-17.

Zaffiri, L., Gardner, J., & Toledo-Pereyra, L. H. (2012). History of antibiotics. From salvarsan to cephalosporins. *Journal of Investigative Surgery*, *25*(2), 67–77. https://doi.org/10.3109/08941939.2012.664099.

Zhanel, G. G., Wiebe, R., Dilay, L., Thomson, K., Rubinstein, E., Hoban, D. J., et al. (2007). Comparative review of the carbapenems. *Drugs*, *67*(7), 1027–1052.

FURTHER READING

EFSA, EFSA (European Food Safety Authority). (2007). Report of the task force on zoonoses data collection including a proposal for a harmonized monitoring scheme of anitmicrobial resistance in Salmonella in fowl (Gallus gallus), turkeys and pigs and Campylobacter jejuni and C. coli in broilers. *The EFSA Journal*. https://doi.org/10.2903/j.efsa.2007.96r.

CHAPTER SIX

Salmonella in Foods: A Reemerging Problem

Alessandra De Cesare[1]
Department of Agricultural and Food Sciences, University of Bologna, Bologna, Italy
[1]Corresponding author: e-mail address: alessandra.decesare@unibo.it

Contents

Abstract

The number of human salmonellosis within the European Union tended to increase since 2013. One of the reasons might be Salmonella Enteritidis rising in laying hens flocks by around 17% in 2015 vs 2014 and by 57% in 2016 vs 2015. The most important sources of food-borne Salmonella outbreaks are still eggs and egg products as well as ready-to-eat foods having a long shelf life. Specific actions are suggested to restart decreasing the number of human salmonellosis: (1) revision of sampling schemes to solve pathogen under detection in both animals and foods; (2) integration of microbiological criteria with fit for purpose performance objectives and food safety objectives; and (3) improvement of epidemiological investigations of human, food, and animal isolates by using whole-genome sequencing in order to effectively track salmonellosis and verify which prevention measures are most effective.

Advances in Food and Nutrition Research, Volume 86
ISSN 1043-4526
https://doi.org/10.1016/bs.afnr.2018.02.007
© 2018 Elsevier Inc.
All rights reserved.

1. CONTEXT

The World Health Organization estimated that *Salmonella enterica* infections from contaminated foods alone constitute a loss of 6.43 million disability adjusted life years worldwide, more than any other enteric pathogen (Kirk et al., 2015). *S. enterica* is a facultative intracellular Gram-negative bacterium, which comprises six subspecies (*S. enterica* subsp. *arizonae*, *S. enterica* subsp. *diarizonae*, *S. enterica* subsp. *enterica*, *S. enterica* subsp. *houtenae*, *S. enterica* subsp. *indica*, and *S. enterica* subsp. *salamae*) (Gayet, Bioley, Rochereau, Paul, & Corthésy, 2017). Among them, *S. enterica* subsp. *enterica* is a food-borne bacterial pathogen having at least 2600 serotypes (Gal-Mor, Boyle, & Grassl, 2014) that contaminate a diversity of foods and are a leading cause of food-borne illnesses and mortality globally (Majowicz et al., 2010).

The Salmonella serotyping system classifies isolates on the basis of the immunological reactions to cell surface antigens, specifically the somatic O and the two variably expressed flagellar H antigens, denoted H1 and H2 (Yoshida et al., 2016). The most recent edition of the White–Kaufmann–Le Minor scheme has identified over 2500 serovars belonging to the five subspecies of *S. enterica* (Grimont & Weill, 2007). However, it is important to note that most of human clinical disease is the result of a select few important human pathogenic serovars (Hendriksen et al., 2011).

Traditionally, serotyping is performed through the phenotypic characterization of the O and H antigens via the slide agglutination test, in which the clumping of cells is observed in response to specific antisera. Although this technique is widely used (Wattiau, Boland, & Bertrand, 2011), it can be time consuming and laborious (Kim et al., 2006; Wattiau et al., 2011; Zhang et al., 2015), and still leave 5%–8% of all Salmonella isolates untypeable (Kim et al., 2006). Whole-genome sequencing (WGS) promises to not only provide the best dataset available to determine pathogen relatedness but also WGS data could be used to derive information about other important characteristics, such as serotype, using in silico workflows (Gilmour, Graham, Reimer, & Van Domselaar, 2013; Ronholm, Nasheri, Petronella, & Pagotto, 2016).

The typhoidal Salmonella serovars *S. enterica* subsp. *enterica* Typhi (S. Typhi) (O:9) and *S. enterica* subsp. *enterica* Paratyphi A (S. Paratyphi) (O:2) exclusively infect humans and cause enteric fever, also referred to as typhoid fever. The nontyphoidal Salmonella serovars *S. enterica* subsp. *enterica* Typhimurium (S. Typhimurium) (O:4) and *S. enterica* subsp. *enterica* Enteritidis

(S. Enteritidis) (O:9) infect both humans and animals and are among the major causal agents of self-limiting gastroenteritis, a local infection that causes diarrhea (Lan et al., 2016).

Nontyphoidal Salmonella serovars are the second most frequent zoonotic agent in the European Union (EU) (EFSA-ECDC, 2017). In Canada, nontyphoidal salmonellosis accounts for more than 88,000 cases of food-borne illness each year and has among the highest incidence rate of any bacterial food-borne pathogen (Thomas et al., 2015). Furthermore, nontyphoidal *S. enterica* is responsible for more than 50% of fresh produce-borne outbreaks, the highest number of food-borne outbreaks of any inspected food commodity in North America (Kozak, MacDonald, Landry, & Farber, 2013). Several research groups have identified relationships between some of the *S. enterica* serotypes and specific foods, which suggest that some food commodities act as reservoirs for particular serotypes (Jackson, Griffin, Cole, Walsh, & Chai, 2013; Kim, 2010; Nüesch-Inderbinen, Cernela, Althaus, Hächler, & Stephan, 2015).

Because of its remarkable genomic diversity, Salmonella is found in complex environmental and ecological niches and survives in harsh environments for long periods (Fatica & Schneider, 2011; Podolak, Enache, Stone, Black, & Elliott, 2010). Reducing the number of Salmonella infections is a complicated problem because Salmonella has many sources and the sources vary by the type of Salmonella (Tessari et al., 2012). The main reservoir of these bacteria is the intestinal tract of humans and warm- and cold-blooded animals (Jakabi et al., 1999), except for fish, molluscs, and crustaceans, which may get contaminated after being fished. Among warm-blooded animals, chickens, geese, turkeys, and ducks are the most important reservoirs. Domestic animals, such as dogs, cats, turtles, and birds, may be carriers and pose great risk mainly to kids (Srisanga et al., 2017).

2. EUROPEAN SALMONELLA MONITORING SYSTEMS IN HUMANS, FOODS, AND ANIMALS

The notification of nontyphoidal salmonellosis in humans is mandatory in most European Member States (MS) as well as Iceland, Norway, and Switzerland, except for six MS where reporting is based on a voluntary system (Belgium, France, Luxembourg, and the Netherlands) or other systems (Spain and the United Kingdom) (EFSA-ECDC, 2017). The surveillance systems for salmonellosis cover the whole population in all MS except four (Belgium, France, the Netherlands, and Spain). The coverage of the surveillance system is estimated to be 48% in France and 64% in the Netherlands, whereas no estimation for population coverage in Belgium and Spain is provided (EFSA-ECDC, 2017). Concerning food-borne outbreaks, the annual reporting of investigated food-borne outbreaks, including salmonellosis, has been mandatory for MS since 2003, according to Directive 2003/99/EC, with the aim of providing data on the epidemiological profile of the outbreaks, the foodstuffs potentially implicated, and the potential causes of the outbreaks.

Monitoring of Salmonella in foods is mainly based on data originating from the reporting obligations of MS under EU Regulation 2073/2005 on microbiological criteria that has been in force since January 1, 2006. Regulation (EC) No. 2073/2005 on microbiological criteria in foodstuffs lays down Salmonella food safety criteria and these should be monitored by individual food business operator in the context of their own HACCP programs. The Salmonella food safety criteria prescribe that Salmonella monitoring results must be compliant with "absence in 25 or 10 g," when products are placed on the market, during their shelf life. Absence is defined by testing 5 or, depending on the food category, 30 sampling units per batch, for specified food categories. Moreover, according to Regulation (EC) No. 1086 that has been in force since December 2011, compliance with "absence in 25 g" is required for the regulated serovars in the context of EU control programs for poultry populations (S. Enteritidis and S. Typhimurium including monophasic S. Typhimurium strains with the antigenic formula 1,4,[5],12: i:-) in batches of fresh poultry meat (including fresh meat from breeding flocks of *Gallus gallus*, laying hens, broilers and breeding, and fattening flocks of turkeys). Regulation (EC) No. 2073/2005 also lays down process hygiene criteria and monitoring of compliance with these criteria is the legal task of the individual food business operator in the context of their own HACCP programs.

According to EU Regulation (EC) No. 2160/2003 and its following amendments, MS have to set up Salmonella National Control Programs (NCP) aimed at reducing the prevalence of Salmonella serovars, which are considered relevant for public health, in certain animal populations. Currently, prevalence targets have been defined for breeding flocks of *G. gallus*, laying hens, broilers and breeding, and fattening turkeys and correspond to the maximum annual percentage of flocks remaining positive for relevant serovars. In particular, the prevalence target is equal to 1% or less for breeding flocks of *G. gallus*, broilers and breeding, and fattening turkeys and to 2% or less for laying hens.

Since the beginning of 2008, commercial flocks of laying hens (*G. gallus*) have been subject to a statutory Salmonella testing program in order to fulfill the requirements of EU legislation. Commission Regulation (EC) No. 1168/2006 as amended by Regulation (EC) No. 517/2011, set out the operator and official sampling requirements. Once birds are in lay, the national control program requires samples to be collected at least every 15 weeks, beginning between 22 and 26 weeks in terms of the age of the flock since hatch. These take the form of boot swabs or feces samples depending on the housing system the birds are kept in.

3. SALMONELLOSIS INCREASES IN HUMANS

Despite the application of EU regulation to keep Salmonella levels under control in both animals and humans, the number of human salmonellosis within the European Union reported by 28 MS tended to increase since 2013 after a decrease from 2011 to 2013. In 2016, a total of 94,530 confirmed salmonellosis cases were reported, resulting in an EU notification rate of 20.4 cases per 100,000 population (Table 1). This was at the same level as in 2015. In 2015, a total of 94,597 confirmed salmonellosis cases were reported, resulting in EU notification rate of 20.9 cases per 100,000 population. This represented a 2.8% increase in the EU notification rate compared with 2014, when 92,012 confirmed salmonellosis cases were reported, resulting in an EU notification rate of 20.7 cases per 100,000 population. This represented a 4.85% increase in the EU notification rate compared with 2013, when a total of 87,753 confirmed salmonellosis cases were reported resulting in an EU notification rate of 20.3 cases per 100,000

Table 1 Reported Confirmed Human Cases of Salmonellosis and Notification Rates Per 100,000 Population in the European Union, 2011–16

Year	Number of Confirmed Human Cases	Rate
2011	96,685	22.7
2012	94,278	21.9
2013	87,753	20.3
2014	92,012	20.7
2015	94,597	20.9
2016	94,530	20.4

Source: ECDC.

Table 2 Reported Salmonellosis Notification Rates Per 100,000 Population in the United States and European Union, 2011–15

Year	US Rate	EU Rate
2011	16.45	22.7
2012	16.37	21.9
2013	15.15	20.3
2014	15.29	20.7
2015	15.74	20.9

Source: CDC and EFSA-ECDC.

population. This represented a 7.34% decrease in the EU notification rate compared with 2012, when 94,278 confirmed salmonellosis cases were reported, resulting in an EU notification rate of 21.9 cases per 100,000 population. This represented a 3.97% decrease in the EU notification rate compared with 2011, when 96,685 confirmed salmonellosis cases were reported, corresponding to a EU notification rate of 22.7 for 100,000 population (Table 1).

The salmonellosis notification rates in the United States ranged between a minimum value of 15.15 for 100,000 population in 2013 to a maximum value of 16.45 for 100,000 population in 2011, whereas in the EU it ranged between a maximum of 22.7 for 100,000 population in 2011 to a minimum of 20.3 in 2013 (Table 2). It is interesting to note that overall, between 2011 and 2015, the salmonellosis notification rates in the EU and United States showed the same trends (Fig. 1).

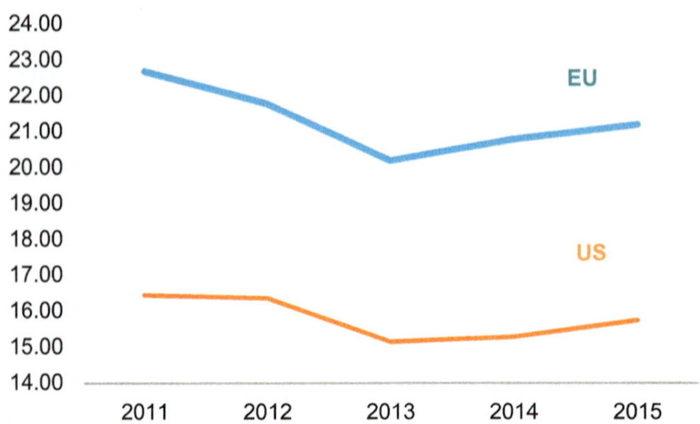

Fig. 1 Trends of EU and US salmonellosis notification rates per 100,000 population between 2011 and 2015. *Source: CDC and EFSA-ECDC.*

4. SALMONELLA CONTAMINATED FOODSTUFFS IN THE EUROPEAN UNION

The total number of food-borne salmonellosis outbreaks was higher in 2016 compared with 2015 in both Europe and United States (Table 3). However, there are no major changes as regard to Salmonella-contaminated foodstuffs year by year. In Europe, the highest levels of noncompliance with Salmonella criteria generally occur in foods of meat origin, which are intended to be cooked before consumption (Table 4). In 2016, the matrices with the high frequencies of noncompliant samples were minced meat and meat preparations from poultry to be eaten cooked representing a potential risk for consumer infection linked to crosscontamination or improper preparation of contaminated meat. By contrast, the percentage of noncompliant samples among fresh poultry meat, for which the food safety criterion considers exclusively S. Enteritidis and S. Typhimurium, was negligible. Some noncompliant samples were also reported for ready-to-eat (RTE) products (minced meat and meat preparations, meat products, and RTE products containing raw eggs), whereas the great majority of MS provided validated data on Salmonella on pig carcasses for compliance with the process hygiene criterion according to Commission Regulation (EU) No. 218/2014. The overall proportions of Salmonella-positive units reported by food business operators in the context of self-checks and those obtained by control authorities were 1.9% and 2.5%, respectively. In all cases where data were provided both by food business operators and control authorities, the proportion of Salmonella-positive units reported by control authorities was higher than the one reported by the food business operators (EFSA-ECDC, 2017).

Table 3 Total Number of Food-Borne Outbreaks (Including Waterborne Outbreaks) Due to Salmonella in the EU and United States, 2012–16

Year	European Union (Source: EFSA)	United States (Source: CDC)
2012	1067	832
2013	953	921
2014	1049	872
2015	1168	826
2016	1533	933

Table 4 Salmonella Occurrence in Foods in Europe, 2016

Food Category	Salmonella Detection in 2016
Broiler meat and its product	Salmonella was detected in 6.39% of the 25,276 units tested. This result is comparable with results in 2015. Salmonella was found in 0.27% of the 1093 units of RTE broiler meat products tested at retail or at processing and including in the large majority of cases cooked and RTE broiler products
Turkey meat and its products	Salmonella was detected in 7.74% of 4250 units of fresh turkey meat. This was higher than in 2015 Salmonella was found in 1 out of 462 (0.22%) RTE turkey meat products. The overall results for 2016 are comparable with 2014 and 2015
Pig meat and its products	Salmonella was detected in 2.38% of 25,049 units of fresh pig meat and this was comparable with 2015 In 2016, 1.93% of the 8641 tested samples of RTE minced meat, meat preparations, and meat products from pig meat were Salmonella positive
Bovine meat and its products	Salmonella was detected in 0.21% of 23,708 samples of fresh bovine meat tested. Only 0.16% of the 1244 units of RTE minced meat, meat preparations, and meat products from bovine meat tested were Salmonella positive
Eggs and egg products	Salmonella was detected in 0.29% of 5782 tested table egg units. These data are similar with what was observed in 2015
Dried seeds	Salmonella was detected in 8.0% of the 525 samples of dried seeds tested in 201. Out of the 675 tested units of sprouted seeds, one sample at processing plant was reported Salmonella positive
Fruit and vegetables	Salmonella was detected in 0.21% of 2429 units of vegetables tested. Most units were tested at retail (81%). Among fruits, of the 1200 tested units, none was positive for Salmonella, and the same was true for the 680 samples reported as "Fruit and vegetables"
Spices and herbs	Salmonella was detected in 1.51% of 1390 units of spices and herbs examined
Live bivalve molluscs and live echinoderms, tunicates, and gastropods	Salmonella was detected in 2% of 199 single samples but none of the sampled batches of live bivalve molluscs and live echinoderms, tunicates, and gastropods

Table 4 Salmonella Occurrence in Foods in Europe, 2016—cont'd

Food Category	**Salmonella Detection in 2016**
Dried infant formulas and dried dietary foods for medical purposes; Milk and whey powder; Unpasteurized fruit and vegetable juices (RTE)	All compliant
Feeding stuffs	Salmonella was detected in 3.9% out of 4750 units of animal- and vegetable-derived feed supplies. In compound feeding stuffs (the finished feed for animals), the prevalence of Salmonella-positive units was 1.2% of 2473 tested samples for poultry, 1.0% of 971 tested samples for cattle, and 0.5% of 1106 tested samples for pigs

In 2016, Salmonella was rarely found in table eggs, in products of vegetable origin and in sprouted seeds (Table 4). Salmonella was, however, found in 1.2% of feed samples for poultry. This makes feed an important source of infection for poultry species and subsequently for the consumer, although the dominant Salmonella serovars found in human cases are rarely identified in animal feed, especially compound feed.

Sprouted seeds as other low moisture foods and ingredients represent a food category of particular concern for *Salmonella* contamination because most low moisture food products require no further cooking and have a long shelf life (Garces-Vega, Jeong, Dolan, & Marks, 2016). Hence, the presence of Salmonella in low-moisture foods can cause extended outbreaks, which affect large numbers of people (Jeong, Marks, & Orta-Ramirez, 2009). Unfortunately, even rigorous hygiene and sanitation practices are insufficient to ensure product safety; therefore, processing interventions are an emerging imperative to reduce the risk of Salmonella in low-moisture products. The dynamics of moisture exchange between the product and the process environment can significantly affect Salmonella thermal resistance (Jeong et al., 2009).

Low-moisture foods are those with water activity (aw) levels lower than 0.70 (Blessington, Mitcham, & Harris, 2012). Such foods include products, which have undergone a lethality step, those that are not subjected to an inactivation step, and those in which ingredients are added after an inactivation step (Farakos et al., 2017). From 2007 to 2012, 22 reported

Salmonella outbreaks caused by low-moisture foods occurred globally, resulting in 2293 cases of infection and 9 deaths (CDC, 2012; EFSA, 2009, 2010; Rodríguez-Urrego et al., 2010; SFI, 2012). From 2010 to January 2015, there have been four outbreaks linked to Salmonella in tree nuts in the United States, one in 2014 involving S. Braenderup in almond butter, two in 2013 linked to S. Stanley in raw cashew cheese and S. Senftenberg in roasted pistachios, and one in 2011 involving S. Enteritidis in pine nuts (Harris, Palumbo, Beuchat, & Danyluk, 2015). The consumption of only one Salmonella cell in a food product may be sufficient to cause illness (D'Aoust & Maurer, 2007).

Salmonella is not a natural inhabitant of the aquatic environment but, several Salmonella serovars are widely distributed in water (sea, estuarine, and river) and in a variety of seafood, with the highest prevalence in molluscs, shrimp, clams, and various fish species (Novoslavskij et al., 2016). The presence of Salmonella in aquaculture environments and products can be explained mainly by hygiene failures during production (Budiati et al., 2013). The reason for high prevalence of Salmonella in filter-feeding organisms is filtration of a large amount of water during their life cycle with accumulation of the pathogen in tissues (Kumar, Surendran, & Thampuran, 2009). Although environmental factors and human activity may influence the prevalence of Salmonella in seafood, contamination of seafood may often occur from contaminated coastal areas and from contaminated surroundings, where seafood is handled (Martinez-Urtaza, Liebana, Garcia-Migura, Perez-Piñeiro, & Saco, 2004). Salmonella also can contaminate water sources because of poor sanitation and incorrect disposal of human and animal waste (Amagliani, Brandi, & Schiavano, 2012).

Concerning table eggs, in 2016, 0.29% of the 5782 tested table egg units were Salmonella positive. These data are similar with what was observed in 2015. However, the most important source of food-borne Salmonella outbreaks is still eggs and egg products. In the last 2 years, different EU MS reported increased target Salmonella serovars flock prevalence in laying hens. In 2015, the odds of flocks being positive for S. Enteritidis increased significantly by around 17% in 2015 vs 2014 and by 57% in 2016 vs 2015 (EFSA-ECDC, 2017).

Despite the increase in the EU flock prevalence of S. Enteritidis in laying hens as well as the documentation of important multistate human outbreaks due to this serovar and related to eggs (ECDC, 2016, 2017a, 2017b, 2017c), the number of Salmonella-positive eggs, as well as the number of isolates serotyped from this source, remain very low, confirming the data reported in the previous years. This finding can be attributed to the fact that Salmonella-positive laying hen flocks produce a small number of contaminated eggs. With a low prevalence of individual egg contamination, large numbers of eggs have to be tested to detect Salmonella and to obtain an accurate measure of the egg contamination rate (Carrique-Mas & Davies, 2008). Although the prevalence of Salmonella in egg and egg products is normally low, the number of human cases associated with these sources can be large, especially because eggs are frequently used to produce pooled dishes that are not properly heat-treated or stored (EFSA, 2014a, 2014b) and because, due to their nutritional and functional properties, eggs are used in different ways to produce and enrich many types of foods.

In table eggs, the low prevalence of Salmonella is coupled with a low contamination level of the pathogen. Frequently the level on the surface of table eggs ranges from 1 to 100 CFU/eggshell rising to 1000 CFU/eggshell only in rare cases (Humphrey, 1994; Humphrey, Whitehead, Gawler, Henley, & Rowe, 1991). In order to detect Salmonella at very low concentration, a sampling plan with high sensitivity needs to be applied. At present no European legislation for official sampling of table eggs exists. There are, however, voluntary sampling plans applied at national level. Pooling is used extensively as a cost-effective sampling strategy to detect positive samples when the prevalence and contamination level of the risk agent are low (Arnold, Carrique-Mas, McLaren, & Davies, 2011; Van Schaik, Stehman, Schukken, Rossiter, & Shin, 2003). In relation to table eggs, sampling plans routinely include pooling of 10 eggs. When polling is made it is assumed that it does not affect the test sensitivity. However, if the group size is large, some positive units may be excessively diluted by negative units and become undetectable in the pool. Pasquali, De Cesare, Valero, Olsen, and Manfreda (2014) assessed the test sensitivity of the reference culture method ISO 6579:2004 and an alternative real-time polymerase chain reaction (PCR) method (Jakočiūnė et al., 2014) applied to eggs and egg products on Salmonella positive pools characterized by different number of eggs and contamination levels. Additionally, they quantified the expected number of sample units to test in order to detect positive Salmonella with 95% of probability, when present, using Monte Carlo simulations.

A total of 270 pools of 15 eggs each were tested. The individual eggshells tested in the pools were spiked with Salmonella ser. Enteritidis at three levels of contamination (1–10 cfu/eggshell = low level; 10–100 cfu/eggshell = medium level; and 100–1000 cfu/eggshell = high level). In 135 pools one inoculated egg was mixed with four uninfected eggshells and in 135 pools one inoculated egg was mixed with nine uninfected eggshells. ISO culture method and real-time PCR detected Salmonella in 122 and 121 samples, respectively, with markedly different sensitivity depending on the level of contamination. ISO 6579 detected Salmonella in 11 (12%), 38 (42%), and 73 (81%) of samples at low, medium, and high contamination level, while real-time PCR tests were positive in 33 (37%), 44 (49%), and 44 (49%) of the same pools. The number of positive samples detected by real-time PCR was significantly higher ($P=0.00014$), with no differences ($P=0.369$) and significantly lower (0.00001) than the number detected by ISO at the lowest, medium, and high levels of contamination, respectively (Table 5). With respect to the different combinations of positive and negative eggs (1/10 to 1/5) and irrespective of the initial inoculum levels, no statistical significant differences were registered between the detection results achieved using ISO method or real-time PCR.

The Monte Carlo simulation estimated 16 pools of 10 eggs each and 8 pools of 9 eggs each as the lowest number of samples to be tested in order to detect Salmonella in positive lots with 95% certainty when ISO 6579 and real-time PCR are used as analytical methods. This underlines the importance of adopt analytical methods with higher sensitivity than ISO method and the need to deeply review the number of eggs to test.

5. SALMONELLA ENTERITIDIS INCREASES IN LAYING HENS

As regard Salmonella in animals, for all poultry categories covered by national control programs, in 2016, as in previous years, overall decreases or at least a stable situation in the prevalence of target Salmonella serovars were documented, with the exception of laying hens (EFSA-ECDC, 2017). The estimated EU target Salmonella serovars flock prevalence in laying hens from 2014 onward, it increased to 0.9% in 2015 and to 1.3% in 2016. The 2016 prevalence was not significantly different compared with the 2015 prevalence ($P=0.111$), but it was higher than 2014 at the limits of significance ($P=0.056$). The estimated odds of laying hen flocks being positive for target serovars decreased significantly by 25%–30% from 2009 to 2012, by 20% in 2013 vs 2012 and by 7% in 2014 vs 2013. Next, the odds of flocks being positive for target serovars increased significantly by 10% in 2015 compared with 2014, and by 40% in 2016 compared with 2015 (EFSA-ECDC, 2017).

The trend for estimated EU S. Enteritidis flock prevalence in laying hens during 2008–16 was similar to the trend described for the target serovars. The prevalence was 3.1% in 2008, which decreased to 0.57% in 2014,

Table 5 Estimation of The Lower Number of Eggs That Need to be Sampled in Order to Detect Salmonella With 95% Certainty on Experimentally Contaminated Table Eggs Tested as Pools Including 5–10 Eggshells by ISO 6579 and Real-Time PCR

Level of Contamination	No. of Eggs Per Pool	Total No. of Tested Eggs	No. of Positive Samples ($N=15$)[a]		No. of Eggs (Pools) to be Sampled	
			ISO 6579	Real-Time PCR	ISO 6579	Real-Time PCR
10^0–10^1 CFU/pool	10	150	6	7	116 (12)	89 (9)
	9	135	2	8	484 (54)	67 (8)
	8	120	2	8	442 (56)	60 (8)
	7	105	0	5	1539–6962[b] (220–995)	109 (16)
	6	90	1	2	748 (125)	333 (56)
	5	75	0	3	1470–4644[b] (294–929)	162 (33)
10^1–10^2 CFU/pool	10	150	5	9	155 (16)	60 (6)
	9	135	7	8	83 (10)	67 (8)
	8	120	7	6	74 (10)	93 (12)
	7	105	5	5	108 (16)	106 (16)
	6	90	7	7	55 (10)	55 (10)
	5	75	7	9	47 (10)	31 (7)
10^2–10^3 CFU/pool	10	150	12	6	35 (4)	117 (12)
	9	135	11	9	38 (5)	56 (7)
	8	120	13	6	23 (3)	93 (12)
	7	105	13	7	20 (3)	65 (10)
	6	90	12	9	21 (4)	37 (7)
	5	75	12	7	18 (4)	46 (10)

[a]The total number of tested pool samples per each pool type was 15.
[b]The results are expressed as a range of eggs to be tested assuming a number of positive samples ranging from 1 (1539; 1470) to 0 (6962; 4644).

and subsequently increased to 0.67% in 2015 and to 1% in 2016. Despite this increase, the prevalence in 2016 was not significantly different compared with 2015 ($P=0.085$), but it was different compared with 2014 ($P=0.0371$). The odds of laying hen flocks in EU being positive for S. Enteritidis decreased significantly by 25%–30% from 2009 to 2012, by 21% in 2013 vs 2012 and by 7% in 2014 vs 2013. In 2015, the odds of flocks being positive for S. Enteritidis increased significantly by around 17% in 2015 vs 2014 and by 57% in 2016 vs 2015 (EFSA-ECDC, 2017).

The trends in monitoring data, especially for S. Enteritidis, raise questions as they indicate a reversal of the declining trend in the EU in humans and poultry. Further cross-sectorial investigations are needed to better understand underlying reasons for the increase. The data suggest that it is pivotal not to underestimate the potential risk posed by S. Enteritidis especially in laying hens, as deteriorating management of the risk could have a direct negative effect on control of Salmonella cases in humans.

Also, some doubts have been raised about the sensitivity of the statutory sampling implemented in commercial laying hen flocks. It has been demonstrated that the sensitivity of the sampling approaches defined as part of the national control programs is influenced by the prevalence of infection within the flocks being sampled and by the type of sampling applied, which depends on the housing system (Arnold, Martelli, McLaren, & Davies, 2014). The improvement of the biosecurity status of farms and better vaccination of flocks, as a direct result of the application of control programs, has probably led to a reduction of the within-flock prevalence, and this could challenge the identification of positive flocks, which is also restrained because of the limits of the laboratory testing methods available (EFSA, 2014a, 2014b). Under detection of positive flocks especially in major exporting European MS, relaxation of effective vaccination programs in some MS once prevalence targets have been achieved, as well as relaxation of farm hygiene controls to reduce costs could have resulted in an increased spread of Salmonella.

The egg laying industry developed laying hen cages in the production housing to make production of eggs commercially more efficient and economical. Consequently, much of the research to generate control measures for Salmonella and improving egg safety were conducted with these types of housing systems. However, in the past couple of decades public animal welfare concerns emerged that initially led to the reduction and/or elimination of conventional caged laying hen housing systems (De Reu et al., 2008; Mench, Sumner, & Rosen-Molina, 2011). This shift and the increased desire from consumers for raw and unprocessed foods, potentially increased the risk of salmonellosis.

It appears that housing type may influence Salmonella infection and subsequent persistence in the house environment but several confounding factors, such as bird stocking density, exposure to varying levels of contaminated feces, dust, and vectors such as rodents, location of eggs (nest box vs outside the nest box), and bird stress level preclude the ability to draw definitive conclusions across independent studies (Gast et al., 2017; Holt et al., 2011; Whiley & Ross, 2015). This leads to a lack of consensus regarding the impact of various housing systems on Salmonella egg contamination (Ricke, 2017). In an European study (De Vylder et al., 2011), S. Enteritidis inoculated seeder hens were introduced to susceptible noninoculated hens housed in either conventional battery cages, furnished cages (contained perches, litter mat, and nest at the back of the cage), aviaries (tilted nest floor, perches at three levels), or floor systems (included nest boxes). The authors noted a trend toward increased transmission among birds occurred for the aviary and floor systems (De Vylder et al., 2011).

Beside S. Enteritidis, other serotypes, like S. Typhimurium and S. Heidelberg have also been considered table egg contaminants and identified in egg-related outbreaks (Foley, Johnson, Ricke, Nayak, & Danzeisen, 2013; Hennessy et al., 2004; Howard, O'Bryan, Crandall, & Ricke, 2012; Martelli & Davies, 2012; Moffatt et al., 2016). However, S. Enteritidis has always been considered the primary infective serotype for its apparent specific capability of transovarian infection and internal egg contamination (Foley et al., 2013; Gantois et al., 2009; Howard et al., 2012). This is true globally, with the exception of Australia, where the most common serovar infecting humans is Typhimurium, with thousands of cases resulting from numerous outbreaks linked to eggs (Moffatt et al., 2017). In Australia most commercially produced eggs are washed to reduce microbial contamination (Gole et al., 2014). Considerable debate exists around egg washing with suggestions it may facilitate shell penetration by S. Typhimurium (Gole et al., 2014), which may offer insight into its capacity for evading postcollection controls and causing outbreaks.

An estimated 67 billion shell eggs are produced each year in the United States and each US citizen consumes around 234 eggs per year (FDA, 2009). Interventions targeting S. Enteritidis in eggs have included elimination of S. Enteritidis from grandparent flocks of egg-layer hens, egg refrigeration requirements, egg trace back programs targeting sources of S. Enteritidis outbreaks, safe handling labels on shell egg products at retail, restrictions on shell egg use in retail establishments and nursing homes, and state-based egg quality assurance programs to reduce S. Enteritidis contamination on egg-laying farms (Wright, Richardson, Mahon, Rothenberg, & Cole, 2016).

On July 9, 2010, FDA implemented the Egg Safety Final Rule (FDA, 2009), requiring producers who maintain more than 50,000 egg-laying hens to routinely test flocks for S. Enteritidis and to take other prevention measures, such as refrigerating eggs on the farm. As these control measures are implemented, more sensitive methods than measuring changes in human S. Enteritidis infection incidence and food-borne disease outbreak rates are needed to assess their impact on food-borne illness; our power to detect changes is significantly reduced as interventions successfully decrease the number of reported outbreaks. Consequently, mathematical models that estimate the proportion of total S. Enteritidis illnesses in the population attributed to specific food sources are needed to explain observed trends and determine changes in sources of illness over time (Wright et al., 2016).

The routes and mechanisms associated with Salmonella infection in laying hens and subsequent contamination of shell eggs is relatively well established and have been extensively described (Finstad, O'Bryan, Marcy, Crandall, & Ricke, 2012; Foley et al., 2013; Gantois et al., 2009). S. Enteritidis is much more resistant then other serotypes to killing by chicken macrophage cells and is much more capable of surviving in egg whites (De Vylder et al., 2013; He, Genovese, Swaggerty, Nisbet, & Kogut, 2012). As WGS progresses and more S. Enteritidis strains have been sequenced, subtle differences in genomic sequences have been linked with distinct phenotypic variability in virulence and survival. These stain differences could make development of control measures more difficult to be universally be applied across all isolates (Ricke, 2017).

As in-depth information on the genome becomes available this will not only aid more precise tracking of the serotype in egg production systems but identify evolutionary relationships and hopefully predictions of functional changes in the genome such as acquisition of antibiotic resistant genes (Ricke, 2017). More detailed genomic information should provide an opportunity to develop a battery of detection targets for distinguishing various isolates. Identification of universal portions of the S. Enteritidis genome also offers potential vaccine genetic targets that would elicit broad spectrum-based protection against all S. Enteritidis strains and depending on the antigen selection non-S. Enteritidis serotypes as well (Ricke, 2017).

6. MICROBIOLOGICAL CRITERIA AND RISK-BASED METRICS: AN INTEGRATED SOLUTION TO KEEP SALMONELLA IN FOODS UNDER CONTROL

In 2002, the Regulation (EC) 178 of the European Parliament and of the Council states that, in order to achieve the general objective of a high level of protection (LOP) of human health and life, food law shall be based on risk analysis. However, the Commission Regulation No. 2073/2005 on microbiological criteria for foodstuffs requires that food business operators ensure that foodstuffs comply with relevant microbiological criteria.

The microbiological criteria define the acceptability of a product, a batch of foodstuffs, or a process, based on the absence, presence, or number of microorganisms, and/or on the quantity of their toxins/metabolites, per unit(s) of mass, volume, area, or batch. In the commission Regulation 2073/2005, the microbiological criteria include the following parameters: (1) food safety criteria, as a mean to define the acceptability of a product or a batch of foodstuff applicable to products placed on the market and (2) process hygiene criteria as a mean indicating the acceptable functioning of the production process.

Salmonella food safety criteria prescribe that Salmonella monitoring results must be compliant with "absence in 25 or 10 g," when products are placed on the market, during their shelf life (Table 6).

The number of units comprising the sample (i.e., *n*) ranges between 5 and 30, for infant formulae, but the number of sample units giving Salmonella presence (i.e., *c*) must be always zero. All food safety criteria refer to Salmonella, except for that for fresh poultry meat targeting S. Enteritidis, S. Typhimurium, and S. Typhimurium monophasic variant strains 1,4,[5],12:i:-. The compliance to all listed food safety criteria must be verified by the ISO reference method 6579 followed by the White–Kaufmann–Le Minor scheme for Salmonella serotyping for fresh poultry meat.

Salmonella process hygiene criteria are regulated for carcasses of pigs, cattle, sheep, goats, horses, broilers, and turkeys (Table 7). The process hygiene criteria are absence in a specific area tested per carcasses of cattle, sheep, goats, horses, and pig; for carcasses of broilers and turkeys, the criterion is Salmonella absence in 25 g of a pooled sample of neck skin. Salmonella isolates collected from broilers and turkeys must be serotyped for identification of S. Enteritidis and Typhimurium. The number of units comprising the sample (i.e., *n*) to verify compliance to the process hygiene criteria is 50, derived in 10 consecutive sampling sessions, whereas the number of sample units that can be positive for Salmonella (i.e., *c*) ranges between 2 for cattle, sheep, goats, and horses and 5 for boilers and turkeys. The analytical method to check compliance to the process hygiene criteria is the ISO reference method 6579 for carcasses after dressing but before chilling for cattle, sheep, goats, horses, and pigs and for carcasses after chilling for broilers and turkeys. When the process hygiene criterion is not achieved, improvements in

Table 6 Salmonella Food Safety Criteria Listed in the Commission Regulation (EC) 2073/2005 on Microbiological Criteria for Foodstuffs

	Sampling Plan		Limits
Food Category	*n*	*c*	*m*
Minced meat and meat preparations intended to be eaten raw	5	0	Absence in 25 g
Minced meat and meat preparations made from poultry meat intended to be eaten cooked	5	0	Absence in 25 g
Minced meat and meat preparations made from other species than poultry meat intended to be eaten cooked	5	0	Absence in 10 g
Mechanically separated meat	5	0	Absence in 10 g
Meat products intended to be eaten raw, excluding products where the manufacturing process or the composition of the product will eliminate the risk	5	0	Absence in 25 g
Meat products made from poultry meat intended to be eaten cooked	5	0	Absence in 25 g
Gelatine and collagen	5	0	Absence in 25 g
Cheese, butter, and cream made from raw milk or milk that undergone a lower heat treatment than pasteurization excluding products when the manufacturer can demonstrate that due to the ripening time and aw of the product there is no Salmonella risk	5	0	Absence in 25 g
Milk powder and whey powder	5	0	Absence in 25 g
Ice cream containing milk ingredients, excluding products where the manufacturing process or the composition of the product will eliminate the Salmonella risk	5	0	Absence in 25 g
Eggs products, excluding products where the manufacturing process or the composition of the product will eliminate the Salmonella risk	5	0	Absence in 25 g
Ready to eat foods containing raw eggs, excluding products where the manufacturing process or the composition of the product will eliminate the Salmonella risk	5	0	Absence in 25 g
Cooked crustaceans and molluscan shellfish	5	0	Absence in 25 g

Table 6 Salmonella Food Safety Criteria Listed in the Commission Regulation (EC) 2073/2005 on Microbiological Criteria for Foodstuffs—cont'd

	Sampling Plan		Limits
Food Category	*n*	*c*	*m*
Live bivalve molluscs and live echinoderms, tunicates, and gastropods	5	0	Absence in 25 g
Sprouted seeds and vegetables ready to eat, excluding sprouts that have received a treatment effective to eliminate Salmonella	5	0	Absence in 25 g
Precut fruit and vegetables (ready to eat)	5	0	Absence in 25 g
Unpasteurized fruit and vegetable juices (ready to eat)	5	0	Absence in 25 g
Dried infant formulae and dried dietary foods for special medical purposes intended for infants below 6 month of age	30	0	Absence in 25 g
Dried follow-on formulae	30	0	Absence in 25 g
Fresh poultry meat from breeding flocks of *Gallus gallus*, laying hens, broilers and breeding, and fattening flocks of turkeys	5	0	Absence in 25 g

Table 7 Salmonella Process Hygiene Criteria in the Commission Regulation (EC) 2073/2005 on Microbiological Criteria for Foodstuffs

	Sampling Plan		Limits		
Food Category	*n*	*c*	*m*	*M*	**Stage where criterion applies**
Carcasses of cattle, sheep, goats, and horses	50	2	Absence in the area tested per carcass		Carcasses after dressing but before chilling
Carcasses of pigs	50	3	Absence in the area tested per carcass		Carcasses after dressing but before chilling
Poultry carcasses of broilers and turkeys	50	5	Absence in 25 g of a pooled sample of neck skin		Carcasses after chilling

slaughter hygiene and review of process controls, origins of animals and of the biosecurity measures in the farms of origin are requested.

Both food safety criteria and process hygiene criteria are not based on risk analysis. However, in 2004 through the activities of Codex Alimentarius Commission and ad hoc expert consultations, FAO and WHO have developed a series of guidelines and report that detail out the various steps in risk analysis, namely risk management, risk assessment, and risk communication. Within this framework risk-based metrics have been defined.

With respect to food-borne pathogens possibly associated to particular foods, risk analysis is a accepted by governments as the framework to (1) estimate the impact of a particular hazard on public health, (2) define an appropriate level of public health protection against that hazard, and (3) establish guidelines to ensure the supply of safe foods (Gorris, 2005). In the framework of risk analysis, the risk estimate, whether an absolute or relative expression, can be used by risk managers, i.e., the competent authorities, to decide on an appropriate course of action. In some cases, the risk to the population does not necessitate action, in others specific measures are needed to reduce the burden of disease. In the latter case, risk managers may choose to set health protection goals and use these to formulate targets to be met by all the relevant supply chains. In the risk analysis framework, the current health status of a population is evaluated conducting a quantitative microbiological risk assessment (QMRA) for a product or a group of products to which a pathogen is associated (Buchanan, Smith, & Long, 2000; Lammerding & Fazil, 2000). A QMRA can give an absolute or a relative indication of the health status, i.e., provide an absolute numerical expression of the risk at population level or a relative or benchmarked expression (e.g., a ranking), respectively.

QMRA studies can be developed on many levels of detail, depending among many others factors on the complexity of the issue, the urgency for obtaining the risk estimate, and the data available (Van Gerwen & Gorris, 2004). What all MRA studies should have in common is that they involve all relevant food products in a country or imported into a country. They should follow the important basic principles of being structured, systematic, transparent, and open studies. They also should provide detailed information that is important to understand the process by which the risk estimate has been assessed as well as the content of the study. Variability and uncertainty should be assessed for each risk estimate. Variability corresponds to the variable nature of a parameter changing over time, over space, or among samples, or to variation among data (e.g., concentration estimates over time). Uncertainty represents an imperfect state of knowledge about a parameter or a model (e.g., whether a concentration estimate is accurate or whether the model for temporal concentration variability correctly represents reality) (Schmidt & Emelko, 2011).

The risk-based metrics formulated by the Codex Alimentarius Commission in 2004 are appropriate level of (human) protection (ALOP), food safety objective (FSO), and performance objective (PO). ALOP is a governmental expression of its national public health goal for food-borne risks, presenting a level above which the risk is unacceptable (Todd, 2004). ALOPs can be expressed as a public health goal in terms of numbers of cases per given number of population over a specific time, for example, 1 in 100,000 per annum, or as risk per serving. Even though the ALOP has originally been introduced as a means of solving trade disputes by comparing the level of risk that is accepted by different countries for the same type of product (WTO, 1995), the feasibility of international comparisons of ALOPs for pathogens between countries has not yet been investigated although it would be of considerable interest (Stringer, 2005).

A FSO has been defined by the CAC (2005) as the level of a hazard (in terms of concentration and/or frequency) that can be tolerated in the final product when it is consumed. Setting an FSO at the moment of consumption is supported by the International Commission on Microbiological Specifications for Foods (ICMSF) as that is the moment when no change in the hazard level can occur anymore and essentially the consumption event is required to have a possible impact on public health (ICMSF, 2002). FSO is proposed to be a metric that gives guidance to food production and preparation of professionals concerning the expected compliance of foods to consumer protection policy regarding a possibly associated hazard (De Swarte & Donker, 2005). By formulation of a FSO, governments communicate to interested private and public parties a more practical form of food safety guidance than the rather abstract ALOP. Guidance is given to food industry (e.g., primary producers, food processors, catering, distribution, and retailers) involved in the production of the food as to the required level of control over the hazard in the food such that the consumers are duly protected. FSOs can then be translated into a set of quantitatively stated requirements that enable appropriate design of product, process, and control measures (Jouve, 1999). In this context, the agro-food industry would use FSOs as means to coordinate risk management in the production process throughout the farm to fork production chain.

Gkogka, Reij, Gorris, and Zwietering (2013) derived ALOP and FSO for Salmonella in raw chicken meat in the Netherlands using publicly available data. Two different risk assessment strategies were followed to this end: an epidemiological approach (i.e., top-down approach) having the current level of risk (current LOP) of the disease salmonellosis at country level as the starting point and a supply chain approach (i.e., bottom-up approach) starting from data on the presence of the hazard (Salmonella) in the food product (Zwietering & Van Gerwen, 2000). The mean estimated LOP for salmonellosis due to chicken meat in the Netherlands was found to be 71 cases per 100,000 people per year (95% CI: 9.9–155, SD 38) deploying the top-down approach model and 87 cases per 100,000 people per year (95% CI: 0.03–904, SD 412) with the bottom-up approach model (Fig. 2).

Since an ALOP expresses the maximum level of illness that is tolerated within a population (Havelaar, Nauta, & Jansen, 2004), it requires the governmental risk manager to judge the degree of confidence in a risk estimate derived either via a risk assessment of food supply chain data or on the basis of epidemiological data. This confidence will affect the ability to set a new ALOP, such that this level is not surpassed (FAO/WHO, 2002). An important decision to be made by risk managers is which upper percentile of the stochastic estimates will be used to set the ALOP. The 95th percentile is

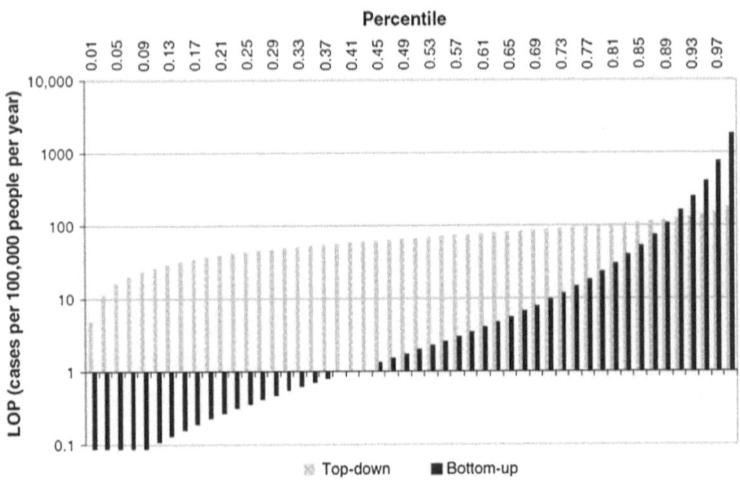

Fig. 2 Detailed characteristics of the level of protection output distributions for chicken mean as obtained with the top-down (*gray bards*) and the bottom-up (*black bars*). *Numbers* on the *y*-axis are presented on a logarithmic scale to facilitate comparisons. *Source: Gkogka, E., Reij, M. W., Gorris, L. G. M., & Zwietering, M. H. (2013). Risk assessment strategies as a tool in the application of the appropriate level of protection (ALOP) and food safety objective (FSO) by risk managers.* International Journal of Food Microbiology, *167(1), 8–28.*

often suggested for such purposes (FAO/WHO, 2002), but other upper percentiles such as the 90th or the 99th may also be likely. A possible option for setting the ALOP could be the 90th percentile, around which the ALOP estimates of the two models in the study by Gkogka et al. (2013) coincide, corresponding to approximately 119 cases per 100,000 people per year.

The percentiles at which the values of the two distributions will coincide will vary depending on the risk unit used to derive the population risk. Using the central limit theorem to estimate the population risk as a normal distribution using the risk per serving simulation data, the top-down ALOP would have been 96 cases per 100,000 people (95% CI: 15–185, SD 44) based on the risk per person and 93 cases per 100,000 people (95% CI: 92.8–93.0, SD 0.047) based on 100,000 people. The estimated arithmetic mean value for the FSO for chicken meat derived by the top-down approach and the bottom-up approach was found to be −4.6 log CFU/g (95% CI: −5.4 to −4.1, SD 0.32) and −6.0 log CFU/g (95% CI: −8.1 to −2.9, SD 1.3), respectively. This FSO can be the pooled concentration of Salmonella from several different types of cross-contaminated or undercooked servings at the time of consumption. The two approaches resulted in very different FSO estimates, both in terms of the mean estimate and the confidence interval, reflecting major differences in the way the FSO was derived. The two distributions coincided around the 90th percentile at −4.3 log CFU/g. If the 90th percentile is chosen, this would mean that for contaminated servings of meat or salad with Salmonella at the time of consumption their pooled concentration can only 10% of the time exceed −4.3 log CFU/g so that the overall health burden does not exceed 119 cases per 100,000 people. Because, conceptually, an FSO should be derived from the ALOP, there is a need for additional milestones that ensure the appropriate frequency and/or concentration of a hazard at specific steps along the food chain. This need has been addressed with the POs that should be based on the FSO. The Codex Alimentarius Commission defines a PO as "the maximum frequency and/or concentration of a hazard in a food at a specified step in the food chain before consumption that provides or contributes to an FSO or ALOP, as applicable."

A PO may be the same as the FSO if the frequency/concentration of the hazard stays at the same level between the point of the PO and FSO. Otherwise, Codex guides the PO to be more or less stringent than the FSO according to the likeliness of the hazard to increase or decrease between the PO and FSO (CAC, 2005). In contrast to the ALOP and FSO, a PO may be established not only by the government but also by the individual food businesses. Thus, insight into the occurrence and behavior of the specific hazard throughout the chain is needed to derive POs at various points along the food chain to obtain the intended FSO (Van der Fels-Klerx, Tromp, Rijgersberg, & Van Asselt, 2008). Moreover, it needs quantification of the relationships between the occurrences at specific steps during production and laying down these relations into a quantitative food chain model. Van der Fels-Klerx et al. (2008) demonstrated how POs for Salmonella at various points in the broiler supply chain can be estimated, starting from preset level of the PO in finished products. The estimations were performed using an analytical transmission model, based on prevalence data collected throughout the food chain in the Netherlands. The end PO was set at 2.5% of the finished products (at the end of processing) being contaminated with Salmonella. The behavior of the pathogen in between critical points of the chain is modeled using a QMRA approach. The QMRA is very resource demanding and it is usually difficult to underpin outcomes of the model estimations with data from the industry. Tuominen, Ranta, and Maijala (2007) developed a QMRA model using the Bayesian probabilistic method for the beef chain to evaluate the capability of different POs to contribute to the ALOP, defined in Finland for beef, beef preparations, and beef products as 10 human Salmonella cases/100,000 population. The model shows that if the *Salmonella* prevalence at the slaughter, domestic cut beef, and retail levels would increase to the level of PO set (i.e., maximum 1%) the ALOP de facto would be exceeded by a factor of roughly two. On the other hand, the zero tolerance applied to microbiological criteria would keep the true Salmonella prevalence at production steps with PO clearly below 1%, and the ALOP would then be achievable. This study demonstrates that POs and microbiological criteria should be estimated as true prevalence and incidences with quantified uncertainties to achieve a sound, transparent scientific based understanding of the risk. This study shows also the POs as tools to keep Salmonella under control and states that POs that are not based on scientific research are not likely to reach the goal (i.e., FSO and/or ALOP) or may be unnecessary stringent (Anthony Tony Cox, 2007).

A clear picture of the approach to follow to define meaningful PO for Salmonella in fresh pork meat intended to be eaten cooked and effective sampling plans to verify the PO achievement is presented (Manfreda et al., 2014). Ten different samplings were conducted along a one-year period at the same pork processing facility. During each sampling the loin chops tested belonged to the same lot, meaning from animals reared in the same house and slaughtered at the same age. For each lot, prevalence of Salmonella in loin chops was evaluated under four different scenarios, throughout the product shelf life (fixed at seventh day): within 2 h from packaging (S1); after delivery at a retailer site shop and storage within a display cabinet set at 4°C up to the fourth or fifth day of the product shelf life (S2); after delivery and storage at retail (i.e., S2) and then transport at car temperature for 45 ± 10 min and storage at 6 ± 1°C, up to the end of the product shelf life (S3); and after delivery and storage at retail (i.e., S2) and then transport at car temperature for 45 ± 10 min and storage at 14 ± 1°C, up to the end of the product shelf life (S4). POs were considered as different target values from Salmonella prevalence. The median of the distribution (50th percentile) was chosen to subsequently derive POs referred to two-class attributes sampling plans ($c = 0$). FSOs allowed the estimation of the maximum percentage of lot units accepted with a 95% probability. Risk management strategies basing on the effect of setting various target levels from prevalence distributions and their effect on POs and FSOs were also assessed. Uncertainty in prevalence was modeled using a Beta distribution. Cumulative distributions are represented in Fig. 3.

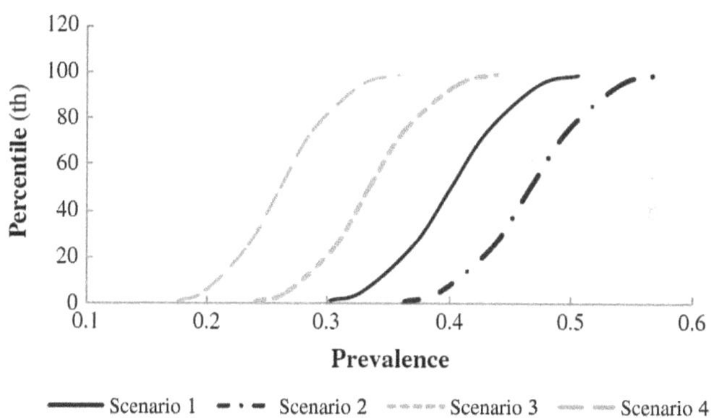

Fig. 3 Cumulative distributions for Salmonella prevalence at packaging (Scenario 1); after delivery at a retailer site shop and storage within a display cabinet set at 4°C up to the fourth or fifth day of the product shelf life (Scenario 2); after delivery and storage at retail and then transport at car temperature for 45 ± 10 min and storage at 6 ± 1°C, up to the end of the product shelf life (Scenario 3); and after delivery and storage at retail and then transport at car temperature for 45 ± 10 min and storage at 14 ± 1°C, up to the end of the product shelf life (Scenario 4). *Source: Manfreda, G., Valero, A., Rodríguez-Lázaro, D., Hernández, M., Pasquali, F., & De Cesare, A. (2014). Performance objectives for Salmonella in fresh pork meat intended to be eaten cooked: How to derive them and verify their achievement.* International Journal of Food Microbiology, 184, *55–59.*

The 50th percentile of each distribution was taken as possible PO. The POs calculated under different scenarios increased between a minimum of 26.10% after final storage at 14°C (Scenario 4) to a maximum of 46.70% of positive samples detected storage at a retailer site at 4°C up to the fourth–fifth day of shelf life (Scenario 2). The number of samples to test in order to verify the compliance to the estimated POs ranged between 5 for samples after storage at retail (Scenario 2) and 10 for samples stored at 14°C before the expiration date (Scenario 4) (Table 8).

Manfreda et al. (2014) showed that the choice of more stringent proportion of contaminated units tolerated (POs) led to an increase in the number of samples needed to accept the lot at 95% CL, that is the established FSO ($c=0$). The reason why different scenarios were considered to derive POs for *Salmonella* in loin chop is the high variability in naturally contaminated lots. In fact, single-point estimations do not reflect the potential growth, which may occur during or at the end of the shelf life of a given product. Instead of using single-point estimates of these variables, distributions characterizing the full range of potential values and their likelihood of occurrence were used as model inputs (Pouillot & Delignette-Muller, 2010). Since the POs are elucidated at a specified point in the food chain before the time of consumption, the PO values calculated in this research after transport and storage at retail as well as at the end of shelf life might be translated into FSOs. However, the assessment of FSOs should be linked to the ALOP for Salmonella in fresh meat intended to be eaten cooked through risk assessment models.

Table 8 Sampling Plans Derived for Salmonella in loin Chops Intended to Comply With the Different POs

Scenario	PO[a] (%)	n[b] ($c=0$)	FSO[c] (%)
1	40.10	6	0.85
2	46.70	5	1.02
3	33.52	8	0.64
4	26.10	10	0.51

[a]PO is assumed to be the maximum allowable proportion of contaminated units in the food lot for each scenario evaluated.
[b]Number of samples needed to accept the PO at 95% CL.
[c]FSO is assumed to be the proportion of contaminated units tolerated by taking n samples from the lot (95% CL).
Source: Manfreda, G., Valero, A., Rodríguez-Lázaro, D., Hernández, M., Pasquali, F., & De Cesare, A. (2014). Performance objectives for Salmonella in fresh pork meat intended to be eaten cooked: How to derive them and verify their achievement. *International Journal of Food Microbiology, 184*, 55–59.

In this study, the PO has been calculated for meat products intended to be eaten cooked. Even if cooking procedures normally destroy Salmonella cells, there is a substantial proportion of food-borne diseases attributed to the food preparation practices used in the domestic environment. The main risk factors include cross-contamination from raw to cooked foods via refrigerators; contaminated hands, cutting boards, and kitchen towels; inadequate refrigeration; improper cooking; inadequate postcooking handling including slow cooling and/or recontamination. Therefore, checking of food-borne pathogens in meat products at the end of the production chain is crucial.

The literature available on FSO and PO definition for Salmonella in specific food matrices might support the in-field implementation of these parameters. In fact, some of the reasons why these risk-based metrics are not being used could be the little guidance on how to establish them (Havelaar et al., 2004) and/or how to implement them in practice linked to each other (Rieu, Duhem, Vindel, & Sanaa, 2007; Stringer, 2005). In the framework of FSO and PO definitions, the BASELINE project (www.baselineeurope.eu) funded by the EC under FP7 suggested a scientific and statistically based approach to derive POs for different food/biological hazard combinations. Such approach has been implemented in a software tool available in the project website (www.baselineeurope.eu). The software shows also how to establish microbiological criteria basing on risk-based metrics and predictive models.

7. MAIN SALMONELLA SEROVARS CIRCULATING IN HUMANS, ANIMALS, AND FOODS

S. Enteritidis dominated among human salmonellosis cases acquired in the EU in 2016. More than half of human reported cases were infected by this serovar. The five most reported serovars in Europe in 2016 have been S. Enteritidis, S. Typhimurium, monophasic S. Typhimurium, S. Infantis and S. Derby (Table 9). Other serovars combined represented 19.6% of the cases. The proportion of S. Enteritidis in humans continued to increase in 2016 compared with 2014 and 2015, the proportion of S. Typhimurium decreased significantly, while its monophasic variant strains 1,4,[5],12:i:- and S. Infantis remained at the same level as in 2015 and 2014 (EFSA-ECDC, 2017). The number of cases acquired in the EU of S. Derby also remained stable during the last 3 years (Table 9). For food and animals, all serotyping data reported by MS in 2016 were collected into the following eight matrices: broilers (5938 isolates, 49.6%), turkeys (1524 isolates, 12.7%), cattle (1482 isolates, 12.4%), broiler meat (1464 isolates, 12.2%), pig meat (814 isolates, 6.8%), pigs (528 isolates, 4.4%), turkey meat (162 isolates, 1.4%), and bovine meat (64 isolates, 0.5%). The most commonly reported serovars in the listed foods were S. Infantis, followed by S. Typhimurium, S. Enteritidis, S. Dublin, and monophasic variants of S. Typhimurium (Table 10). All these serovars, except S. Dublin, were reported among the most frequent from human cases. S. Derby, which was ranked as the fifth most common serovar isolated from humans (acquired in EU), was seventh in the ranking of veterinary isolates (390 isolates; 3.3%) after S. Mbandaka (416 isolates; 3.5%) (EFSA-ECDC, 2017).

Table 9 Top Five Serovars Associated to Reported Cases of Human Salmonellosis Acquired in the EU, 2014–16

	2016		2015		2014	
Serovar	**Cases**	**%**	**Cases**	**%**	**Cases**	**%**
Enteritidis	26,240	59.0	25,258	56.7	25,474	54.6
Typhimurium	6049	13.6	7228	16.1	8625	18.5
Monophasic Typhimurium 1,4,[5],12:i:-	2088	4.7	2303	5.1	1775	3.8
Infantis	1030	2.3	1094	2.4	1163	2.5
Derby	325	19.6	300	0.7	447	1.0

Source: EFSA.

Table 10 Top Five Serovars Associated to Broilers, Broiler Meat, Turkeys, Turkey Meat, Pigs, Pig Meat, Cattle, and Bovine Meat in the EU, 2014–16

	2016		2015		2014	
Serovar	**Isolates**	**%**	**Isolates**	**%**	**Isolates**	**%**
Infantis	4344	36.3	3397	23.3	2834	21
Typhimurium	1551	13.0	3409	23.4	3010	22.3
Enteritidis	807	6.7	1136	7.8	1397	10.4
Dublin	600	5.0	858	5.9	1021	4.5
Monophasic Typhimurium 1,4,[5],12:i:-	589	4.9	na	—	na	—

na: not available.
Source: EFSA.

For S. Enteritidis, which was first-ranked serovar reported from human cases in the EU, the number of isolates serotyped and reported in the context of the national control programs in 2016 was comparable with the number of isolated reported in previous years, thus not showing a decrease. S. Enteritidis was by far the most prominent serovar reported among the Salmonella isolates from laying hen flocks, accounting for more than 40% of the isolates from this source. The importance of laying hens as a major source of S. Enteritidis is confirmed by the recent multistate outbreaks due to this serovar and related to the egg production chain (Dallman et al., 2016; ECDC, 2016, 2017a, 2017b, 2017c; Inns et al., 2017). S. Enteritidis was also reported to a certain extent from broiler flocks and broiler meat.

The second most reported serovar in human cases was S. Typhimurium. S. Typhimurium was the second most reported serovar from pig herds and the first most common serovar from pig meat. Lastly, it was also the most reported serovar from cattle herds and the second most common serovar from bovine meat. Considering the pig chain, the data showed S. Typhimurium to be widely prevalent along the entire pig chain. It was reported a lesser extent from poultry and their meat. The pig chain was also the principal source for monophasic variants of S. Typhimurium, which was the most common serovar reported in pig herds and the second-ranked serovar from pig meat. This observation may be explained by the fact that this serovar has developed some adaptive mechanisms, such as resistance to heavy metals, which allow it to grow and proliferate in pig herds even when some other Salmonella serovars do not normally persist (Petrovska et al., 2016). The persistence of this serovar, as well as of S. Typhimurium is favored by the immune deficiency of weaned pigs and the continuous contamination of pig holdings.

S. Infantis has emerged as the fourth most common serovar causing human salmonellosis in Europe in 2016 (EFSA-ECDC, 2017). In the European Union, for broiler and turkey flocks a significant increase in the number of isolates of S. Infantis was reported in 2016 compared with 2015 (EFSA-ECDC, 2017). This serovar has been able to massively spread along the entire broiler production chain and is remarkably persistent on farms once it has become established. Depopulation is the measure prescribed for breeding flocks positive for this serovar but some MS do not this control measure (EFSA-ECDC, 2017). S. Infantis is an important public health concern not only for its frequent isolation from humans but also because of its high levels of multidrug resistance (Hindermann et al., 2017), the successful spread of certain clones of the serovar, and finally, its extensive isolation from different poultry sources (EFSA-ECDC, 2017).

Finally, S. Derby has been recognized as the fifth most common serovar reported from human cases of salmonellosis acquired in the EU. On the food-animal end, S. Derby was most commonly reported from pigs and pig meat and to a lesser extent from poultry and cattle. However, for poultry samples, in the last 2 years (i.e., 2015 and 2016), the number of samples and notifications of S. Derby have doubled compared with those reported in 2010, when the control programs had just started. However, overall, a significant decrease of S. Derby isolates was recorded in 2016.

EFSA constructed a "pyramid plot" for each serovar of interest to show for each source the frequency of reporting between animal and food (meat) sources. S. Enteritidis accounted for less than 10% of all Salmonella isolates reported from broiler flocks (considering data from the poultry national control programs and all data from other matrices) but more than 20% of all isolates from broiler meat. Similarly, for turkeys, pigs, and cattle, the specific proportion of reported S. Enteritidis among the isolates was less than 5%, whereas for bovine meat and turkey meat that specific proportion was higher than 10%. For bovine meat and turkey meat reporting of distinct serovars serotyped is not a legal mandatory reporting requirement, hampering any drawing of conclusions from these data. The "pyramid plot" showed that about 25%–30% of all isolates notified from pigs and pig meat during 2016 were monophasic variants of S. Typhimurium. As already described for S. Typhimurium, these data confirmed that monophasic variants of S. Typhimurium are prevalent along the entire pig production chain. For the other sources considered, the percentage of isolation of this serovar was lower than 5%.

8. FROM SEROTYPING TO WGS: A NEW ERA IN SALMONELLA EPIDEMIOLOGICAL INVESTIGATIONS

Salmonella epidemiological investigations have been classically performed by isolation in culture media, confirmation, and typing. Confirmation of the identity of Salmonella isolates has been done by using biochemical tests and PCR based on detection of Salmonella genes, like *fimA* (Cohen, Mechanda, & Lin, 1996), *hilA* (Guo, Chen, Beuchat, & Brackett, 2000), *invA* (Malorny, Hoorfar, Bunge, & Helmuth, 2003), *ttr* (Malorny et al., 2004), and *ssaN* (Chen et al., 2010). Other markers and combinations thereof have been developed for use in real-time-PCR (Postollec, Falentin, Pavan, Combrisson, & Sohier, 2011) and other detection platforms, such as loop-mediated isothermal amplification (Kokkinos, Ziros, Bellou, & Vantarakis, 2014).

Typing of Salmonella isolates has been started using serotyping, based on allelic variation in somatic and flagellar genes and has been conducted, with at least four laboratory methods: Salmonella genoserotyping assay (Yoshida et al., 2014); Salmonella serogenotyping assay; Check&Trace Salmonella; and xMAP Salmonella serotyping assay. These commercial kits can identify over 100 of the most common *S. enterica* serovars (Yoshida et al., 2016). Beside serotyping, pulsed-field gel electrophoresis (PFGE) has been the gold standard of molecular subtyping tool in discriminating between Salmonella strains for epidemiological investigations (Petersen et al., 2011). A drawback of PFGE is that it is unable to separate very closely related strains because the low rate of genetic variation does not significantly impact the electrophoretic mobility of a restriction fragment (Foley, Zhao, & Walker, 2007).

WGS has displaced both serotyping and PFGE as the de facto standard for the complete characterization of bacterial pathogens, including Salmonella, in both ongoing surveillance and outbreak investigations (Deng, den Bakker, & Hendriksen, 2016; Franz, Gras, & Dallman, 2016) and is currently being utilized in reference laboratories worldwide. Antimicrobial resistance (McDermott et al., 2016; Tyson et al., 2015; Zhao et al., 2015), serovar (Ingle et al., 2016; Yoshida, Kruczkiewicz, et al., 2016), and the results of other traditional subtyping schemes, such as multilocus sequence typing (MLST) (Sheppard, Jolley, & Maiden, 2012), can be accurately predicted in silico through the analysis of bacterial genome sequences. However, identifying bacterial isolates that are most likely to cause disease in humans, based on the genome sequence alone, is a more complex task.

Salmonella Syst-OMICS is a consortium to develop metadata systems for combining Salmonella phenotypic and genomic data to develop linkages among Salmonella isolates from a wide range of sources and conduct comparative analyses of specific virulence and antibiotic genes across Salmonella serotypes (Emond-Rheault et al., 2017). Studies of *S. enterica* population structure in humans, animals, food, and the environment are central to understand the biodiversity, evolution, ecology, and epidemiology of this pathogen. However, studies describing the genetic structure of Salmonella populations are commonly based on isolates drawn overwhelmingly from clinical collections (Hoffmann et al., 2014). This approach has resulted in a limited view of Salmonella's evolutionary history (Perry & Wright, 2014).

In Salmonella as in many other bacterial pathogens, there is limited knowledge on how genome content, rearrangements, and the complement of genes including those acquired by horizontal gene transfer contribute to strain-specific phenotypes, including virulence (Casadevall, 2017). Various studies have sought to resolve the population structure of Salmonella using complementary subtyping methods including PFGE, multiple loci VNTR analysis (MLVA), seven-gene housekeeping schemes, whole-genome multilocus sequence typing (wgMLST) profiles, pan- and core genome studies, and CRISPR analysis to define molecular signatures, pathogen subtypes, and the potential for pathogenicity (Liu, Chen, & Chiou, 2016; Rouli, Merhej, Fournier, & Raoult, 2015; Shariat & Dudley, 2014). Next-generation sequencing coupled with whole-genome comparison is well positioned to become the gold standard subtyping method, as it offers previously unmatched resolution for phylogenetic analysis, and rapid subtyping during investigation of food contamination and outbreaks (Ashton et al., 2016; Bekal et al., 2016).

Public health laboratories are in need of tools that can analyze WGS data to generate a type of portable genetic fingerprint (genotype) for use in discriminating among closely related strains for interlaboratory perspective disease surveillance and outbreak investigation (Liu et al., 2016). The single-nucleotide polymorphism (SNP)-based method is a widely used approach in which WGS data are employed for high-resolution subtyping of bacterial strains (Bekal et al., 2016; Taylor et al., 2015). To apply the SNP-based approach, a reference genome sequence is required for calling SNPs from WGS data of strains. A potential drawback is that the use of different reference genomes between studies would result in different SNP profiles, making it difficult to compare results between studies.

wgMLST, an extension of traditional MLST (Maiden et al., 1998), is a genome wide gene-by-gene comparison approach (Maiden et al., 2013) which has been applied to analyze WGS data for detection of disease clusters and outbreak investigation (de Been et al., 2015; Jackson et al., 2016; Jonathan, Michael, & Adam, 2016). To make the wgMLST scheme a standard subtyping tool, a pan-genome allele database with 395 genomes of *S. enterica* serovar Enteritidis has been developed by Liu et al. (2016). wgMLST profiles generated from that common pan-genome allele database can be portable and comparable across laboratories. Performance of wgMLST is equivalent to that of the SNP-based approach (Been et al., 2015; Raphael et al., 2016). One great advantage is that the wgMLST profile consists of serial digital numbers in numeric order that represent alleles of the target genes. Thus, wgMLST is far less computationally intensive than an SNP-based approach for using WGS data to investigate genetic relatedness among bacterial strains. A webserver (http://wgmlst.imst.nsysu.edu.tw)

has been set up with the database and the tools, allowing users to upload WGS data to generate wgMLST profiles and to perform cluster analysis of wgMLST profiles.

Laing, Whiteside, and Gannon (2017) examined a quality filtered set of 4893 Salmonella genomes downloaded from GenBank and identified a pan-genome of 25.3 Mbp, a strict core of 1.5 Mbp present in all genomes, and a conserved core of 3.2 Mbp found in at least 96% of the genomes investigated. In addition, they identified 404 species-specific regions, within which a minimum set of two was required to unambiguously identify a genome as being part of the species *S. enterica.* These species-specific regions were found to have functions related to the propagation in and colonization of the host, including the utilization of sialic acid in intestinal mucus, secretion systems for attachment to the host, and the killing of other host microbiota. Within subspecies enterica, the species-specific regions were found most frequently in serovar Enteritidis. Each of the six subspecies (i.e., *enterica, salamae, arizonae, diarizonae, houtenae,* and *indica*) was found to have genomic regions specific to it; however, the number of subspecies-specific regions appeared to be correlated with the level of sampling of the diversity within the subspecies. No serovar had pan-genome regions that were present in all of its representative genomes and absent in all other serovar genomes; however, each serovar did have genomic regions that were universally present among all constituent members, and statistically predictive of the serovar. The genomic regions identified by Laing et al. (2017) are predictive of the species *S. enterica,* its six subspecies and the serovar groups within subspecies enterica and can help to predict the strain groups that pose the most significant health threats to humans or that can persist in specific environments.

Leekitcharoenphon, Nielsen, Kaas, Lund, and Aarestrup (2014) evaluated WGS for typing of S. Typhimurium and compared pan-genome tree, k-mer tree, nucleotide difference tree, and SNP tree for WGS data analysis. The outcome of each approach was evaluated in relation to the association of the isolates to specific outbreaks. The pan-genome tree clustered 65% of the S. Typhimurium isolates according to the predefined epidemiology, the k-mer tree 88%, the nucleotide difference tree 100%, and the SNP tree 100% of the strains within S. Typhimurium. The resulting outcome of the four phylogenetic analyses was also compared to PFGE reveling that WGS typing achieved the greater performance than the traditional method.

In recent years, multiple applications for the in silico determination of Salmonella serovars from WGS data have been developed (Achtman et al.,

2012; Yoshida, Gurnik, et al., 2016; Zhang et al., 2015). Achtman et al. (2012) suggested that the serovar of an isolate could be inferred from MLST (Achtman et al., 2012). MLST assigns unique alleles to different sequences across 400–500 bp fragments of specified housekeeping genes (loci). The alleles assigned across all the loci are used to define the individual sequence types (ST), converting a large amount of data into an easily defined single number (Maiden et al., 1998). In the MLST serotyping scheme developed for Salmonella, seven housekeeping gene fragments are typed and the individual ST or their larger clonal complexes are then linked to Salmonella serovars. While MLST is not strictly an in silico analysis, the MLST data can be mined directly from WGS data using bioinformatic pipelines (Achtman et al., 2012; Ashton et al., 2016). Applications such as SeqSero (Zhang et al., 2015) and the Salmonella in silico typing resource (SISTR) (Yoshida, Kruczkiewicz, et al., 2016), have utilized an approach in which the gene sequences encoding the individual somatic and flagellar antigens are used to determine an isolate's serovar. Yachison et al. (2017) assessed and compared SeqSero, SISTR, and MLST for serovar prediction to traditional serotyping techniques using a set of 813 Salmonella verified clinical and laboratory isolates. Successful results were obtained for 94.8%, 88.2%, and 88.3% of the isolates tested using SISTR, SeqSero, and MLST, respectively, indicating all would be suitable for maintaining historical records, surveillance systems, and communication structures currently in place and the choice of the platform used will ultimately depend on the users need. Results also pointed to the need to reframe serotyping in the genomic era as a test to understand the genes that are carried by an isolate, one which is not necessarily congruent with what is antigenically expressed.

9. CONCLUSIONS AND FUTURE PROSPECTIVE

Human salmonellosis within the EU tended to increase since 2013. This increase has been mainly attributed to S. Enteritidis but other serotypes, like infantis, significantly increased in broiler and turkey flocks in 2016. Moreover, on December 1, 2017, an outbreak of Salmonella Agona infections among infants has been identified (Jourdan-da et al., 2018). The implicated food is baby milk distributed in 66 countries, and we are still counting the cases.

Reducing the number of Salmonella infections is a complicated problem because Salmonella has many sources and the sources vary by the type of Salmonella. Furthermore, Salmonella continues to genetically evolve and has the potential to become more recalcitrant to certain control practices, such as vaccines or antimicrobials. To reduce incidence, we need interventions that target the types of Salmonella that are increasing or staying the same. To better figure out the sources of people's illnesses different strategies might help. Those indicated in this chapter are (1) better sampling, especially in relation to table eggs; (2) integration between microbiological criteria and addition metrics (i.e., POs and FSOs) estimated as true prevalence and incidences with quantified uncertainties in order to achieve a sound, transparent scientific-based understanding of the risk; and (3) extended application of WGS to human, food, and animal isolates because it seems the most scientific and cost-effective analytical method to track salmonellosis and verify which prevention measures work.

The application of these strategies might help to keep Salmonella infections under control only within a framework of strong cooperation between the European countries. The ongoing S. Agona outbreak well shows that Salmonella spreads in complex food supply networks. Therefore, information provided through RASF, both official and informal, are needed in both detecting the outbreaks and ensuring that public health actions are timely as possible.

REFERENCES

Achtman, M., Wain, J., Weill, F. X., Nair, S., Zhou, Z., Sangal, V., et al. (2012). Multilocus sequence typing as a replacement for serotyping in Salmonella enterica. *PLoS Pathogens*, *8*(6), e1002776.

Amagliani, G., Brandi, G., & Schiavano, G. F. (2012). Incidence and role of Salmonella in seafood safety. *Food Research International*, *45*(2), 780–788.

Anthony Tony Cox, L. (2007). Does concern-driven risk management provide a viable alternative to QRA? *Risk Analysis*, *27*(1), 27–43.

Arnold, M. E., Carrique-Mas, J. J., McLaren, I., & Davies, R. H. (2011). A comparison of pooled and individual bird sampling for detection of Salmonella in commercial egg laying flocks. *Preventive Veterinary Medicine*, *99*(2), 176–184.

Arnold, M. E., Martelli, F., McLaren, I., & Davies, R. H. (2014). Estimation of the sensitivity of environmental sampling for detection of Salmonella in commercial layer flocks post-introduction of national control programmes. *Epidemiology & Infection*, *142*(5), 1061–1069.

Ashton, P. M., Nair, S., Peters, T. M., Bale, J. A., Powell, D. G., Painset, A., et al. (2016). Identification of Salmonella for public health surveillance using whole genome sequencing. *PeerJ*, *4*, e1752.

Bekal, S., Berry, C., Reimer, A. R., Van Domselaar, G., Beaudry, G., Fournier, E., et al. (2016). Usefulness of high-quality core genome single-nucleotide variant analysis for subtyping the highly clonal and the most prevalent Salmonella enterica serovar Heidelberg clone in the context of outbreak investigations. *Journal of Clinical Microbiology*, *54*(2), 289–295.

Blessington, T., Mitcham, E. J., & Harris, L. J. (2012). Survival of Salmonella enterica, Escherichia coli O157: H7, and Listeria monocytogenes on inoculated walnut kernels during storage. *Journal of Food Protection*, *75*(2), 245–254.

Buchanan, R. L., Smith, J. L., & Long, W. (2000). Microbial risk assessment: Dose–response relations and risk characterization. *International Journal of Food Microbiology, 58*(3), 159–172.

Budiati, T., Rusul, G., Wan-Abdullah, W. N., Arip, Y. M., Ahmad, R., & Thong, K. L. (2013). Prevalence, antibiotic resistance and plasmid profiling of Salmonella in catfish (*Clarias gariepinus*) and tilapia (*Tilapia mossambica*) obtained from wet markets and ponds in Malaysia. *Aquaculture, 37*, 127–132.

CAC Codex Alimentarius Commission. (2005). *The 15th Edition of CAC procedural manual.* Available from ftp://ftp.fao.org/codexPublications/ProcManuals/Manual_15e.pdf.

Carrique-Mas, J., & Davies, R. H. (2008). Bacteriological detection of Salmonella enteritidis in eggs: A review. *Revue Scientifique et Technique, 27*(3), 657.

Casadevall, A. (2017). The pathogenic potential of a microbe. *mSphere, 2*(1), e00015–17.

CDC (Centers for Disease Control, Prevention). (2012). *Foodborne Outbreak Online Database (FOOD).* http://wwwn.cdc.gov/foodborneoutbreaks/.

Chen, J., Zhang, L., Paoli, G. C., Shi, C., Tu, S. I., & Shi, X. (2010). A real-time PCR method for the detection of Salmonella enterica from food using a target sequence identified by comparative genomic analysis. *International Journal of Food Microbiology, 137*(2), 168–174.

Cohen, H. J., Mechanda, S. M., & Lin, W. (1996). PCR amplification of the fimA gene sequence of Salmonella typhimurium, a specific method for detection of Salmonella spp. *Applied and Environmental Microbiology, 62*(12), 4303–4308.

D'Aoust, J. Y., & Maurer, J. (2007). Salmonella species. In *Food microbiology: Fundamentals and Frontiers* (3rd ed., pp. 187–236). American Society of Microbiology.

Dallman, T., Inns, T., Jombart, T., Ashton, P., Loman, N., Chatt, C., et al. (2016). Phylogenetic structure of European Salmonella Enteritidis outbreak correlates with national and international egg distribution network. *Microbial Genomics, 2*(8), 1–8.

De Been, M., Pinholt, M., Top, J., Bletz, S., Mellmann, A., Van Schaik, W., ... & Corander, J. (2015). Core genome multilocus sequence typing scheme for high-resolution typing of Enterococcus faecium. Journal of Clinical Microbiology, 53(12), 3788–3797.

De Reu, K., Messens, W., Heyndrickx, M., Rodenburg, T. B., Uyttendaele, M., & Herman, L. (2008). Bacterial contamination of table eggs and the influence of housing systems. *World's Poultry Science Journal, 64*(1), 5–19.

De Swarte, C., & Donker, R. A. (2005). Towards an FSO/ALOP based food safety policy. *Food Control, 16*(9), 825–830.

De Vylder, J., Dewulf, J., Van Hoorebeke, S., Pasmans, F., Haesebrouck, F., Ducatelle, R., et al. (2011). Horizontal transmission of Salmonella Enteritidis in groups of experimentally infected laying hens housed in different housing systems. *Poultry Science, 90*(7), 1391–1396.

De Vylder, J., Raspoet, R., Dewulf, J., Haesebrouck, F., Ducatelle, R., & Van Immerseel, F. (2013). Salmonella Enteritidis is superior in egg white survival compared with other Salmonella serotypes. *Poultry Science, 92*(3), 842–845.

Deng, X., den Bakker, H. C., & Hendriksen, R. S. (2016). Genomic epidemiology: Whole-genome-sequencing-powered surveillance and outbreak investigation of foodborne bacterial pathogens. *Annual Review of Food Science and Technology, 7*, 353–374.

ECDC (European Centre for Disease Prevention and Control). (2016). *Multi-country outbreak of Salmonella Enteritidis phage type 8 MLVA type 2-9-7-3-2 and 2-9-6-3-2 infections, 27 October* (p. 2016). Stockholm: ECDC.

ECDC (European Centre for Disease Prevention and Control). (2017a). *Multi-country outbreak of Salmonella Enteritidis phage types 56 and 62, MLVA profile 2-11-3-3-2 and 2-12-3-3-2 infections 20 July 2017, Stockholm, Sweden.* 7 pp. Available online: https://ecdc.europa.eu/sites/portal/files/d ocuments/rapid-risk-assessment-multi-country-outbreak-Salmonella-Enteritidis.pdf.

ECDC (European Centre for Disease Prevention and Control). (2017b). *Re-emerging multi-country WGS-defined outbreak of Salmonella Enteritidis, MLVA type 2-12-7-3-2 and 2-14-7-3-2, 3 February 2017. Stockholm, Sweden.* 6 pp. Available online https://ecdc.europa.eu/en/publications-data/re-emerging-multi-country-wgsdefined-outbreak-salmonella-enteritidis-mlva-type-2.

ECDC (European Centre for Disease Prevention and Control). (2017c). *Tularaemia: Factsheet for health professionals.* Last updated 15 July 2017. Available online https://ecdc.europa.eu/en/tularaemia/facts.

EFSA (European Food Safety Authority). (2009). *The Community Summary Report on Food-borne Outbreaks in the European Union in 2007.* http://www.efsa.europa.eu/en/efsajournal/pub/271r.htm.

EFSA (European Food Safety Authority). (2010). *Trends and sources of zoonoses and zoonotic agents and food-borne outbreaks in the European Union in 2008.* http://www.efsa.europa.eu/en/efsajournal/pub/1496.htm.

EFSA (European Food Safety Authority). (2014a). Analysis of the baseline survey on the prevalence of Listeria monocytogenes in certain ready-to-eat foods in the EU, 2010–2011. Part B: Analysis of factors related to prevalence and exploring compliance. *EFSA Journal, 12*(8), 3810. 73 pp.

EFSA (European Food Safety Authority). (2014b). Update of the technical specifications for harmonised reporting of food-borne outbreaks through the European Union reporting system in accordance with Directive 2003/99/EC. *EFSA Journal, 12*(3), 3598. 25 pp.

EFSA (European Food Safety Authority) and ECDC (European Centre for Disease Prevention and Control). (2017). The European Union summary report on trends and sources of zoonoses, zoonotic agents and food-borne outbreaks in 2016. *EFSA Journal, 15*(12), 5077. 228 pp.

Emond-Rheault, J. G., Jeukens, J., Freschi, L., Kukavica-Ibrulj, I., Boyle, B., Dupont, M. J., et al. (2017). A syst-OMICS approach to ensuring food safety and reducing the economic burden of salmonellosis. *Frontiers in Microbiology, 8*, 1–8.

FAO/WHO. (2002). *Principles and guidelines for incorporating microbiological risk assessment in the development of food safety standards, guidelines and related texts.* Report of a Joint FAO/WHO Consultation, Kiel, Germany, 18–22 March 2002. Rome/Geneva: Food and Agriculture Organization of the United Nations/World Health Organization, ISBN: 92-5-104845-2.

Farakos, S. M. S., Pouillot, R., Johnson, R., Spungen, J., Son, I., Anderson, N., et al. (2017). A quantitative assessment of the risk of human salmonellosis arising from the consumption of almonds in the United States: The impact of preventive treatment levels. *Journal of Food Protection, 80*(5), 863–878.

Fatica, M. K., & Schneider, K. R. (2011). Salmonella and produce: Survival in the plant environment and implications in food safety. *Virulence, 2*(6), 573–579.

FDA Food and Drug Administration, HHS. (2009). Prevention of Salmonella enteritidis in shell eggs during production, storage, and transportation. Final rule. *Federal Register, 74*(130), 33029.

Finstad, S., O'Bryan, C. A., Marcy, J. A., Crandall, P. G., & Ricke, S. C. (2012). Salmonella and broiler processing in the United States: Relationship to foodborne salmonellosis. *Food Research International, 45*(2), 789–794.

Foley, S. L., Johnson, T. J., Ricke, S. C., Nayak, R., & Danzeisen, J. (2013). Salmonella pathogenicity and host adaptation in chicken-associated serovars. *Microbiology and Molecular Biology Reviews,* 77(4), 582–607.

Foley, S. L., Zhao, S., & Walker, R. D. (2007). Comparison of molecular typing methods for the differentiation of Salmonella foodborne pathogens. *Foodborne Pathogens and Disease, 4*(3), 253–276.

Franz, E., Gras, L. M., & Dallman, T. (2016). Significance of whole genome sequencing for surveillance, source attribution and microbial risk assessment of foodborne pathogens. *Current Opinion in Food Science*, *8*, 74–79.

Gal-Mor, O., Boyle, E. C., & Grassl, G. A. (2014). Same species, different diseases: How and why typhoidal and non-typhoidal Salmonella enterica serovars differ. *Frontiers in Microbiology*, *5*, 391.

Gantois, I., Ducatelle, R., Pasmans, F., Haesebrouck, F., Gast, R., Humphrey, T. J., et al. (2009). Mechanisms of egg contamination by Salmonella Enteritidis. *FEMS Microbiology Reviews*, *33*(4), 718–738.

Garces-Vega, F., Jeong, S., Dolan, K., & Marks, B. (2016). Modeling Salmonella inactivation in low moisture foods: Using parameter estimation to improve model performance. *Procedia Food Science*, 7, 41–46.

Gast, R. K., Guraya, R., Jones, D. R., Guard, J., Anderson, K. E., & Karcher, D. M. (2017). Colonization of internal organs by Salmonella serovars Heidelberg and Typhimurium in experimentally infected laying hens housed in enriched colony cages at different stocking densities. *Poultry Science*, *96*(5), 1402–1409.

Gayet, R., Bioley, G., Rochereau, N., Paul, S., & Corthésy, B. (2017). Vaccination against salmonella infection: The mucosal way. *Microbiology and Molecular Biology Reviews*, *81*(3), e00007-17.

Gilmour, M. W., Graham, M. W. G. M., Reimer, A., & Van Domselaar, G. (2013). Public health genomics and the new molecular epidemiology of bacterial pathogens. *Public Health Genomics*, *16*(1–2), 25–30.

Gkogka, E., Reij, M. W., Gorris, L. G. M., & Zwietering, M. H. (2013). Risk assessment strategies as a tool in the application of the appropriate level of protection (ALOP) and food safety objective (FSO) by risk managers. *International Journal of Food Microbiology*, *167*(1), 8–28.

Gole, V. C., Chousalkar, K. K., Roberts, J. R., Sexton, M., May, D., Tan, J., et al. (2014). Effect of egg washing and correlation between eggshell characteristics and egg penetration by various Salmonella Typhimurium strains. *PLoS One*, *9*(3), e90987.

Gorris, L. G. (2005). Food safety objective: An integral part of food chain management. *Food Control*, *16*(9), 801–809.

Grimont, P. A., & Weill, F. X. (2007). Antigenic formulae of the Salmonella serovars. *WHO collaborating centre for reference and research on Salmonella*, *9*, 1–161.

Guo, X., Chen, J., Beuchat, L. R., & Brackett, R. E. (2000). PCR detection of Salmonella enterica serotype montevideo in and on raw tomatoes using primers derived from hilA. *Applied and Environmental Microbiology*, *66*(12), 5248–5252.

Harris, L. J., Palumbo, M., Beuchat, L. R., & Danyluk, M. D. (2015). Outbreaks of foodborne illness associated with the consumption of tree nuts, peanuts, and sesame seeds [Table and references]. In Outbreaks from tree nuts, peanuts, and sesame seeds. http://ucfoodsafety.ucdavis.edu/Nuts_and_Nut_Pastes/.

Havelaar, A. H., Nauta, M. J., & Jansen, J. T. (2004). Fine-tuning food safety objectives and risk assessment. *International Journal of Food Microbiology*, *93*(1), 11–29.

He, H., Genovese, K. J., Swaggerty, C. L., Nisbet, D. J., & Kogut, M. H. (2012). A comparative study on invasion, survival, modulation of oxidative burst, and nitric oxide responses of macrophages (HD11), and systemic infection in chickens by prevalent poultry Salmonella serovars. *Foodborne Pathogens and Disease*, *9*(12), 1104–1110.

Hendriksen, R. S., Vieira, A. R., Karlsmose, S., Lo Fo Wong, D. M., Jensen, A. B., Wegener, H. C., et al. (2011). Global monitoring of Salmonella serovar distribution from the World Health Organization global foodborne infections network country data Bank: Results of quality assured laboratories from 2001 to 2007. *Foodborne Pathogens and Disease*, *8*(8), 887–900.

Hennessy, T. W., Cheng, L. H., Kassenborg, H., Ahuja, S. D., Mohle-Boetani, J., Marcus, R., et al. (2004). Egg consumption is the principal risk factor for sporadic Salmonella serotype Heidelberg infections: A case-control study in FoodNet sites. *Clinical Infectious Diseases*, *38*(Suppl 3), S237–S243.

Hindermann, D., Gopinath, G., Chase, H., Negrete, F., Althaus, D., Zurfluh, K., et al. (2017). Salmonella enterica serovar infantis from food and human infections, Switzerland, 2010–2015: Poultry-related multidrug resistant clones and an emerging esbl producing clonal lineage. *Frontiers in Microbiology*, *8*, 1322.

Hoffmann, M., Zhao, S., Pettengill, J., Luo, Y., Monday, S. R., Abbott, J., et al. (2014). Comparative genomic analysis and virulence differences in closely related Salmonella enterica serotype Heidelberg isolates from humans, retail meats, and animals. *Genome Biology and Evolution*, *6*(5), 1046–1068.

Holt, P. S., Davies, R. H., Dewulf, J., Gast, R. K., Huwe, J. K., Jones, D. R., et al. (2011). The impact of different housing systems on egg safety and quality 1. *Poultry Science*, *90*(1), 251–262.

Howard, Z. R., O'Bryan, C. A., Crandall, P. G., & Ricke, S. C. (2012). Salmonella Enteritidis in shell eggs: Current issues and prospects for control. *Food Research International*, *45*(2), 755–764.

Humphrey, T. J. (1994). Contamination of egg shell and contents with Salmonella enteritidis: A review. *International Journal of Food Microbiology*, *21*(1–2), 31–40.

Humphrey, T. J., Whitehead, A., Gawler, A. H. L., Henley, A., & Rowe, B. (1991). Numbers of Salmonella enteritidis in the contents of naturally contaminated hens' eggs. *Epidemiology & Infection*, *106*(3), 489–496.

ICMSF. (2002). *International commission on microbiological specifications for foods. Book 7. Microbiological testing in food safety management.* NY: Kluwer Academic/Plenum Publishers.

Ingle, D. J., Valcanis, M., Kuzevski, A., Tauschek, M., Inouye, M., Stinear, T., et al. (2016). In silico serotyping of E. coli from short read data identifies limited novel O-loci but extensive diversity of O:H serotype combinations within and between pathogenic lineages. *Microbial Genomics*, *2*(7), 1–14.

Inns, T., Ashton, P. M., Herrera-Leon, S., Lighthill, J., Foulkes, S., Jombart, T., et al. (2017). Prospective use of whole genome sequencing (WGS) detected a multi-country outbreak of Salmonella Enteritidis. *Epidemiology & Infection*, *145*(2), 289–298.

Jackson, B. R., Griffin, P. M., Cole, D., Walsh, K. A., & Chai, S. J. (2013). Outbreak-associated Salmonella enterica serotypes and food commodities, United States, 1998–2008. *Emerging Infectious Diseases*, *19*(8), 1239.

Jackson, B. R., Tarr, C., Strain, E., Jackson, K. A., Conrad, A., Carleton, H., et al. (2016). Implementation of nationwide real-time whole-genome sequencing to enhance listeriosis outbreak detection and investigation. *Reviews of Infectious Diseases*, *63*(3), 380–386.

Jakabi, M., Buzzo, A. A., Ristori, C. A., Tavechio, A. T., Sakuma, H., Paula, A. M. R. D., et al. (1999). Observações laboratoriais sobre surtos alimentares de Salmonella sp, ocorridos na Grande São Paulo, no periódo de 1994 a 1997. *Revista do Instituto Adolfo Lutz*, 47–51.

Jakočiūnė, D., Pasquali, F., da Silva, C. S., Löfström, C., Hoorfar, J., Klein, G., et al. (2014). Enumeration of salmonellae in table eggs, pasteurized egg products, and egg-containing dishes by using quantitative real-time PCR. *Applied and Environmental Microbiology*, *80*(5), 1616–1622.

Jeong, S., Marks, B. P., & Orta-Ramirez, A. (2009). Thermal inactivation kinetics for salmonella Enteritidis PT30 on almonds subjected to moist-air convection heating. *Journal of Food Protection*, *72*(8), 1602–1609.

Jonathan, S. B., Michael, G., & Adam, M. (2016). Whole-genome sequencing detection of ongoing contamination at a restaurant, Rhode Island, USA, 2014. *Emerging Infectious Diseases*, *22*, 1474–1476.

Jourdan-da, S. N., Fabre, L., Robinson, E., Fournet, N., Nisavanh, A., Bruyand, M., et al. (2018). Ongoing nationwide outbreak of Salmonella Agona associated with internationally distributed infant milk products, France, December 2017. *Euro Surveill*, 23(*2*). pii: 17-00852.

Jouve, J. L. (1999). Establishment of food safety objectives. *Food Control*, *10*(4), 303–305.

Kim, S. (2010). Salmonella serovars from foodborne and waterborne diseases in Korea, 1998–2007: Total isolates decreasing versus rare serovars emerging. *Journal of Korean Medical Science*, *25*(12), 1693–1699.

Kim, S., Frye, J. G., Hu, J., Fedorka-Cray, P. J., Gautom, R., & Boyle, D. S. (2006). Multiplex PCR-based method for identification of common clinical serotypes of Salmonella enterica subsp. enterica. *Journal of Clinical Microbiology*, *44*(10), 3608–3615.

Kirk, M. D., Pires, S. M., Black, R. E., Caipo, M., Crump, J. A., Devleesschauwer, B., et al. (2015). World Health Organization estimates of the global and regional disease burden of 22 foodborne bacterial, protozoal, and viral diseases, 2010: A data synthesis. *PLoS Medicine*, *12*(12), e1001921.

Kokkinos, P. A., Ziros, P. G., Bellou, M., & Vantarakis, A. (2014). Loop-mediated isothermal amplification (LAMP) for the detection of Salmonella in food. *Food Analytical Methods*, 7, 512–526.

Kozak, G. K., MacDonald, D., Landry, L., & Farber, J. M. (2013). Foodborne outbreaks in Canada linked to produce: 2001 through 2009. *Journal of Food Protection*, *76*(1), 173–183.

Kumar, R., Surendran, P. K., & Thampuran, N. (2009). Distribution and genotypic characterization of Salmonella serovars isolated from tropical seafood of Cochin, India. *Journal of Applied Microbiology*, *106*(2), 515–524.

Laing, C. R., Whiteside, M. D., & Gannon, V. P. (2017). Pan-genome analyses of the species Salmonella enterica, and identification of genomic markers predictive for species, subspecies, and serovar. *Frontiers in Microbiology*, *8*, 1345.

Lammerding, A. M., & Fazil, A. (2000). Hazard identification and exposure assessment for microbial food safety risk assessment. *International Journal of Food Microbiology*, *58*(3), 147–157.

Lan, N. P. H., Phuong, T. L. T., Huu, H. N., Thuy, L., Mather, A. E., Park, S. E., et al. (2016). Invasive non-typhoidal Salmonella infections in Asia: Clinical observations, disease outcome and dominant serovars from an infectious disease hospital in Vietnam. *PLoS Neglected Tropical Diseases*, *10*(8), e0004857.

Leekitcharoenphon, P., Nielsen, E. M., Kaas, R. S., Lund, O., & Aarestrup, F. M. (2014). Evaluation of whole genome sequencing for outbreak detection of Salmonella enterica. *PLoS One*, *9*(2), e87991.

Liu, Y.-Y., Chen, C.-C., & Chiou, C.-S. (2016). Construction of a pan-genome allele database of Salmonella enterica Serovar Enteritidis for molecular subtyping and disease cluster identification. *Frontiers in Microbiology*, 7, 2010.

Maiden, M. C., Bygraves, J. A., Feil, E., Morelli, G., Russell, J. E., Urwin, R., et al. (1998). Multilocus sequence typing: A portable approach to the identification of clones within populations of pathogenic microorganisms. *Proceedings of the National Academy of Sciences*, *95*(6), 3140–3145.

Maiden, M. C., Van Rensburg, M. J. J., Bray, J. E., Earle, S. G., Ford, S. A., Jolley, K. A., et al. (2013). MLST revisited: The gene-by-gene approach to bacterial genomics. *Nature Reviews Microbiology*, *11*(10), 728–736.

Majowicz, S. E., Musto, J., Scallan, E., Angulo, F. J., Kirk, M., O'brien, S. J., et al. (2010). The global burden of nontyphoidal Salmonella gastroenteritis. *Clinical Infectious Diseases*, *50*, 882–889.

Malorny, B., Hoorfar, J., Bunge, C., & Helmuth, R. (2003). Multicenter validation of the analytical accuracy of Salmonella PCR: Towards an international standard. *Applied and Environmental Microbiology*, *69*(1), 290–296.

Malorny, B., Paccassoni, E., Fach, P., Bunge, C., Martin, A., & Helmuth, R. (2004). Diagnostic real-time PCR for detection of Salmonella in food. *Applied and Environmental Microbiology*, *70*(12), 7046–7052.

Manfreda, G., Valero, A., Rodríguez-Lázaro, D., Hernández, M., Pasquali, F., & De Cesare, A. (2014). Performance objectives for Salmonella in fresh pork meat intended to be eaten cooked: How to derive them and verify their achievement. *International Journal of Food Microbiology*, *184*, 55–59.

Martelli, F., & Davies, R. H. (2012). Salmonella serovars isolated from table eggs: An overview. *Food Research International*, *45*(2), 745–754.

Martinez-Urtaza, J., Liebana, E., Garcia-Migura, L., Perez-Piñeiro, P., & Saco, M. (2004). Characterization of Salmonella enterica serovar Typhimurium from marine environments in coastal waters of Galicia (Spain). *Applied and Environmental Microbiology*, *70*(7), 4030–4034.

McDermott, P. F., Tyson, G. H., Kabera, C., Chen, Y., Li, C., Folster, J. P., et al. (2016). Whole-genome sequencing for detecting antimicrobial resistance in nontyphoidal Salmonella. *Antimicrobial Agents and Chemotherapy*, *60*(9), 5515–5520.

Mench, J. A., Sumner, D. A., & Rosen-Molina, J. T. (2011). Sustainability of egg production in the United States—The policy and market context 1. *Poultry Science*, *90*(1), 229–240.

Moffatt, C. R., Musto, J., Pingault, N., Combs, B., Miller, M., Stafford, R., et al. (2017). Recovery of Salmonella enterica from Australian layer and processing environments following outbreaks linked to eggs. *Foodborne Pathogens and Disease*, *14*(8), 478–482.

Moffatt, C. R., Musto, J., Pingault, N., Miller, M., Stafford, R., Gregory, J., et al. (2016). Salmonella Typhimurium and outbreaks of egg-associated disease in Australia, 2001 to 2011. *Foodborne Pathogens and Disease*, *13*(7), 379–385.

Novoslavskij, A., Terentjeva, M., Eizenberga, I., Valciņa, O., Bartkevičs, V., & Bērziņš, A. (2016). Major foodborne pathogens in fish and fish products: A review. *Annals of Microbiology*, *66*(1), 1–15.

Nüesch-Inderbinen, M., Cernela, N., Althaus, D., Hächler, H., & Stephan, R. (2015). Salmonella enterica Serovar Szentes, a rare serotype causing a 9-month outbreak in 2013 and 2014 in Switzerland. *Foodborne Pathogens and Disease*, *12*(11), 887–890.

Pasquali, F., De Cesare, A., Valero, A., Olsen, J. E., & Manfreda, G. (2014). Improvement of sampling plans for Salmonella detection in pooled table eggs by use of real-time PCR. *International Journal of Food Microbiology*, *184*, 31–34.

Perry, J. A., & Wright, G. D. (2014). Forces shaping the antibiotic resistome. *BioEssays*, *36*(12), 1179–1184.

Petersen, R. F., Litrup, E., Larsson, J. T., Torpdahl, M., Sørensen, G., Müller, L., et al. (2011). Molecular characterization of Salmonella Typhimurium highly successful outbreak strains. *Foodborne Pathogens and Disease*, *8*(6), 655–661.

Petrovska, L., Mather, A. E., AbuOun, M., Branchu, P., Harris, S. R., Connor, T., et al. (2016). Microevolution of monophasic Salmonella Typhimurium during epidemic, United Kingdom, 2005–2010. *Emerging Infectious Diseases*, *22*(4), 617.

Podolak, R., Enache, E., Stone, W., Black, D. G., & Elliott, P. H. (2010). Sources and risk factors for contamination, survival, persistence, and heat resistance of Salmonella in low-moisture foods. *Journal of Food Protection*, *73*(10), 1919–1936.

Postollec, F., Falentin, H., Pavan, S., Combrisson, J., & Sohier, D. (2011). Recent advances in quantitative PCR (qPCR) applications in food microbiology. *Food Microbiology*, *28*(5), 848–861.

Pouillot, R., & Delignette-Muller, M. L. (2010). Evaluating variability and uncertainty separately in microbial quantitative risk assessment using two R packages. *International Journal of Food Microbiology*, *142*(3), 330–340.

Raphael, B. H., Baker, D. J., Nazarian, E., Lapierre, P., Bopp, D., Kozak-Muiznieks, N. A., et al. (2016). Genomic resolution of outbreak-associated Legionella pneumophila serogroup 1 isolates from New York State. *Applied and Environmental Microbiology*, *82*(12), 3582–3590.

Ricke, S. C. (2017). Insights and challenges of salmonella infection of laying hens. *Current Opinion in Food Science*, *18*, 43–49.

Rieu, E., Duhem, K., Vindel, E., & Sanaa, M. (2007). Food safety objectives should integrate the variability of the concentration of pathogen. *Risk Analysis*, *27*(2), 373–386.

Rodríguez-Urrego, J., Herrera-León, S., Echeita-Sarriondia, A., Soler, P., Simon, F., & Mateo, S. (2010). Nationwide outbreak of Salmonella serotype Kedougou associated with infant formula, Spain, 2008. *Eurosurveillance*, *15*(22), 19582.

Ronholm, J., Nasheri, N., Petronella, N., & Pagotto, F. (2016). Navigating microbiological food safety in the era of whole-genome sequencing. *Clinical Microbiology Reviews*, *29*(4), 837–857.

Rouli, L., Merhej, V., Fournier, P. E., & Raoult, D. (2015). The bacterial pangenome as a new tool for analysing pathogenic bacteria. *New Microbes and New Infections*, 7, 72–85.

Safe Food International (SFI). (2012). *Food/Water Borne Illness Outbreaks*. http://regionalnews.safefoodinternational.org/page/Food%2FWater+Borne+Illness+Outbreaks.

Schmidt, P. J., & Emelko, M. B. (2011). QMRA and decision-making: Are we handling measurement errors associated with pathogen concentration data correctly? *Water Research*, *45*(2), 427–438.

Shariat, N., & Dudley, E. G. (2014). CRISPRs: Molecular signatures used for pathogen subtyping. *Applied and Environmental Microbiology*, *80*(2), 430–439.

Sheppard, S. K., Jolley, K. A., & Maiden, M. C. (2012). A gene-by-gene approach to bacterial population genomics: Whole genome MLST of Campylobacter. *Genes*, *3*(2), 261–277.

Srisanga, S., Angkititrakul, S., Sringam, P., Le Ho, P. T., Vo, A. T., & Chuanchuen, R. (2017). Phenotypic and genotypic antimicrobial resistance and virulence genes of Salmonella enterica isolated from pet dogs and cats. *Journal of Veterinary Science*, *18*(3), 273–281.

Stringer, M. (2005). Summary report: Food safety objectives—Role in microbiological food safety management. *Food Control*, *16*(9), 775–794.

Taylor, A. J., Lappi, V., Wolfgang, W. J., Lapierre, P., Palumbo, M. J., Medus, C., et al. (2015). Characterization of foodborne outbreaks of Salmonella enterica serovar Enteritidis with whole-genome sequencing single nucleotide polymorphism-based analysis for surveillance and outbreak detection. *Journal of Clinical Microbiology*, *53*(10), 3334–3340.

Tessari, E. N. C., Kanashiro, A. M. I., Stoppa, G. F., Luciano, R. L., De Castro, A. G. M., & Cardoso, A. L. S. (2012). Important aspects of Salmonella in the poultry industry and in public health. In *Salmonella—A dangerous foodborne pathogen*. InTech.

Thomas, M. K., Murray, R., Flockhart, L., Pintar, K., Fazil, A., Nesbitt, A., et al. (2015). Estimates of foodborne illness-related hospitalizations and deaths in Canada for 30 specified pathogens and unspecified agents. *Foodborne Pathogens and Disease*, *12*(10), 820–827.

Todd, E. C. (2004). Microbiological safety standards and public health goals to reduce foodborne disease. *Meat Science*, *66*(1), 33–43.

Tuominen, P., Ranta, J., & Maijala, R. (2007). Studying the effects of POs and MCs on the Salmonella ALOP with a quantitative risk assessment model for beef production. *International Journal of Food Microbiology*, *118*(1), 35–51.

Tyson, G. H., McDermott, P. F., Li, C., Chen, Y., Tadesse, D. A., Mukherjee, S., et al. (2015). WGS accurately predicts antimicrobial resistance in Escherichia coli. *Journal of Antimicrobial Chemotherapy*, *70*(10), 2763–2769.

Van der Fels-Klerx, H. J., Tromp, S., Rijgersberg, H., & Van Asselt, E. D. (2008). Application of a transmission model to estimate performance objectives for Salmonella in the broiler supply chain. *International Journal of Food Microbiology, 128*(1), 22–27.

Van Gerwen, S. J., & Gorris, L. G. (2004). Application of elements of microbiological risk assessment in the food industry via a tiered approach. *Journal of Food Protection, 67*(9), 2033–2040.

Van Schaik, G., Stehman, S. M., Schukken, Y. H., Rossiter, C. R., & Shin, S. J. (2003). Pooled fecal culture sampling for Mycobacterium avium subsp. paratuberculosis at different herd sizes and prevalence. *Journal of Veterinary Diagnostic Investigation, 15*(3), 233–241.

Wattiau, P., Boland, C., & Bertrand, S. (2011). Methodologies for Salmonella enterica subsp. enterica subtyping: Gold standards and alternatives. *Applied and Environmental Microbiology*, 77(22), 7877–7885.

Whiley, H., & Ross, K. (2015). Salmonella and eggs: From production to plate. *International Journal of Environmental Research and Public Health, 12*(3), 2543–2556.

Wright, A. P., Richardson, L., Mahon, B. E., Rothenberg, R., & Cole, D. J. (2016). The rise and decline in Salmonella enterica serovar Enteritidis outbreaks attributed to egg-containing foods in the United States, 1973–2009. *Epidemiology & Infection, 144*(4), 810–819.

WTO. (1995). *World Trade Organization. Agreement on the application of sanitary and phytosanitary measures (SPS Agreement).* Available from http://www.wto.org/english/tratop_e/sps_e/spsagr_e.htm.

Yachison, C. A., Yoshida, C., Robertson, J., Nash, J. H., Kruczkiewicz, P., Taboada, E. N., et al. (2017). The validation and implications of using whole genome sequencing as a replacement for traditional serotyping for a national Salmonella reference laboratory. *Frontiers in Microbiology, 8*, 1044.

Yoshida, C., Gurnik, S., Ahmad, A., Blimkie, T., Murphy, S. A., Kropinski, A. M., et al. (2016). Evaluation of molecular methods for identification of Salmonella serovars. *Journal of Clinical Microbiology, 54*(8), 1992–1998.

Yoshida, C. E., Kruczkiewicz, P., Laing, C. R., Lingohr, E. J., Gannon, V. P., Nash, J. H., et al. (2016). The Salmonella in silico typing resource (SISTR): An open web-accessible tool for rapidly typing and subtyping draft Salmonella genome assemblies. *PLoS One*, 11(1), e0147101.

Yoshida, C., Lingohr, E. J., Trognitz, F., MacLaren, N., Rosano, A., Murphy, S. A., et al. (2014). Multi-laboratory evaluation of the rapid genoserotyping array (SGSA) for the identification of Salmonella serovars. *Diagnostic Microbiology and Infectious Disease, 80*(3), 185–190.

Zhang, S., Yin, Y., Jones, M. B., Zhang, Z., Kaiser, B. L. D., Dinsmore, B. A., et al. (2015). Salmonella serotype determination utilizing high-throughput genome sequencing data. *Journal of Clinical Microbiology, 53*(5), 1685–1692.

Zhao, S., Tyson, G. H., Chen, Y., Li, C., Mukherjee, S., Young, S., et al. (2015). Whole-genome sequencing analysis accurately predicts antimicrobial resistance phenotypes in Campylobacter spp. *Applied and Environmental Microbiology, 82*(2), 459–466.

Zwietering, M. H., & Van Gerwen, S. J. C. (2000). Sensitivity analysis in quantitative microbial risk assessment. *International Journal of Food Microbiology, 58*(3), 213–221.

FURTHER READING

Dallman, T., Inns, T., Jombart, T., Ashton, P., Loman, N., Chatt, C., et al. (2006). Sampling the antibiotic resistome. *Science, 311*(5759), 374–377.

CHAPTER SEVEN

Listeria monocytogenes in Foods

Kieran Jordan[1], Olivia McAuliffe
Teagasc Food Research Centre, Cork, Ireland
[1]Corresponding author: e-mail address: kieran.jordan@teagasc.ie

Contents

Abstract

Listeria monocytogenes causes listeriosis, a rare foodborne disease with a mortality rate of 20%–30%. The elderly and immunocompromised are particularly susceptible to listeriosis. *L. monocytogenes* is ubiquitous in nature and can contaminate food-processing environments, posing a threat to the food chain. This is particularly important for ready-to-eat foods as there is no heat treatment or other antimicrobial step between production and consumption. Thus, occurrence and control of *L. monocytogenes* are important for industry and public health. Advances in whole-genome sequence

Advances in Food and Nutrition Research, Volume 86
ISSN 1043-4526
https://doi.org/10.1016/bs.afnr.2018.02.006
© 2018 Elsevier Inc.
All rights reserved.

technology are facilitating the investigation of disease outbreaks, linking sporadic cases to outbreaks, and linking outbreaks internationally. Novel control methods, such as bacteriophage and bacteriocins, can contribute to a reduction in the occurrence of *L. monocytogenes* in the food-processing environment, thereby reducing the risk of food contamination and contributing to a reduction in public health issues.

1. INTRODUCTION

Listeria monocytogenes is a foodborne pathogen that causes listeriosis, a relatively rare but potentially fatal gastrointestinal illness. In a global estimation, Maertens de Noordhout et al. (2014) estimated that the mortality rate was 24%, while Scallan et al. (2011) determined that, at 99%, it has the highest hospitalization rate among the foodborne diseases. In 2016, there were 2536 confirmed human cases of listeriosis in the European Union (EU), a notification rate of 0.47 cases per 100,000 population. This represents a 9.3% increase in 2015, and a continuing statistically significant increasing trend of listeriosis from 2008 to 2016 (European Commission, 2017). The incidence of listeriosis in the United States is about 0.24/100,000 population (Centers for Disease Control, 2017).

L. monocytogenes is ubiquitous in the environment, being found in soil, water, and feces. It also has the ability to survive in the human body, crossing the intestinal barrier, the blood–brain barrier, and the fetoplacental barrier, infecting organs such as the brain or uterus, thereby causing severe life-threatening infections such as meningitis, encephalitis, spontaneous abortion, or miscarriage. Healthy individuals are normally not susceptible to *L. monocytogenes*, but it can have severe implications for those with compromised immune systems, such as the elderly, newborns, and pregnant women (Buchanan, Gorris, Hayman, Jackson, & Whiting, 2017).

Being ubiquitous in the environment, *L. monocytogenes* contamination of the food-processing environment occurs. Once in the food-processing environment, it can survive for long periods of time in the seemingly hostile environment, partially due to its ability to endure various stresses, such as sanitizers, pH, and temperature (Moorhead & Dykes, 2004; Zhang et al., 2011), and its ability to form biofilm (Cruz & Fletcher, 2011; Latorre et al., 2010). If measures are not taken to control it in the food-processing environment, it can persist, creating a potential cross-contamination route to the food.

As the public health consequences of listeriosis are so serious, occurrence of *L. monocytogenes* in the food-processing environment and the possible cross-contamination of food creates two major problems for the food industry: first, the public health issue (as outlined earlier) and second the challenge to control it (the potential recalls of food, the costs of adequate testing, etc.). In particular, *L. monocytogenes* is a problem for the ready-to-eat (RTE) food industry as there is no heat or other antimicrobial step between production and consumption.

The focus of this chapter is on the occurrence of *L. monocytogenes* in the food-processing environment, the consequences of that occurrence, and exploring options for its reduction.

2. PUBLIC HEALTH ISSUES

2.1 Listeriosis Outbreaks

Despite the efforts of the food industry and regulatory authorities to prevent and control *L. monocytogenes*, outbreaks of listeriosis occur. An outbreak is defined as two or more people being ill after consuming the same food. It is important to keep in mind that the majority of the *L. monocytogenes* cases are sporadic, rather than being part of an outbreak. Some recent outbreaks of listeriosis in the EU and United States are listed in Table 1.

2.2 Food Recalls/Withdrawals Due to *L. monocytogenes*

The differentiation between a "recall" and a "withdrawal" is not clear. In some cases the terms are interchangeable, while in others "recall" is related to a food safety issue, and "withdrawal" refers to less serious issues, for example, with labeling. Alternatively, "recall" refers to involving the consumer, whereas "withdrawal" refers to the withholding of food in the distribution chain (not including the consumer). For the purposes of this chapter, the terms are used interchangeably.

As mentioned, *L. monocytogenes* is a public health hazard that can lead to incidences of listeriosis. For that reason, the occurrence of *L. monocytogenes* in food (or in the United States, the occurrence in the food-processing environment) is treated as a very serious issue by regulatory authorities. If such contamination is detected either before or after product release, then a product recall/withdrawal, either voluntary or compulsory, may be instigated. Such recall/withdrawal can have major consequences, especially where a

Table 1 Reported *Listeria monocytogenes* Outbreaks in the EU (2013–2015) and in the United States (2013–2016)

Year	Food Vehicle	Reporting Country	Cases	Deaths
2013	Not available	Austria[a]	7	0
2013	Cheese	Belgium	2	0
2013	Pig meat and products thereof	Belgium	2	0
2013	Crustaceans, shellfish, molluscs, and products thereof	France	3	0
2013	Vegetables and juices and other products thereof	Germany	3	1
2013	n.a.	The Netherlands	2	0
2013	n.a.	Sweden	2	0
2013	Meat and meat products	Sweden	34	0
2013	n.a.	UK	3	0
2013	Crustaceans, shellfish, molluscs, and products thereof	UK[a]	7	2
2013	Hummus	USA—California	28	3
2013	n.a.	USA—Florida	9	4
2013	n.a.	USA—Massachusetts	2	0
2013	Cheese-le frere	USA—Multistate	6	1
2013	Latin-style soft cheese	USA—Multistate	8	1
2013	Mexican-style cheese, pasteurized	USA—Multistate	9	1
2013	Frozen vegetables	USA—Multistate	10	3
2013	Hummus	USA—Multistate	8	1
2013	n.a.	USA—Rhode Island	4	2
2014	Bovine meat and products thereof	Belgium	2	0
2014	Fish and fish products	Denmark	6	0
2014	Other foods	Denmark	41	0
2014	Mixed food	Denmark	6	0
2014	Unknown	Denmark	8	0
2014	Mixed food	Germany	2	0

Table 1 Reported *Listeria monocytogenes* Outbreaks in the EU (2013–2015) and in the United States (2013–2016)—cont'd

Year	Food Vehicle	Reporting Country	Cases	Deaths
2014	Unknown	Germany[a]	4	0
2014	Unknown	Malta	2	0
2014	Vegetables and juices and other products thereof	Spain	3	0
2014	Unknown	Spain	2	0
2014	Other or mixed red meat and products thereof	Sweden	4	0
2014	Fish and fish products	Sweden	17	0
2014	Unknown	Sweden	5	0
2014	Buffet meals	UK	4	0
2014	Fresh curd cheese	USA—California and Maryland	8	
2014	n.a.	USA—Maine	2	0
2014	Peaches, unspecified; nectarine	USA—Multistate	2	1
2014	Mung bean sprouts	USA—Multistate	5	2
2014	Caramel apple	USA—Multistate	35	7
2014	Raw milk	USA—Multistate	2	1
2014	Smoked fish	USA—Multistate	4	0
2014	n.a.	USA—New York	2	2
2014	n.a.	USA—New York	2	0
2014	Sprouts	USA—Virginia	2	0
2014	Mexican-style cheese, pasteurized	USA—Washington	3	1
2014	Milkshake	USA—Washington	2	0
2015	Unknown	Denmark	2	0
2015	Buffet meals	Finland	24	0
2015	Mixed food	Germany	159	0
2015	Unknown	Germany[b]	6	0
2015	Unknown	Greece	2	2

Continued

Table 1 Reported *Listeria monocytogenes* Outbreaks in the EU (2013–2015) and in the United States (2013–2016)—cont'd

Year	Food Vehicle	Reporting Country	Cases	Deaths
2015	Pig meat and products thereof	Italy	12	2
2015	Unknown	Latvia[a]	4	0
2015	Fish and fish products	The Netherlands	3	0
2015	Mixed food	Portugal	3	0
2015	Vegetables and juices and other products thereof	Spain	3	0
2015	Mixed food	Sweden	13	0
2015	Unknown	Sweden	2	0
2015	Lettuce, prepackaged	USA—Multistate	19	1
2015	American cheese, pasteurized	USA—New York	2	1
2015	Sour cream	USA—Oregon	2	0
2016	n.a.	USA—Multistate	5	1
2016	Frozen foods	USA—Multistate		3
2016	Salads	USA—Multistate		1
2016	Artisanal soft cheese, unpasteurized	USA—Multistate	10	2

[a]Two outbreaks.
[b]Three outbreaks.
n.a., Not available.

product is used as an ingredient by other companies. Economic loss combined with reputational damage can be detrimental for companies. Table 2 shows some of the recalls of food that were undertaken in 2017 in the United States, and demonstrates the number of foods and food companies involved. Where products are used as ingredients by other companies, recalls can be very extensive as in the cheese recall (Anonymous, 2017a) and the frozen food recall which resulted in hundreds of products being recalled (Anonymous, 2017b).

2.3 The Role of Whole-Genome Sequencing in Listeriosis Outbreaks

In more recent years, with the advances in sequencing technologies, whole-genome sequencing (WGS) has become an important tool for routine

Table 2 Food Recalls Due to *L. monocytogenes* From February to September 2017 in the United States (https://www.fda.gov/Safety/Recalls/ArchiveRecalls/2017/default.htm)

Month	Product Description
October	Egg Salad Sandwiches, Ham Salad Sandwiches, and Seafood Stuffing
September	Egg Salad Sandwiches, Ham Salad Sandwiches, and Seafood Stuffing; Deli Chicken Salad Sandwich; Fajita blend, Stir fry vegetable, Vegetable kabob, and more
August	Frozen organic dark sweet pitted cherry products; Protein Bars
July	Protein Bars; Matcha Vanilla Oats
June	Hummus; Rabbit and Macaw diets; Baked crunchy chick peas; Almond butter, Cashew butter; Trail Mixes; Cashews, Almonds; Granola and muesli products; Collagen protein bars and bites; Macadamia nuts; Tropical Medley Mix; Grain-free granola products; MacroBars and Thrive Bars; Soybean sprouts; Salad and Slaw kits containing leafy greens; Snack kits containing vegetables; Queso Fresco
May	Cashews; Macadamia Nuts; Queso Fresco; Various burritos; White cheese (2); Spinach; Chicken & Waffle Sandwich; Pancakes, waffles, toast; Cashew Butter
April	Smoked Fish; Sweet Peas; Frozen Peas
March	Beans & Cheese Burritos; Edamame (Soybeans); Cheese (3); Ouleout and Miranda soft raw milk cheese; Monterey Jack Cheese with Jalapeno Peppers; Muenster Cheese; Szechuan Stir Fry
February	Cheese and cheese-containing gift boxes; Butternut Spirals; Stuffed mushrooms; Stuffed mushrooms, fruit and cheese; Colby Cheese and Colby Jack Cheese; Pimento Spread (2); Soureliette Cheese, Tomme Brebis Fedou Cheese; Frozen Ajiaco (vegetables mix)

The number of recalls for a product is given in parentheses.

surveillance to maximize discrimination of isolates and for tracking of listeriosis outbreaks. The Centers for Disease Control (CDC) have applied WGS to their epidemiology investigations since September 2013. What began as a 1-year collaborative pilot project between the CDC, the US Food and Drug Administration, the US Department of Agriculture, the National Center for Biotechnology Information, and state and local health departments (Jackson et al., 2016) has now become standard practice for CDC outbreak investigations. By combining WGS with patient data regarding the foods consumed and the prevalence and behavior of *L. monocytogenes* in those foods, public health officials can detect clusters of listeriosis cases and perhaps limit the possibility of an outbreak, link cases to a likely source of contamination, and potentially identify previously unrecognized sources of contamination. Other jurisdictions have since followed suit. In 2015, the French National Reference Centre for *Listeria* agency implemented WGS and subsequent core genome multilocus sequence typing (cgMLST) as a typing method for *L. monocytogenes* and compared it with the PFGE standard method. The analysis, published in 2017, showed the usefulness and feasibility of WGS for *L. monocytogenes* surveillance and its value over PFGE. The cgMLST detected clusters not detected by PGFE, which enabled elimination of several pseudoclusters defined by PFGE and detection of closely related isolates with different PFGE profiles caused by phage insertions or deletions. It also identified clusters of cases associated with persistent food production environmental contamination that were previously unrecognized (Moura et al., 2017). Overall, the WGS approach led to increased discrimination of isolates, leading to detection of more clusters of related isolates at an earlier stage than PFGE. Recent studies have reported the implementation of WGS in the investigation of a number of large listeriosis outbreaks (Chen et al., 2017; Comandatore et al., 2017; Kleta et al., 2017). WGS has potential in food safety, for example, in rapid identification and characterization of organisms, or enhanced integration of information from human and animal sources, linking apparently sporadic cases of listeriosis to an outbreak (FAO, 2016). Rapidly declining costs will lead to more widespread use of WGS in food safety.

3. METHODS FOR ANALYSIS OF *L. MONOCYTOGENES*

3.1 Methodologies of Sampling for *L. monocytogenes*

To facilitate the control of *L. monocytogenes* in the food-processing environment, particularly in high-risk areas where there is the risk of cross-contamination to the food, an appropriate food-processing environment monitoring program is an advantage (Beno et al., 2016). In the EU, regulation 2073-2005 places the responsibility for the production of safe food on the food business owner. The European Union Reference Laboratory (EURL) on *L. monocytogenes* has published a guidance document on sampling that can help with controlling *L. monocytogenes* (Beaufort et al., 2014). Sampling programs should target areas where contamination would occur, for example, drains, floors, wet areas, hard-to-clean niches in the equipment, doors, windows, and air handling systems. Additionally, samples should not be taken directly after cleaning/disinfection as sampling in this manner would severely decrease the chances of finding *L. monocytogenes.* In order to obtain the most accurate representation of the contamination present, sampling plans must attempt to obtain as many positive samples as possible so that positive areas can be targeted with more rigorous hygiene measures. End-product testing is a useful part of controlling *L. monocytogenes.* However, it is not sufficient on its own to control *L. monocytogenes* as low numbers are difficult to detect in large batches where not all units of the batch will be tested. Food production environment testing should be undertaken in association with end-product testing.

3.2 Methodologies for Sample Analysis of *L. monocytogenes*

There are many conventional and rapid methods available for the detection and enumeration of *L. monocytogenes.* It is not the focus of this chapter to assess the advantages/disadvantages of the various methods. Standard methods for the analysis of foods are generally by enrichment as the numbers present are too low for direct detection by molecular or immunological methods. As a consequence, enumeration is not possible, and the results are qualitative. There have been publications for *Salmonella* (Krämer et al., 2011) and *E. coli* O157:H7 and O26 (Lawal, Burgess, McCabe, Whyte, & Duffy, 2015; Mancusi & Trevisani, 2014) showing that a short enrichment time (5–8 h) can be used for quantification purposes; however, the dynamics of enrichment preclude this approach to quantification of *L. monocytogenes* (Ottesen et al., 2016).

If the sample is enriched, as recommended by the standard method (International Standardisation Organisation [ISO] 11290-1, -2: 2017), polymerase chain reaction (PCR) can be used to detect the pathogen in the enriched culture, while at the same time plating the enriched culture to get a valid result from the standard method. In this way, the time-to-result can be reduced by several days using PCR (for in-house use), while a valid result can be obtained simultaneously using the standard method (Dalmasso et al., 2014). Alternatively, immunological tests can be used for analysis of the enriched culture (Gasanov, Hughes, & Hansbro, 2005). It is important to be aware that such combinations are not yet incorporated into most standard methods, although using the ISO standard methods for validation of alternative methods (ISO 16140-1:2016, ISO 16140-2:2016), the use of such methods is not ruled out.

The ISO standard method for detection of *L. monocytogenes* is ISO 11290-1:2017, and for the enumeration is ISO 11290-2:2017. The detection method is a two-step enrichment, using half Fraser broth (containing half the antibiotic concentration) and full Fraser broth (containing the full concentration of antibiotics), taking a total of 3 days to complete. The selective plating medium used for both methods is Agar Listeria according to Ottaviani and Agosti and any other equivalent selective media, which takes a further 2 days incubation. Following this, a further 2 days is required for confirmation of any suspect positive isolates, resulting in 7 days to get a confirmed positive result. The Bacteriological Analytical Manual (BAM) detection method uses a buffered Listeria enrichment broth incubated for 24–48 h enrichment, followed by plating and confirmation.

Alternative methods validated according to ISO 16140-1:2016 and ISO 16140-2:2016 are used, most notably AOAC International- and/or Association Française de Normalisation (AFNOR, en: French Standardization Association)-validated methods. Alternative methods based on different technologies, including molecular and immunological techniques, are also used. Molecular methods, including DNA hybridization and real-time PCR, result in a more rapid detection of *L. monocytogenes*, although these have the disadvantage that by direct detection the sensitivity is reduced, differentiation of live and dead cells is not feasible, and there is no bacterial isolate for further characterization. One advantage of molecular methods is that they provide confirmation of *L. monocytogenes* as they target virulence genes such as *actA* or *hly*. Immunological methods are based on the antibody–antigen reaction, where antibodies specific for *L. monocytogenes* are used, for example, in flow cytometry assays (Kennedy & Wilkinson, 2016). Enzyme-linked immunosorbent assay incorporates fluorescent or colorimetric detection, or a method combining immunoassay techniques to real-time immunoquantitative PCR (Rajkovic et al., 2012).

4. CHARACTERIZATION OF *L. MONOCYTOGENES* ISOLATES OBTAINED

Once an isolate is obtained from food, comparison of the isolate to clinical isolates or food-processing isolates or other food isolates is important. Such comparison can facilitate identification of foodborne disease outbreaks, source attribution studies, or tracking routes of contamination.

4.1 Differentiation of *L. monocytogenes* Isolates

4.1.1 Serotyping

Traditionally, *L. monocytogenes* is divided into 13 serotypes using antisera. The vast majority (about 95%) of foodborne listeriosis is caused by serotypes 1/2a, 1/2b, and 4b. The serotyping method is subjective, labor intensive, and not very discriminating. In an attempt to overcome the first two disadvantages, a serogrouping PCR method was developed (Doumith, Buchrieser, Glaser, Jacquet, & Martin, 2004).

4.1.2 Serogrouping

The PCR method developed by Doumith et al. (2004) does not differentiate *L. monocytogenes* into all of the serotypes. It differentiates them into serogroups as follows: serogroup 1 (serotypes 1/2a, 1/2c, 3a, and 3c), serogroup 2 (serotypes 1/2c and 3c), serogroup 3 (serotypes 1/2b, 3b, 4b, 4d, and 4e), and serogroup 4 (serotypes 4b, 4d, and 4e). Serotypes 1/2a, 1/2b, and 4b are differentiated into different serogroups, and 100% correlation between these serotypes and the serogroups has been demonstrated (Leong et al., 2017). A combination of serogrouping and serotyping can also be used to facilitate determination of the actual serotype (Fox, Hunt, O'Brien, & Jordan, 2011).

4.1.3 Sequence Type

Multilocus sequence typing (MLST) can be used to characterize the isolates using the DNA sequences of seven housekeeping genes, ABC transporter (*abcZ*), beta-glucosidase (*bglA*), catalase (*cat*), succinyl diaminopimelate desuccinylase (*dapE*), D-amino acid aminotransferase (*dat*), L-lactate dehydrogenase (*ldh*), and histidine kinase (*IhkA*). For each housekeeping gene, the different sequences in a bacterial species are assigned as distinct alleles and, for each isolate, the alleles for each housekeeping gene define the allelic profile or sequence type (ST). MLST databases (http://bigsdb.web.pasteur.fr/; pubmlst.org; mlst.net), containing interrogation and analysis software, include the reference allele sequences and STs which facilitate a query of allele sequences obtained from an organism. A limitation of MLST is that it only uses approximately 0.1% of the genomic sequence to assign an ST and so lacks discriminatory power to differentiate bacterial strains, which limits its use in epidemiological investigations. Multivirulence-locus sequence typing is a similar principle focusing on virulence genes (Chen, Zhang, & Knabel, 2007).

4.1.4 Clonal Complex

In terms of evolutionary biology, a clonal complex (CC) can be defined as a group of bacterial isolates that have descended from a common recent ancestor and accumulate differences among themselves by a predominantly mutational process (Cantinelli et al., 2013). The group generally includes the ancestral genotype and strains with minor variations/alleles at various phylogenetically informative loci. In many bacterial species, MLST is used as a reference method for clonal group definition. In *L. monocytogenes*, an MLST scheme based on seven housekeeping genes was developed and allowed for the recognition of highly prevalent CCs (Chenal-Francisque et al., 2011; Ragon et al., 2008). The term "epidemic clone (EC)" has also been applied to *L. monocytogenes*. This refers to genetically similar isolates involved in either geographically and temporally distant listeriosis outbreaks or large, single listeriosis outbreaks (Cantinelli et al., 2013).

4.1.5 Lineages

L. monocytogenes consists of four evolutionary lineages—lineage I (serotype 4b), lineage II, lineage III, and lineage IV. Most *L. monocytogenes* isolates associated with human clinical cases belong to lineages I (serotypes 1/2b and 4b) and II (serotype 1/2a). Lineage II strains are associated with foods and are associated with the farm environment, whereas most human listeriosis outbreaks are associated with lineage I isolates.

4.1.6 Pulsotype

There is an international standard for the experimental procedures of PFGE (PulseNet, 2017), but there are no standards for naming of the PFGE clusters obtained. Therefore, the designation of a pulsotype is associated with a single laboratory, or a group of laboratories that reach agreement on a naming system.

4.1.7 Ribotype

Although ribotyping does not have the discriminatory power of PFGE, it is a rapid and specific DNA-based subtyping method that is widely used in clinical diagnostics and analysis of microbial communities in food, water, and beverages. Bacterial DNA is cut with restriction enzymes into smaller fragments (more than 300–500 fragments, 1–30 kb in size) than with PFGE. The fragments are separated according to their size by agarose gel electrophoresis, which is followed by hybridization with a labeled 16S or 23S rRNA probe.

Thus, only the fragments coding for such rRNA are visualized and then analyzed. The resulting pattern is digitized and used to identify the origin of the DNA by comparison with reference organisms in a computer database (De Cesare, Mioni, & Manfreda, 2007).

4.1.8 Whole-Genome Sequencing

Generally, WGS allows for highly improved discriminatory power as well as characterization of evolutionary relatedness of isolates, which is not possible with PFGE. In addition, WGS has technical advantages over PFGE and many other subtyping methods such as the potential for a higher level of automation, a simpler integrated work flow, reduced time of analysis, and generation of highly standardized and compatible data even with different sequencing platforms.

4.1.9 cgMLST; wgMLST

With the development of WGS, whole-genome MLST (wgMLST), basically doing MLST on the entire genome, and cgMLST, MLST on the core genome which consists of about 80% of the genome, are being established to utilize a greater percentage of the genome than MLST (Maiden, Caugant, Feavers, Achtman, & Spratt, 2013; Ruppitsch et al., 2015; http://bigsdb.web.pasteur.fr/listeria).

4.2 Subgrouping of *L. monocytogenes* Isolates

Beyond the species level, subtyping of *L. monocytogenes* strains can be used to track putative routes of contamination throughout the processing environment, and to give some indication of the source of such contamination. The decision on the method to use can be based on discriminatory power, reproducibility, speed, cost, and laboratory capacity, although DNA fingerprinting methods, such as PFGE, are best.

4.2.1 Pulsed-Field Gel Electrophoresis

Pulsed-field gel electrophoresis (PFGE) is the "gold standard" method for assessing *L. monocytogenes* strain relatedness. Briefly, the principal of PFGE is as follows: bacteria are embedded in agarose plugs in which the cells are lysed in order to release the DNA, which is then cut into large fragments by restriction enzymes and separated in a horizontal agarose gel using pulsed-field migration. This results in DNA fragment patterns or pulsotypes which differ from one strain to the other depending on the number and size of DNA fragments.

The PulseNet International network (www.pulsenetinternational.org) proposes a standardized PFGE protocol for the study of *L. monocytogenes*. For example, PFGE was used to identify the route of contamination of farmhouse Cheddar cheese from the outside to the inside of the cheese processing facility and finally to the cheese (Dalmasso & Jordan, 2013). The transfer of *L. monocytogenes* strains from dairy farms to associated cheese processing facility has also been demonstrated using PFGE (Ho, Lappi, & Wiedmann, 2007).

4.2.2 Other Subtyping Methods

There are many other subtyping methods that have been used to differentiate strains of *L. monocytogenes*, including ribotyping (Gasanov et al., 2005), MLST (Salcedo, Arreaza, Alcalá, de la Fuente, & Vázquez, 2003), amplified fragment length polymorphism (Graves, Swaminathan, & Hunter, 2007), random amplified polymorphic DNA (Chambel et al., 2007), REP-PCR (Zunabovic, Domig, Pichler, & Kneifel, 2012), and Fourier-transform infrared spectroscopy (Davis & Mauer, 2011). WGS of *L. monocytogenes* isolates has already been discussed.

5. OCCURRENCE OF *L. MONOCYTOGENES*

5.1 Food and the Food-Processing Environment

There are many surveys published on the prevalence of *L. monocytogenes* in food and food-processing environments. Frequently, studies involving the food-processing environment also include food samples so that cross-contamination issues can be studied. However, comparison of the results from one survey to another is not always appropriate. The following variables can influence the prevalence observed:

(1) Different methodologies for sampling are used, for example, the swab size and the area that is swabbed (which can vary from 10 cm^2 to 1 m^2).

(2) Different methodologies for *L. monocytogenes* analysis are used, for example, the ISO, BAM, or alternative methods.

(3) Different frequencies of repeated facility testing, for example, in some cases a number of facilities are surveyed on one occasion, whereas in other cases one facility is surveyed on several occasions and in some other cases, several facilities are surveyed on several occasions.

(4) A facility that has been shown to be positive is targeted, thus biasing the results.

(5) Different sample numbers and different sampling locations can influence the results.

In surveys where the results are comparable, the occurrence of *L. monocytogenes* in the food-processing environment is variable, while the occurrence on food is also variable, but is generally around 5%. Food-processing environments can become contaminated rapidly with *L. monocytogenes* (Bolocan et al., 2016), particularly if measures are not taken to control it. The source of processing environment contamination can, to some extent, be determined by PFGE analysis of isolates from different locations. For example, an isolate from raw materials with a similar PFGE profile to a food-processing environment isolate indicates that the contamination may have come from the raw material (Rückerl et al., 2014), although the food-processing environment contaminating the raw material cannot be ruled out. Similarly, identification of a similar PFGE type inside a food-processing facility and in the area outside the food-processing facility can indicate a potential source of contamination from the outside (Fox et al., 2011), although again transfer from the processing environment to outside cannot be ruled out.

5.2 Persistence of *L. monocytogenes* in the Processing Environment

Persistence of *L. monocytogenes* in a processing environment is generally defined as repeated isolation of an indistinguishable pulsotype from the same facility for longer than 6 months (Ferreira, Wiedmann, Teixeira, & Stasiewicz, 2014; Fox et al., 2011). This indicates that the strain with that pulsotype can persist in the processing environment, despite the hygiene procedures of the facility. It is possible that repeated occurrence of a strain in a processing environment may result from repeated contamination of the processing facility from an outside source, but even in that situation it is necessary for the strain to survive and persist outside. The basis of such persistence is unknown. A genetic marker for persistence has not been identified. Some candidate genes for a genetic marker include *qacH*, SSI, and biofilm forming genes. However, persistent strains that do not have these genes have been identified and transient strains that do not persist have been shown to have these genes. An alternative hypothesis is that the harborage sites and niches where persistent strains survive give them protection from the cleaning procedures (for review, see Carpentier & Cerf, 2011).

5.3 Occurrence of *L. monocytogenes* at Retail Level

Awareness about the presence of *L. monocytogenes* at retail level is relevant because it is the last step before the product reaches the consumer. For that reason, it is important to evaluate the prevalence of *L. monocytogenes* at retail level. Recently conducted risk assessments for *L. monocytogenes* in deli meats indicated that the majority of listeriosis cases and deaths associated with deli meats are probably due to contamination of products at retail. Endrikat et al. (2010) estimated that 83% of human listeriosis cases and deaths attributable to deli meats are due to retail-sliced products, and Pradhan et al. (2010) performed a risk assessment using product-specific growth kinetic parameters that indicated that 63%–84% of human listeriosis deaths linked to deli ham and turkey can be attributed to contamination at retail. Occurrence and cross-contamination at retail level are not as frequent as processing environment studies, but are obviously an important source of listeriosis. Comparing surveys on prevalence of *L. monocytogenes* at retail level has the same limitations as comparing surveys at processing level, as shown in Table 3.

In 2010–2011, a European Union-wide baseline survey on the prevalence of *L. monocytogenes* at retail level was undertaken (European Food Safety Authority, 2013). Similar methodologies were used to determine the prevalence of *L. monocytogenes* in packaged (not frozen) hot or cold-smoked or gravad fish, packaged heat-treated meat products, and soft or semisoft cheeses in 26 member states and 1 nonmember state. A total of 3053 batches of fish, 3530 batches of deli-meat, and 3452 batches of cheese were analyzed at the end of their shelf-life for detection and enumeration of *L. monocytogenes*. A prevalence of 10.3% was determined for the fish samples, while the prevalence on meat and cheese was 2.07% and 0.47%, respectively. The number of samples with a *L. monocytogenes* count exceeding the level of 100 CFU/g at the end of shelf-life was 1.7%, 0.43%, and 0.06% for fish, meat, and cheese samples, respectively.

Surveys conducted during a long period or on thousands of samples usually result in more valuable data on the prevalence and persistence of *L. monocytogenes* and can give the FBOs a greater opportunity to improve their hygiene practices, focusing on specific issues, for example, staff workflows and sanitizing regimes (Leong et al., 2017; Murugesan et al., 2015; Ortiz et al., 2010; Sala et al., 2016; Taguchi et al., 2017) (Table 4).

Table 3 Some Surveys on the Occurrence of *L. monocytogenes* in Food-Processing Environments, Conducted Between 2015 and 2017

Detection Method	Country	No. Samples (No. Companies)	Sample, Swab Type	Survey Period	Reference
50 mL BPW, 1 mL + 25 mL HF broth, 30°C, 24 h. 100°μL from tubes w/black media in 10 mL FF, 37°C, 24 h. 100°μl on chromogenic agar. 16S, PFGE, serogrouping PCR, RAPD-PCR, biofilm (SS), fluorescence microscopy	Spain	270 environmental samples (21)	Sponges moistened with LPT neutralizing broth, 200 cm^2	2010–2011	Rodriguez-Lopez, Saa-Ibusquiza, Mosquera-Fernandez, and Lopez-Cabo (2015)
Bacterial Analytical Manual protocol. Conf: sigB AT sequencing. PFGE	USA	183 raw milk samples, 4430 environmental samples (9)	3M Sponges	2013–2016	Beno et al. (2016)
EN ISO 11290/2000 A1/2005. Gram staining and catalase, oxidase, and motility tests, VITEK 2, confirmation PCR, antibiotics susceptibility test with VITEK 2. Antimicrobial agents	Romania	97 swabs (1)	Cotton swabs. Analyzed in groups of five if from the same area	2015?	Sala et al. (2016)
EN ISO 11290-1	Romania	226 environmental and raw materials samples (1)	Sponge swabs	2012–2013	Bolocan et al. (2015)
EN ISO 11290-1, EN ISO 11290-2: 2004, serotyping, ribotyping, PFGE	Japan	100 retail food samples (55), 87 production swabs and samples (2)	Pickled vegetables, cotton swabs (10 × 10 cm)	2013–2015	Taguchi et al. (2017)

Continued

Table 3 Some Surveys on the Occurrence of *L. monocytogenes* in Food-Processing Environments, Conducted Between 2015 and 2017—cont'd

Detection Method	Country	No. Samples (No. Companies)	Sample, Swab Type	Survey Period	Reference
EN ISO 11290-1. Confirmation: PCR. Serogroup, serotype, PFGE	Ireland	5869 (54)	Food samples, sponge swabs, liquid	2013–2015	Leong et al. (2017)
EN ISO 11290-1. *L.* spp. PCR, virulence genes PCR, serogroup, antibiotic susceptibility, PFGE	Portugal	20 food and 60 swabs (10)	RTEMP, no swab description in the methods	2015?	Henriques, Gama, and Fraqueza (2017)
EN ISO 11290-1:1996/Amd 1:2004 and EN ISO 11290-2:1998/Amd 1:2004	Italy	45—2008/2009 (21), 255—2009/2010 (32), 654—2010/2013 (48)	Sausages, salami and soppresse samplings from the start to the end of production. 197 swabs analyzed for Lm presence	2008–2013	Roccato et al. (2017)
Enrichment + mini VIDAS	USA	255 environmental samples: NFCS (1)	Cotton swabs + sponge swabs	2012–2013	Murugesan, Kucerova, Knabel, and Laborde (2015)
ISO 18593, confirmation: 16S—MLST, serogroup	Brazil	437 (5 dairy + retail)	500 mL milk, brine; 500 g cheese; swabs and cotton swabs	12/2013 to 07/2014	Oxaran et al. (2017)
US Food and Drug Administration Bacteriological Analytical Manual standards (4 h + 20 h enrichment, Oxford plates). Confirmation iap PCR. Serotyping, PFGE	Taiwan	Plant A: 1248 environmental samples and 16 food samples. Plant B: 736 environmental samples and 16 food samples (2)	Tilapia sashimi. Cotton swabs, 10 × 10 cm	2-year period	Chen et al. (2016)

Due to the different methodologies used, comparison of the results for occurrence is not appropriate. n.a., Not available.

Table 4 Some Retail Surveys on the Occurrence of *L. monocytogenes* in Food, Conducted Between 2015 and 2017

Detection Method	Country	No. Samples (No. Areas)	Sample Type	Survey Period	Reference
EN ISO 11290	Czech Republic	387	Cheese	2007–2016	Gelbíčová, Zuzana, Koláčková, and Karpíšková (2017)
EN ISO 11290-1 + API	India	480 (5 markets)	Vegetables	2013–2014	Mritunjay and Kumar (2017)
EN ISO 11290-1,2	Czech Republic	339	Vegetables	2014	Vojkovská et al. (2017)
EN ISO 11290-1,2	UK	862	Meat pies	2013	McLauchlin et al. (2016)
EN ISO 11290-1,2	Portugal	120 (19 companies)	RTE meat-based food	2011–2013	Henriques et al. (2017)
EN ISO 11290-1,2	Spain	2864	Food	2006–2012	Doménech, Jimenez - Belenguer, Amoros, Ferrus, and Escriche (2015)
EN ISO 11290-1,2	Italy	778 (12 cities)	Smoked fish	2011	Acciari et al. (2017)
EN ISO 11290-1,2	Poland	301 (retail)	Smoked fish	2014–2016	Wieczorek and Osek (2017)
EN ISO 11290-1:2004	Nigeria	555 (markets)	RTE vegetables	2012–2013	Ajayeoba, Atanda, Obadina, Bankole, and Adelowo (2016)
Enrichment + PCR	China	200 (retail)	Frozen meat products	n.a.	Tao, Chen, Bie, Lu, and Lu (2017)

Continued

Table 4 Some Retail Surveys on the Occurrence of *L. monocytogenes* in Food, Conducted Between 2015 and 2017—cont'd

Detection Method	Country	No. Samples (No. Areas)	Sample Type	Survey Period	Reference
GB 4789.30-2010	China	648 (retail dairy farms)	Raw milk, meat, others	2013–2014	Wang et al. (2017)
GB 4789.30-2010 + MPN	China	1036 (134 retail)	Variety	2012–2014	Wu et al. (2015)
McClain and Lee (1988)	India	457 (15 cities)	Raw milk	2014–2015	Sharma et al. (2017)
FDA-BAM; MDA-LM	Thailand	200	Variety	2013	Vongkamjan, Fuangpaiboon, Turner, and Vuddhakul (2016)
MPN + API + BAX PCR	USA	27,389 (retail)	Variety	2010–2013	Luchansky et al. (2017)
One enrichment + RAPIDEC	Singapore	475 (retail)	RTE salad	2011–2015	Chau et al. (2017)
Listeria Précis + others	Nigeria	193 (2 fish markets)	Seafood	1-Year study	Esther, Isiaku, and Kolawole (2017)
VIDAS kit + API	Chile	850 (retail)	Variety	2008–2009	Montero et al. (2015)

Due to the different methodologies used, comparison of the results for occurrence is not appropriate.

6. REGULATIONS REGARDING THE OCCURRENCE OF *L. MONOCYTOGENES* IN FOOD

Regulations regarding the occurrence of *L. monocytogenes* in food differ in different jurisdictions. Broadly speaking, there are three different categories, (i) no regulations at all, (ii) presence of *L. monocytogenes* is deemed unsafe at all times, and (iii) up to 100 CFU *L. monocytogenes*/g is allowed in certain circumstances. In general, companies exporting food must comply with the relevant regulations in the country they export to.

In the United States, the regulation in place requires absence of *L. monocytogenes* in 5 × 25 g of food and in the food-processing environment (Anonymous, 2014a). The food is deemed "unsafe" if *L. monocytogenes* is detected. These strict policies pose a serious challenge to food producers and companies that are exporting to the United States and can lead to extensive recalls/withdrawals of food.

The current legislation for *L. monocytogenes* in the EU, Regulation (EC) No 2073/2005 (European Commission, 2005), sets the criteria that foods must comply with regarding *L. monocytogenes*. It requires absence (10 × 25 g samples) for foods intended for infants and special medical purposes. Presence at different levels depending on the ability of the food to support growth of the bacterium is allowed in other foods. For RTE foods unable to support the growth of *L. monocytogenes*, the numbers should be <100 CFU/g throughout the shelf-life of the product (5 × 25 g samples). For RTE foods able to support growth, *L. monocytogenes* must be absent in 5 × 25 g samples at the time the food leaves the production plant or it may not exceed 100 CFU/g throughout its shelf-life (5 × 25 g samples). If the ability of a food to support growth has not been determined, it is assumed that growth will occur, and the criterion of absence is applied. There are similar regulations in Canada (Anonymous, 2011a) and in Australia/New Zealand (Anonymous, 2014b).

Further discussion on regulations in different jurisdictions is reviewed in a special issue of Food Control published in 2011 (Anonymous, 2011b).

7. GROWTH OF *L. MONOCYTOGENES* ON FOOD

The survival and growth of *L. monocytogenes* in food depends on factors intrinsic to the food, for example, pH and water activity, and extrinsic factors such as relative humidity, storage temperature, and packing material.

Processing techniques used in food production, temperature changes, and the physiological state of cells can all cause variations of survival and growth of *L. monocytogenes* in food. Previously stressed cells exposed to sublethal conditions can cause *L. monocytogenes* to be more resistant to additional stressors (Lin & Chou, 2004; Lou & Yousef, 1997).

Where occurrence of *L. monocytogenes* is permitted in food under defined circumstances, the ability of the food to support its growth is important, and it is necessary to determine this ability. This can be done by an assessment of the pH and water activity (a_w) of the food; it is considered that foods with a pH $\leq$ 4.4, an $a_w \leq 0.92$, or with a combination of pH $\leq$ 5.0 and $a_w \leq 0.94$ cannot support growth (European Commission, 2005).

Alternatively, predictive modeling can be used. There are many predictive modeling programs available, where, based on the pH, water activity, temperature of incubation, and other factors, the growth of *L. monocytogenes* can be predicted (for example, "ComBase" (Anonymous, 2017c; Baranyi & Tamplin, 2004), "Food Spoilage and Safety Predictor" (Anonymous, 2014c), and "Pathogen Modeling Program" (Anonymous, 2015)). It is important to remember that such predictions are only an indication of the potential for growth and should not be used as a definitive result. If growth is predicted, there could be other characteristics of the food that would inhibit growth, such as competing microflora, that are not accounted for in the models. For example, using ComBase, Schvartzman, Belessi, Butler, Skandamis, and Jordan (2011) determined that in 40% of cases where growth in cheese was predicted, no growth actually occurred in the cheese. Finally, a determination of actual growth in food can be made by challenge studies (where food is deliberately inoculated), or determination of growth in naturally contaminated food. The EU and other jurisdictions have published guidelines for undertaking challenge studies to determine the ability of food to support the growth of *L. monocytogenes* (Anonymous, 2014b; Beaufort et al., 2014). Challenge studies can be used to determine the growth potential of the organism or to determine the growth rate. A different type of study is required in each of these circumstances.

As many RTE foods are traditionally produced in local regions using variable formulations which may have an impact on the growth of *L. monocytogenes*, studies to determine the ability of each food to support the growth of *L. monocytogenes* must be done. Any changes in the processing method or ingredients, either due to the desire to extend the shelf-life of a product or to address the consumer's demand for the reduction of preservatives in their food, may lead to a change in growth potential (Rivera et al., 2017).

Therefore, challenge studies must be undertaken with each newly formulated food. In cases where growth potential is demonstrated ($\geq$0.5 log increase in numbers from day 0 to day end), the initial numbers and the growth rate determine if the numbers will exceed the limit of 100 CFU/g during shelf-life. The EURL Lm Technical Guidance document (Beaufort et al., 2014) includes a section on undertaking challenge studies to determine growth rate. The major differences between the challenge studies to determine growth potential and the challenge studies to determine growth rate are that when testing growth rate, each strain must be tested individually, sampling must be undertaken on at least 10 occasions, and food storage must be carried out at a uniform temperature.

8. NOVEL METHODS FOR CONTROL OF *L. MONOCYTOGENES* IN FOOD

8.1 Bacteriophage as Novel Control Agents

Bacteriophages are naturally occurring viruses of bacteria which harness the host cell's replication machinery, resulting in host cell lysis and death. Due to the targeted killing action toward specific hosts, bacteriophages have been proposed as biocontrol candidates for *L. monocytogenes* in the food environment. There are many advantages to using phages in a biocontrol capacity. Phages are specific and therefore there is little collateral damage to the natural microbiota of product or environment to be treated. They also are self-replicating, simple and inexpensive to produce, and safe to use, as they have no effect on mammalian cells. Cocktails of live whole phages have been developed which can control *L. monocytogenes* populations in various food matrices and on food preparation surfaces. In 2006, the United States Food and Drug Administration (FDA) approved the use of the LMP-102 phage preparation from Intralytix as an additive for the control of *L. monocytogenes* on RTE foods such as meat and poultry products (Bren, 2007). Listex P100, a phage that targets *L. monocytogenes*, was also approved by the FDA and the United States Department of Agriculture (USDA) for the control of the pathogen in meat and cheese products (Carlton, Noordman, Biswas, De Meester, & Loessner, 2005). Studies on the application of live phages have shown their biocontrol efficacy in a broad range of foods including meat, fish, dairy, and plant foods (Guenther, Huwyler, Richard, & Loessner, 2009). In a study of the broad host range phages A511 and P100, it was found that either phage could bring about a reduction in *L. monocytogenes* numbers by up to 5 log units on most foods tested. An even more dramatic increase was observed in liquid foodstuffs, such as chocolate milk. The study showed that the amounts of phage needed for efficacy varied depending on the food matrix, but that in order to obtain optimum efficiency, concentrations of 10^8 PFU/g of food were required (Guenther et al., 2009). Other studies in this area have demonstrated synergistic activity between bacteriophage and other treatments. Combined phage and nisin treatments reduced bacterial populations of *L. monocytogenes* on Honeydew melons more significantly than with nisin treatments alone (Leverentz, Conway, Janisiewicz, & Camp, 2004).

Another potential approach to the use of phages as biocontrol agents is the application of phage endolysins. Endolysins are enzymes encoded by the phage that degrade the peptidoglycan in the bacterial cell wall, thus allowing release of the progeny phage. As purified proteins, endolysins can also act on the peptidoglycan when added externally. This phenomenon of "lysis from without" has shown to be effective at killing Gram-positive bacteria such as *L. monocytogenes*, but not Gram-negatives due to the presence of the outer membrane. Studies have demonstrated the potential of lysins for *Listeria* biocontrol in fresh dairy products (Gaeng, Scherer, Neve, & Loessner, 2000), but the engineered nature of the lysin-producing strain raises some safety concerns and further work on this area is required to overcome this and other challenges.

8.2 Bacteriocins as Novel Control Agents

Bacteriocins are ribosomally synthesized peptides or proteins produced by certain bacteria which are active at inhibiting various other bacterial groups (Gálvez, Abriouel, López, & Ben Omar, 2007). They have advantages as bioprotective agents since they are generally produced by food-grade organisms, demonstrate activity against a wide range of pathogenic and spoilage bacteria, and are generally pH- and heat-stable (Cotter, Hill, & Ross, 2005). The use of bacteriocins during the food manufacturing process can reduce economic losses due to food spoilage and prevent transfer of pathogens through the food chain while satisfying consumer demand for minimally processed fresh-tasting foods.

To date, nisin is the only bacteriocin that has been approved by the World Health Organization for use as a food preservative. The class I bacteriocin nisin has been used as an effective biopreservative in dairy products for many years. Pediocin PA-1 is a class IIa bacteriocin that shows a particularly strong activity against *L. monocytogenes* (Rodriguez, Martinez, Horn, & Dodd, 2003).

Other bacteriocins have also demonstrated efficacy against *L. monocytogenes* including lacticin 3147 (Morgan, Galvin, Ross, & Hill, 2001), divergicin M35 (Tahiri et al., 2009), enterocin AS-48 (Ananou et al., 2005), and piscicosin CS526 (Azuma, Bagenda, Yamamoto, Kawai, & Yamazaki, 2007). While there are many different modes of action, most bacteriocins act by forming a pore in the cell membrane disrupting the membrane potential and causing cell death. Bacteriocinogenic strains can be used either directly as starter cultures, as adjunct or cocultures in combination with a starter culture, or as purified products extracted from the producing cultures (Gálvez et al., 2007).

There are strict regulatory requirements for use of bacteriocins in food preservation. For example, they must not have any negative effect on the food properties, they must be stable during food storage, be economically feasible, and should have no medical use. The development of strains that are highly tolerant or resistant to bacteriocins may decrease the efficiency of their use as biopreservatives. Resistance of some *L. monocytogenes* to bacteriocins, and subsequent growth of these resistant strains, has been shown (Lourenço, Kamnetz, Gadotti, & Diez-Gonzalez, 2017).

8.3 Future Perspectives on Bacteriocins and Bacteriophage

Since a single bacteriocin-based or bacteriophage-based approach is unlikely to control safety issues in foods, it is most likely that a combination of novel biotechnologies will be exploited. The most promising results include a mixture of natural antagonistic bacteria and their bacteriocins, or a combination of antagonistic bacteria, bacteriocins, and bacteriophages (Vijayakumar & Muriana, 2017), or the utilization of bacteriocins and bacteriophages (Figueiredo & Almeida, 2017).

9. CONCLUDING REMARKS

Due to its ubiquitous nature, its ability to contaminate food and food-processing environments, and its ability to cause severe life-threatening disease, *L. monocytogenes* is a concern for industry and public health authorities. Vigilance with regard to its occurrence in the food-processing environment can contribute to a reduction in cross-contamination to food. Allied with novel methods to control its growth in food, the burden of *L. monocytogenes* to industry and public health authorities can be reduced.

REFERENCES

Acciari, V. A., Torresi, M., Iannetti, L., Scattolini, S., Pomilio, F., Decastelli, L., et al. (2017). *Listeria monocytogenes* in smoked salmon and other smoked fish at retail in Italy: Frequency of contamination and strain characterization in products from different manufacturers. *Journal of Food Protection, 80*(2), 271–278. https://doi.org/10.4315/0362-028X.JFP-15-599.

Ajayeoba, T. A., Atanda, O. O., Obadina, A. O., Bankole, M. O., & Adelowo, O. O. (2016). The incidence and distribution of *Listeria monδcytogenes* in ready-to-eat vegetables in South-Western Nigeria. *Food Science & Nutrition, 4*(1), 59–66. https://doi.org/10.1002/fsn3.263.

Ananou, S., Garriga, M., Hugas, M., Maqueda, M., Martinez-Bueno, M., Galvez, A., et al. (2005). Control of *Listeria monocytogenes* in model sausages by enterocin AS-48. *International Journal of Food Microbiology, 103*, 179–190.

Anonymous. (2011a). *Policy on* Listeria monocytogenes *in ready-to-eat (RTE) foods*. Available at: https://www.canada.ca/en/health-canada/services/food-nutrition/legislation-guidelines/policies/policy-listeria-monocytogenes-ready-eat-foods-2011.html. Accessed 10 January 2018.

Anonymous. (2011b). Special issue: *Listeria regulation. Food Control, 22*(9), 1477–1550.

Anonymous. (2014a). *10240.4 verification activities for the* Listeria monocytogenes (Lm) *regulation and the ready-to-eat (RTE) sampling program*. Washington, DC: United States Department of Agriculture–Food Safety and Inspection Service. Available at: https://www.fsis.usda.gov/wps/wcm/connect/b8cd03ed-222c-4cef-ad92-3647e3be6c53/10240.4.pdf?MOD=AJPERES. Accessed 10 January 2018.

Anonymous. (2014b). *Guidance on the application of microbiological criteria for* Listeria monocytogenes *in RTE food*. The Australian and New Zealand Food Standards System, Food Standards Australia New Zealand. Available at: http://www.foodstandards.gov.au/foodsafety/standards/Pages/Microbiological-limits-for-food-(Standard-1.6.1).aspx. Accessed 10 January 2018.

Anonymous. (2014c). *Food spoilage and safety predictor (FSSP)*. Available at: http://fssp.food.dtu.dk/. Accessed 10 January 2018.

Anonymous. (2015). *Pathogen modeling program (PMP) online*. Available at: https://pmp.errc.ars.usda.gov/PMPonline.aspx. Accessed 10 January 2018.

Anonymous. (2017a). *Anatomy of a cheese recall*. Available at: https://www.theatlantic.com/health/archive/2017/02/anatomy-of-a-cheese-recall/517053/. Accessed 9 January 2018.

Anonymous. (2017b). *Updated: CRF frozen foods expands voluntary recall to include all frozen vegetable and fruit products due to possible health risk*. Available at: https://www.prnewswire.com/news-releases/crf-frozen-foods-expands-voluntary-recall-to-include-all-frozen-vegetable-and-fruit-products-due-to-possible-health-risk-300261539.html. Accessed 9 January 2018.

Anonymous. (2017c). *ComBase*. Available at: https://www.combase.cc/index.php/en/. Accessed 10 January 2018.

Azuma, T., Bagenda, D. K., Yamamoto, T., Kawai, Y., & Yamazaki, K. (2007). Inhibition of *Listeria monocytogenes* by freeze-dried piscicocin CS526 fermentate in food. *Letters in Applied Microbiology, 44*, 138–144.

Baranyi, J., & Tamplin, M. L. (2004). ComBase: A common database on microbial responses to food environments. *Journal of Food Protection, 67*(9), 1967–1971. Retrieved from http://www.ncbi.nlm.nih.gov/pubmed/15453591.

Beaufort, A., Bergis, H., Lardeux, A.-L., Polet, M., Botteldoorn, N., Papageorgiou, G., et al. (2014). Technical guidance document for conducting shelf-life studies on *Listeria monocytogenes* in ready-to-eat foods. In *EURL Lm technical guidance document*: European Union Reference Laboratory for *Listeria monocytogenes*. Available at: https://ec.europa.eu/food/sites/food/files/safety/docs/biosafety_fh_mc_technical_guidance_document_listeria_in_rte_foods.pdf. Accessed 10 January 2018.

Beno, S. M., Stasiewicz, M. J., Andrus, A. D., Raylea, R. D., Kent, D. J., Martin, N. H., et al. (2016). Development and validation of pathogen environmental monitoring programs for small cheese processing facilities. *Journal of Food Protection*, *79*(12), 2095–2106. https://doi.org/10.4315/0362-028X.JFP-16-241.

Bolocan, A. S., Nicolau, A. I., Alvarez-Ordóñez, A., Borda, D., Oniciuc, E. A., Stessl, B., et al. (2016). Dynamics of *Listeria monocytogenes* colonisation in a newly-opened meat processing facility. *Meat Science*, *113*, 26–34.

Bolocan, A. S., Oniciuc, E. A., Alvarez-Ordóñez, A., Wagner, M., Rychli, K., Jordan, K., et al. (2015). Putative cross-contamination routes of *Listeria monocytogenes* in a meat processing facility in Romania. *Journal of Food Protection*, *78*(9), 1664–1674. https://doi.org/10.4315/0362-028X.JFP-14-539.

Bren, L. (2007). Bacteria-eating virus approved as food additive. *FDA Consumer*, *41*, 20–22.

Buchanan, R. L., Gorris, L. G. M., Hayman, M. M., Jackson, T. C., & Whiting, R. C. (2017). A review of *Listeria monocytogenes*: An update on outbreaks, virulence, dose-response, ecology, and risk assessments. *Food Control*, *75*, 1–13. https://doi.org/10.1016/j.foodcont.2016.12.016.

Cantinelli, T., Chenal-Francisque, V., Diancourt, L., Frezal, L., Leclercq, A., Wirth, T., et al. (2013). "Epidemic clones" of *Listeria monocytogenes* are widespread and ancient clonal groups. *Journal of Clinical Microbiology*, *51*(11), 3770–3779. https://doi.org/10.1128/JCM.01874-13.

Carlton, R. M., Noordman, W. H., Biswas, B., De Meester, E. D., & Loessner, M. J. (2005). Bacteriophage P100 for control of *Listeria monocytogenes* in foods: Genome sequence, bioinformatic analyses, oral toxicity study, and application. *Regulatory Toxicology and Pharmacology*, *43*, 301–312.

Carpentier, B., & Cerf, O. (2011). Review—Persistence of *Listeria monocytogenes* in food industry equipment and premises. *International Journal of Food Microbiology*, *145*(1), 1–8. https://doi.org/10.1016/j.ijfoodmicro.2011.01.005.

Centers for Disease Control. (2017). *Information for health professionals and laboratories*. Available at: https://www.cdc.gov/listeria/technical.html. Accessed 9 January 2018.

Comandatore, F., Corbella, M., Andreoli, G., Scaltriti, E., Aguzzi, M., Gaiarsa, S., et al. (2017). Genomic characterization helps dissecting an outbreak of listeriosis in Northern Italy. *PLoS Currents Outbreaks* Edition 1. https://doi.org/10.1371/currents.outbreaks.633fd8994e9f06f31b3494567c7e504c.

Chambel, L., Sol, M., Fernandes, I., Barbosa, M., Zilhão, I., Barata, B., et al. (2007). Occurrence and persistence of *Listeria* spp. in the environment of ewe and cow's milk cheese dairies in Portugal unveiled by an integrated analysis of identification, typing and spatial-temporal mapping along production cycle. *International Journal of Food Microbiology*, *116*, 52–63. https://doi.org/10.1016/j.ijfoodmicro.2006.12.035.

Chau, M. L., Aung, K. T., Hapuarachchi, H. C., Sze, P., Lee, V., Lim, P. Y., et al. (2017). Microbial survey of ready-to-eat salad ingredients sold at retail reveals the occurrence and the persistence of *Listeria monocytogenes* sequence types 2 and 87 in pre-packed smoked salmon. *BMC Microbiology*, *17*(46), 1–13. https://doi.org/10.1186/s12866-017-0956-z.

Chen, Y., Luo, Y., Carleton, H., Timme, R., Melka, D., Muruvanda, T., et al. (2017). Whole genome and core genome multilocus sequence typing and single nucleotide polymorphism analyses of *Listeria monocytogenes* isolates associated with an outbreak linked to cheese, United States, 2013. *Applied and Environmental Microbiology*, *83*(15), e00633–17, 1–15. https://doi.org/10.1128/AEM.00633-17.

Chen, B.-Y., Wang, C.-Y., Wang, C.-L., Fan, Y.-C., Weng, I.-T., & Chou, C.-H. (2016). Prevalence and persistence of *Listeria monocytogenes* in ready-to-eat tilapia sashimi processing plants. *Journal of Food Protection*, *79*(11), 1898–1903. https://doi.org/10.4315/0362-028X.JFP-16-149.

Chen, Y., Zhang, W., & Knabel, S. J. (2007). Multi-virulence-locus sequence typing identifies single nucleotide polymorphisms which differentiate epidemic clones and outbreak strains of *Listeria monocytogenes*. *Journal of Clinical Microbiology, 45*(3), 835–846.

Chenal-Francisque, V., Lopez, J., Cantinelli, T., Caro, V., Tran, C., Leclercq, A., et al. (2011). Worldwide distribution of major clones of *Listeria monocytogenes*. *Emerging Infectious Diseases, 17*(6), 1110–1112. https://doi.org/10.3201/eid1706.101778.

Cotter, P. D., Hill, C., & Ross, R. P. (2005). Bacteriocins: Developing innate immunity for food. *Nature Reviews. Microbiology, 3*, 777–788.

Cruz, C. D., & Fletcher, G. C. (2011). Prevalence and biofilm-forming ability of *Listeria monocytogenes* in New Zealand mussel (Perna canaliculus) processing plants. *Food Microbiology, 28*(7), 1387–1393. https://doi.org/10.1016/j.fm.2011.06.014.

Dalmasso, M., & Jordan, K. (2013). Process environment sampling can help to reduce the occurrence of *Listeria monocytogenes* in food processing facilities. *Irish Journal of Agricultural and Food Research, 52*(1), 93–100.

Dalmasso, M., Sorin Bolocan, A., Hernandez, M., Kapetanakou, A., Kuchta, T., Manios, S., et al. (2014). Comparison of polymerase chain reaction methods and plating for analysis of enriched cultures of *Listeria monocytogenes* when using the ISO11290-1 method. *Journal of Microbiological Methods, 98*, 8–14.

Davis, R., & Mauer, L. J. (2011). Subtyping of *Listeria monocytogenes* at the haplotype level by Fourier transform infrared (FT-IR) spectroscopy and multivariate statistical analysis. *International Journal of Food Microbiology, 150*(2–3), 140–149. https://doi.org/10.1016/j.ijfoodmicro.2011.07.024.

De Cesare, A., Mioni, R., & Manfreda, G. (2007). Prevalence of *Listeria monocytogenes* in fresh and fermented Italian sausages and ribotyping of contaminating strains. *International Journal of Food Microbiology, 120*, 124–130.

Doménech, E., Jimenez -Belenguer, A., Amoros, J. A., Ferrus, M. A., & Escriche, I. (2015). Prevalence and antimicrobial resistance of *Listeria monocytogenes* and *Salmonella* strains isolated in ready-to-eat foods in Eastern Spain. *Food Control, 47*, 120–125. https://doi.org/10.1016/j.foodcont.2014.06.043.

Doumith, M., Buchrieser, C., Glaser, P., Jacquet, C., & Martin, P. (2004). Differentiation of the major *Listeria monocytogenes* serovars by multiplex PCR. *Journal of Clinical Microbiology, 42*(8), 3819–3822. https://doi.org/10.1128/JCM.42.8.3819.

Endrikat, S., Gallagher, D., Pouillot, R., Hicks Quesenberry, H., Labarre, D., Schroeder, C. M., et al. (2010). A comparative risk assessment for *Listeria monocytogenes* in prepackaged versus retail-sliced deli meat. *Journal of Food Protection, 73*(4), 612–619. https://doi.org/10.4315/0362-028X-73.4.612.

Esther, A. E., Isiaku, S. A., & Kolawole, B. (2017). Listeria species in seafoods from two major fish markets in Lagos, Nigeria. *Covenant Journal of Physical and Life Sciences, 5*(1), 52–58.

European Commission. (2005). Commission Regulation (EC) N0. 2073/2005 of 15 November 2005 on microbiological criteria for foodstuffs. *Official Journal of the European Communities, 338*(2073), 1–26. https://doi.org/10.1016/B978-0-12-385007-2.00012-7.

European Commission. (2017). The European Union summary report on trends and sources of zoonoses, zoonotic agents and food-borne outbreaks in 2016. *EFSA Journal, 15*(12), 5077. 1–228. https://doi.org/10.2903/j.efsa.2017.5077.

European Food Safety Authority. (2013). Analysis of the baseline survey on the prevalence of *Listeria monocytogenes* in certain ready-to-eat foods in the EU, 2010–2011 part A: *Listeria monocytogenes* prevalence estimates. *EFSA Journal, 11*(6), 3241. https://doi.org/10.2903/j.efsa.2013.3241.

Ferreira, V., Wiedmann, M., Teixeira, P., & Stasiewicz, A. M. J. (2014). Listeria monocytogenes persistence in food-associated environments: Epidemiology, strain characteristics, and implications for public health. *Journal of Food Protection, 77*(1), 150–170. https://doi.org/10.4315/0362-028X.JFP-13-150.

Figueiredo, A. C. L., & Almeida, R. C. C. (2017). Antibacterial efficacy of nisin, bacteriophage P100 and sodium lactate against *Listeria monocytogenes* in ready-to-eat sliced pork ham. *Brazilian Journal of Microbiology, 48*(4), 1–6. https://doi.org/10.1016/j.bjm.2017.02.010.

Food and Agriculture Organization (FAO). (2016). *Applications of whole genome sequencing in food safety management*. Rome: FAO.

Fox, E., Hunt, K., O'Brien, M., & Jordan, K. (2011). *Listeria monocytogenes* in Irish farmhouse cheese processing environments. *International Journal of Food Microbiology, 145*, S39–S45. https://doi.org/10.1016/j.ijfoodmicro.2010.10.012.

Gaeng, S., Scherer, S., Neve, H., & Loessner, M. J. (2000). Gene cloning and expression and secretion of *Listeria monocytogenes* bacteriophage-lytic enzymes in *Lactococcus lactis*. *Applied and Environmental Microbiology, 66*, 2951–2958.

Gálvez, A., Abriouel, H., López, R. L., & Ben Omar, N. (2007). Bacteriocin-basedstrategies for food biopreservation. *International Journal of Food Microbiology, 120*, 51–70.

Gasanov, U., Hughes, D., & Hansbro, P. M. (2005). Methods for the isolation and identification of *Listeria* spp. and *Listeria monocytogenes*: A review. *FEMS Microbiology Reviews, 29*, 851–875.

Gelbíčová, T., Zuzana, T., Koláčková, I., & Karpíšková, R. (2017). A survey on prevalence and sources of *Listeria monocytogenes* in ripened and steamed cheeses from the retail market in the Czech Republic. *Journal of Food and Nutrition Research, 56*(1), 42–47.

Graves, L. M., Swaminathan, B., & Hunter, S. B. (2007). Subtyping *Listeria monocytogenes*. In T. E. Ryser & E. H. Marth (Eds.), *Listeria, listeriosis and food safety*. Boca Raton: CRC Press, Taylor & Francis Group.

Guenther, S., Huwyler, D., Richard, S., & Loessner, M. J. (2009). Virulent bacteriophage for efficient biocontrol of *Listeria monocytogenes* in ready-to-eat foods. *Applied and Environmental Microbiology, 75*, 93–100.

Henriques, A. R., Gama, L. T., & Fraqueza, M. J. (2017). Tracking *Listeria monocytogenes* contamination and virulence-associated characteristics in the ready-to-eat meat-based food products industry according to the hygiene level. *International Journal of Food Microbiology, 242*, 101–106. https://doi.org/10.1016/j.ijfoodmicro.2016.11.020.

Ho, A. J., Lappi, V. R., & Wiedmann, M. (2007). Longitudinal monitoring of *Listeria monocytogenes* contamination patterns in a farmstead dairy processing facility. *Journal of Dairy Science, 90*(5), 2517–2524.

Jackson, B. R., Tarr, C., Strain, E., Jackson, K. A., Conrad, A., Carleton, H., et al. (2016). Implementation of nationwide real-time whole-genome sequencing to enhance listeriosis outbreak detection and investigation. *Clinical Infectious Diseases: An Official Publication of the Infectious Diseases Society of America, 63*(3), 380–386. https://doi.org/10.1093/cid/ciw242.

Kennedy, D., & Wilkinson, M. W. (2016). Application of flow cytometry to the detection of pathogenic bacteria. *Current Issues in Molecular Biology, 23*, 21–38. https://doi.org/10.21775/cimb.023.021.

Kleta, S., Hammerl, J., Dieckmann, R., Malorny, B., Borowiak, M., Halbedel, S., et al. (2017). Molecular tracing to find source of protracted invasive listeriosis outbreak, southern Germany, 2012–2016. *Emerging Infectious Diseases, 23*(10), 1680–1683. https://doi.org/10.3201/eid2310.161623.

Krämer, N., Löfström, C., Vigre, H., Hoorfar, J., Bunge, C., & Malorny, B. (2011). A novel strategy to obtain quantitative data for modelling: Combined enrichment and real-time PCR for enumeration of salmonellae from pig carcasses. *International Journal of Food Microbiology, 145*, S86–S95.

Latorre, A. A., Van Kessel, J. S., Karns, J. S., Zurakowski, M. J., Pradhan, A. K., Boor, K. J., et al. (2010). Biofilm in milking equipment on a dairy farm as a potential source of bulk tank milk contamination with *Listeria monocytogenes*. *Journal of Dairy Science*, *93*(6), 2792–2802. https://doi.org/10.3168/jds.2009-2717.

Lawal, D., Burgess, C., McCabe, E., Whyte, P., & Duffy, G. (2015). Development of a quantitative real time PCR assay to detect and enumerate *Escherichia coli* O157 and O26 serogroups in bovine recto-anal swabs. *Journal of Microbiological Methods*, *114*, 9–15.

Leong, D., NicAogáin, K., Luque-Sastre, L., McManamon, O., Hunt, K., Alvarez-Ordonez, A., et al. (2017). A 3-year multi-food study of the presence and persistence of *Listeria monocytogenes* in 54 small food businesses in Ireland. *International Journal of Food Microbiology*, *249*(16), 18–26. https://doi.org/10.1016/j.ijfoodmicro.2017.02.015.

Leverentz, B., Conway, W. S., Janisiewicz, W., & Camp, M. J. (2004). Optimizing concentration and timing of a phage spray application to reduce *Listeria monocytogenes* on honeydew melon tissue. *Journal of Food Protection*, *67*, 1682–1686.

Lin, Y.-D., & Chou, C.-C. (2004). Effect of heat shock on thermal tolerance and susceptibility of *Listeria monocytogenes* to other environmental stresses. *Food Microbiology*, *21*(5), 605–610. https://doi.org/10.1016/j.fm.2003.10.007.

Lou, Y., & Yousef, A. E. (1997). Adaptation to sublethal environmental stresses protects *Listeria monocytogenes* against lethal preservation factors. *Applied and Environmental Microbiology*, *63*(4), 1252–1255.

Lourenço, A., Kamnetz, M. B., Gadotti, C., & Diez-Gonzalez, F. (2017). Antimicrobial treatments to control *Listeria monocytogenes* in queso fresco. *Food Microbiology*, *64*, 47–55. https://doi.org/10.1016/j.fm.2016.12.014.

Luchansky, J. B., Chen, Y., Porto-Fett, A. C. S., Pouillot, E., Shoyer, B. A., Johnson-Derycke, R., et al. (2017). Survey for *Listeria monocytogenes* in and on ready-to-eat foods from retail establishments in the United States (2010 through 2013): Assessing potential changes of pathogen prevalence and levels in a decade. *Journal of Food Protection*, *80*(6), 903–921. https://doi.org/10.4315/0362-028X.JFP-16-420.

Maertens de Noordhout, C., Devleesschauwer, B., Angulo, F. J., Verbeke, G., Haagsma, J., Kirk, M., et al. (2014). The global burden of listeriosis: A systematic review and meta-analysis. *The Lancet Infectious Diseases*, *14*(11), 1073–1082. https://doi.org/10.1016/S1473-3099(14)70870-9.

Maiden, M., Caugant, D., Feavers, I., Achtman, M., & Spratt, B. (2013). *MLST multi locus sequence typing*. Available from: http://www.mlst.net. Accessed 10 January 2018.

Mancusi, R., & Trevisani, M. (2014). Enumeration of verocytotoxigenic *Escherichia coli* (VTEC) O157 and O26 in milk by quantitative PCR. *International Journal of Food Microbiology*, *184*, 121–127.

McClain, D., & Lee, W. H. (1988). Development of USDA-FSIS method for isolation of Listeria monocytogenes from raw meat & poultry. *Journal of the Association of Analytical Chemists*, *71*, 660–664.

McLauchlin, J., Aird, H., Charlett, A., Elviss, N., Fox, A., Kaye, M., et al. (2016). Assessment of the microbiological quality of meat pies from retail sale in England 2013. *Journal of Food Protection*, *79*(5), 781–788. https://doi.org/10.4315/0362-028X.JFP-15-535.

Montero, D., Bodero, M., Riveros, G., Lapierre, L., Gaggero, A., Vidal, R. M., et al. (2015). Molecular epidemiology and genetic diversity of *Listeria monocytogenes* isolates from a wide variety of ready-to-eat foods and their relationship to clinical strains from listeriosis outbreaks in Chile. *Frontiers in Microbiology*, *6*, 384. https://doi.org/10.3389/fmicb.2015.00384. https://doi.org/10.3389/fmicb.2015.00384.

Moorhead, S. M., & Dykes, G. A. (2004). Influence of the sigB gene on the cold stress survival and subsequent recovery of two *Listeria monocytogenes* serotypes. *International Journal of Food Microbiology*, *91*(1), 63–72. https://doi.org/10.1016/S0168-1605(03)00332-5.

Morgan, S. M., Galvin, M., Ross, R. P., & Hill, C. (2001). Evaluation of a spray-dried lacticin 3147 powder for the control of *Listeria monocytogenes* and *Bacillus cereus* in a range of food systems. *Letters in Applied Microbiology*, *33*(5), 387–391. https://doi.org/10.1046/j.1472-765X.2001.01016.x.

Moura, A., Tourdjman, M., Leclercq, A., Hamelin, E., Laurent, E., Fredriksen, N., et al. (2017). Real-time whole-genome sequencing for surveillance of *Listeria monocytogenes*, France. *Emerging Infectious Diseases*, *23*(9), 1462–1470. https://doi.org/10.3201/eid2309.170336.

Mritunjay, S. K., & Kumar, V. (2017). A study on prevalence of microbial contamination on the surface of raw salad vegetables. *3 Biotech*, 7(1), 1–9. https://doi.org/10.1007/s13205-016-0585-5.

Murugesan, L., Kucerova, Z., Knabel, S. J., & Laborde, L. F. (2015). Predominance and distribution of a persistent *Listeria monocytogenes* clone in a commercial fresh mushroom processing environment. *Journal of Food Protection*, *78*(11), 1988–1998. https://doi.org/10.4315/0362-028X.JFP-15-195.

Ortiz, S., Ló Pez, V., Villatoro, D., Ló Pez, P., Dá, J. C., & Martínez-Suá Rez, J. V. (2010). A 3-year surveillance of the genetic diversity and persistence of *Listeria monocytogenes* in an Iberian pig slaughterhouse and processing plant. *Foodborne Pathogens and Disease*, 7(10), 1177–1184. https://doi.org/10.1089/fpd.2010.0535.

Ottesen, A., Grim, C., Hanes, D., Reed, E., Brown, E., Ryan, G., et al. (2016). Enrichment dynamics of *Listeria monocytogenes* and the associated microbiome from naturally contaminated ice cream linked to a listeriosis outbreak. *BMC Microbiology*, *16*(1), 275.

Oxaran, V., Hwa, S., Lee, I., Chaul, L. T., Corassin, C. H., Barancelli, G. V., et al. (2017). *Listeria monocytogenes* incidence changes and diversity in some Brazilian dairy industries and retail products. *Food Microbiology*, *68*, 16–23. https://doi.org/10.1016/j.fm.2017.06.012.

Pradhan, A. K., Ivanek, R., Gröhn, Y. T., Bukowski, R., Geornaras, I., Sofos, J. N., et al. (2010). Quantitative risk assessment of listeriosis-associated deaths due to *Listeria monocytogenes* contamination of deli meats originating from manufacture and retail. *Journal of Food Protection*, *73*(4), 620–630. https://doi.org/10.4315/0362-028X-73.4.620.

PulseNet. 2017. Available at: http://www.pulsenetinternational.org/. Accessed March 12, 2018.

Ragon, M., Wirth, T., Hollandt, F., Lavenir, R., Lecuit, M., Le Monnier, A., et al. (2008). A new perspective on *Listeria monocytogenes* evolution. *PLoS Pathogens*, *4*(9), e1000146. https://doi.org/10.1371/journal.ppat.1000146.

Rajkovic, A., El Moualij, B., Fikri, Y., Dierick, K., Zorzi, W., Heinen, E., et al. (2012). Detection of *C. botulinum* neurotoxins A and B in milk by ELISA and immuno-PCR at higher sensitivity than mouse bio-assay. *Food Analytical Methods*, *5*, 319–326.

Rivera, D., Toledo, V., Reyes-Jara, A., Navarrete, P., Tamplin, M., Kimura, B., et al. (2017). Approaches to empower the implementation of new tools to detect and prevent foodborne pathogens in food processing. *Food Microbiology*. in press. https://doi.org/10.1016/j.fm.2017.07.009.

Roccato, A., Uyttendaele, M., Barrucci, F., Cibin, V., Favretti, M., Cereser, A., et al. (2017). Artisanal Italian salami and soppresse: Identification of control strategies to manage microbiological hazards. *Food Microbiology*, *61*, 5–13. https://doi.org/10.1016/j.fm.2016.07.010.

Rodriguez, J. M., Martinez, M. I., Horn, N., & Dodd, H. M. (2003). Heterologous production of bacteriocins by lactic acid bacteria. *International Journal of Food Microbiology*, *80*, 101–116.

Rodriguez-Lopez, P., Saa-Ibusquiza, P., Mosquera-Fernandez, M., & Lopez-Cabo, M. (2015). *Listeria monocytogenes*-carrying consortia in food industry. Composition, subtyping and numerical characterisation of mono-species biofilm dynamics on stainless steel. *International Journal of Food Microbiology*, *206*, 84–95.

Rückerl, I., Muhterem-Uyar, M., Muri-Klinger, S., Wagner, K. H., Wagner, M., & Stessl, B. (2014). *L. monocytogenes* in a cheese processing facility: Learning from contamination scenarios over three years of sampling. *International Journal of Food Microbiology, 189*, 98–105. https://doi.org/10.1016/j.ijfoodmicro.2014.08.001.

Ruppitsch, W., Pietzka, A., Prior, K., Bletz, S., Fernandez, H. L., Allerberger, F., et al. (2015). Defining and evaluating a core genome multilocus sequence typing scheme for whole-genome sequence-based typing of *Listeria monocytogenes*. *Journal of Clinical Microbiology, 53*(9), 2869–2876. https://doi.org/10.1128/JCM.01193-15.

Sala, C., Morar, A., Tîrziu, E., Nichita, I., Imre, M., & Imre, K. (2016). Environmental occurrence and antibiotic susceptibility profile of *Listeria monocytogenes* at a slaughterhouse raw processing plant in Romania. *Journal of Food Protection, 79*(10), 1794–1797. https://doi.org/10.4315/0362-028X.JFP-16-052.

Salcedo, C., Arreaza, L., Alcalá, B., de la Fuente, L., & Vázquez, J. A. (2003). Development of a multilocus sequence typing method for analysis of *Listeria monocytogenes* clones. *Journal of Clinical Microbiology, 41*(2), 757–762. https://doi.org/10.1128/JCM.41.2.757.

Scallan, E., Hoekstra, R. M., Angulo, F. J., Tauxe, R. V., Widdowson, M.-A., Roy, L., et al. (2011). Foodborne illness acquired in the United States—Major pathogens. *Emerging Infectious Diseases, 17*(1), 7–15. Retrieved from http://wwwnc.cdc.gov/eid/article/17/1/p1-1101_article.

Schvartzman, M. S., Belessi, C., Butler, F., Skandamis, P. N., & Jordan, K. N. (2011). Effect of pH and water activity on the growth limits of *Listeria monocytogenes* in a cheese matrix at two contamination levels. *Journal of Food Protection, 74*(11), 1805–1813. https://doi.org/10.4315/0362-028X.JFP-11-102.

Sharma, S., Sharma, V., Dahiya, D. K., Khan, A., Mathur, M., & Sharma, A. (2017). Prevalence, virulence potential, and antibiotic susceptibility profile of *Listeria monocytogenes* isolated from bovine raw milk oamples obtained from Rajasthan, India. *Foodborne Pathogens and Disease, 14*(3), 132–140. https://doi.org/10.1089/fpd.2016.2118.

Taguchi, M., Kanki, M., Yamaguchi, Y., Inamura, H., Koganei, Y., Sano, T., et al. (2017). Prevalence of *Listeria monocytogenes* in retail lightly pickled vegetables and its successful control at processing plants. *Journal of Food Protection, 80*(3), 467–475. https://doi.org/10.4315/0362-028X.JFP-16-062.

Tahiri, I., Desbiens, M., Kheadr, E., Lacroix, C., & Fliss, I. (2009). Comparison of different application strategies of divergicin M35 for inactivation of *Listeria monocytogenes* in cold-smoked wild salmon. *Food Microbiology, 26*, 783–793.

Tao, T., Chen, Q., Bie, X., Lu, F., & Lu, Z. (2017). Investigation on prevalence of *Listeria* spp. and *Listeria monocytogenes* in animal-derived foods by multiplex PCR assay targeting novel genes. *Food Control, 73*, 704–711. https://doi.org/10.1016/j.foodcont.2016.09.026.

Vijayakumar, P., & Muriana, P. (2017). Inhibition of *Listeria monocytogenes* on ready-to-eat meats using bacteriocin mixtures based on mode-of-action. *Foods, 6*(22), 1–13. https://doi.org/10.3390/foods6030022.

Vojkovská, H., Myšková, P., Gelbíčová, T., Skočková, A., Koláčková, I., & Karpíšková, R. (2017). Occurrence and characterization of food-borne pathogens isolated from fruit, vegetables and sprouts retailed in the Czech Republic. *Food Microbiology, 63*, 147–152. https://doi.org/10.1016/j.fm.2016.11.012.

Vongkamjan, K., Fuangpaiboon, J., Turner, M. P., & Vuddhakul, V. (2016). Various ready-to-eat products from retail stores linked to occurrence of diverse *Listeria monocytogenes* and *Listeria* spp. isolates. *Journal of Food Protection, 79*(2), 239–245. https://doi.org/10.4315/0362-028X.JFP-15-361.

Wang, W., Zhou, X., Suo, Y., Deng, X., Cheng, M., Shi, C., et al. (2017). Prevalence, serotype diversity, biofilm-forming ability and eradication of *Listeria monocytogenes* isolated from diverse foods in Shanghai, China. *Food Control, 73*, 1068–1073. https://doi.org/10.1016/j.foodcont.2016.10.025.

Wieczorek, K., & Osek, J. (2017). Prevalence, genetic diversity and antimicrobial resistance of *Listeria monocytogenes* isolated from fresh and smoked fish in Poland. *Food Microbiology, 64*, 164–171. https://doi.org/10.1016/j.fm.2016.12.022.

Wu, S., Wu, Q., Zhang, J., Chen, M., Yan, Z., & Hu, H. (2015). *Listeria monocytogenes* prevalence and characteristics in retail raw foods in China. *PLoS One, 10*(8), e0136682. https://doi.org/10.1371/journal.pone.0136682.

Zhang, Q., Feng, Y., Deng, L., Feng, F., Wang, L., Zhou, Q., et al. (2011). SigB plays a major role in *Listeria monocytogenes* tolerance to bile stress. *International Journal of Food Microbiology, 145*(1), 238–243. https://doi.org/10.1016/j.ijfoodmicro.2010.12.028.

Zunabovic, M., Domig, K. J., Pichler, I., & Kneifel, W. (2012). Monitoring transmission routes of Listeria spp. in smoked salmon production with repetitive element sequence-based PCR techniques. *Journal of Food Protection, 75*(3), 504–511. https://doi.org/10.4315/0362-028X.JFP-11-341.

FURTHER READING

Burall, L. S., Simpson, A. C., & Datta, A. R. (2011). Evaluation of a serotyping scheme using a combination of an antibody-based serogrouping method and a multiplex PCR assay for identifying the major serotypes of *Listeria monocytogenes*. *Journal of Food Protection, 74*(3), 403–409. https://doi.org/10.4315/0362-028X.JFP-10-355.

Carlton, R. M. (1999). Phage therapy: Past history and future prospects. *Archivum Immunologiae et Therapiae Experimentalis, 47*, 267–274.

McAuliffe, O., & Jordan, K. N. (2012). Biotechnological approaches for control of *Listeria monocytogenes* in foods. *Current Biotechnology, 1*(4), 267–280. https://doi.org/10.2174/2211550111201040267.

Moura, A., Criscuolo, A., Pouseele, H., Maury, M. M., Leclercq, A., Tarr, C., et al. (2016). Whole genome-based population biology and epidemiological surveillance of *Listeria monocytogenes*. *Nature Microbiology, 2*(2), 16185. https://doi.org/10.1038/nmicrobiol.2016.185.

Vongkamjan, K., Benjakul, S., Kim Vu, H. T., & Vuddhakul, V. (2017). Longitudinal monitoring of *Listeria monocytogenes* and *Listeria* phages in seafood processing environments in Thailand. *Food Microbiology, 66*, 11–19. https://doi.org/10.1016/j.fm.2017.03.014.

CHAPTER EIGHT

Campylobacter in the Food Chain

Lourdes García-Sánchez, Beatriz Melero, Jordi Rovira[1]
Biotechnology and Food Science Department, University of Burgos, Burgos, Spain
[1]Corresponding author: e-mail address: jrovira@ubu.es

Contents

Advances in Food and Nutrition Research, Volume 86
ISSN 1043-4526
https://doi.org/10.1016/bs.afnr.2018.04.005
© 2018 Elsevier Inc.
All rights reserved.

Abstract

Currently *Campylobacter* is the most commonly reported zoonosis in developed and developing countries. In the European Union, the number of reported confirmed cases of human campylobacteriosis was 246,307 in 2016, which represents 66.3 cases per 100,000 population. The genus *Campylobacter* includes 31 species with 10 subspecies. Within the genus *Campylobacter, C. jejuni* subsp. *jejuni* and *C. coli* are most frequently associated with human illness. Mainly, the infection is sporadic and self-limiting, although some cases of outbreaks have been also reported and some complications such as Guillain–Barré syndrome might appear sporadically. Although campylobacters are fastidious microaerophilic, unable to multiply outside the host and generally very sensitive, they can adapt and survive in the environment, exhibiting aerotolerance and resistance to starvation. Many mechanisms are involved in this, including pathogenicity, biofilm formation, and antibiotic resistant pathways. This chapter reviews the sources, transmission routes, the mechanisms, and strategies used by *Campylobacter* to persist in the whole food chain, from farm to fork. Additionally, different strategies are recommended for application along the poultry food chain to avoid the public health risk associated with this pathogen.

1. THE ORGANISM

1.1 History

The history of the genus *Campylobacter* starts with the first description by Theodor Escherich in 1886, of a nonculturable spiral form bacteria associated with the stools of children suffering diarrhea. In the following years several publications appeared, describing the occurrence of such "spirilla" in cases of enteric diseases such as "cholera-like" and "dysentery" (Kist, 1986).

In 1913, McFadyean and Stockman isolated a *Vibrio*-like bacterium from aborted ovine fetuses. Six years later, Smith and Taylor (1919) isolated a spirilla bacterium from aborted bovine fetuses and named it as *Vibrio fetus*. In 1931, *Vibrio jejuni* was named after isolation in cows and calves with intestinal disorders (Jones, Orcutt, & Little, 1931). *Vibrio coli* was named and detected in 1944 from swine with dysentery (Doyle, 1948).

Although *Campylobacter* was assigned as a veterinary disease for more than 40 years, it was not until the 1970s that campylobacters were recognized as human pathogens. This microorganism was first isolated in humans from blood cultures from women who had aborted (Vinzent, Dumas, & Picard, 1947). However, the first documented human infection due to this spiral bacterium occurred in 1938 in a milk-associated outbreak among prisoners in the United States (Levi, 1946). In 1963 these "related vibrios" were renamed by Sebald and Veron as *Campylobacter* due to differences between

Vibrio and the new genus in DNA base composition, growth requirements, and metabolism (Sebald & Veron, 1963).

Elisabeth King was committed to find a methodology to culture this microorganism from feces because she believed that the few cases reported underestimated the actual prevalence of the disease (Butzler, 2004). The development of a special filtration technique, used in veterinary medicine in the early 1970s, allowed Butzler to isolate *Campylobacter* from human stools of patients with diarrhea and high fever (Butzler, Dekeyser, Detrain, & Dehaen, 1973). However, the main step toward its successful cultivation was achieved when a selective supplement comprising a mixture of vancomycin, polymyxin B, and trimethoprim was added to a basal medium. This development was a crucial step in the evaluation of the *Campylobacter* epidemiology and their clinical role (Dekeyser, Gossuin-Detrain, Butzler, & Sternon, 1972; Skirrow, 1977).

1.2 Taxonomy

The taxonomy of the genus *Campylobacter* has been extensively revised since 1963. Veron and Chatelain (1973) proposed four species within the genus *Campylobacter* after a taxonomy study: *C. fetus, C. coli, C. jejuni*, and *C. sputorum* with two subspecies, *C. sputorum* subsp. *sputorum* and *C. sputorum* subsp. *bubulus*. Due to the development of new methods and a selective supplement to isolate campylobacters (Butzler et al., 1973; Skirrow, 1977), the number of *Campylobacter*-like organisms (CLO) isolated from different sources increased. However, some of these CLO were classified subsequently as novel genera, species, or variants of previously defined species (Vandamme, 2000).

Currently the immediate family is that of *Campylobacteriaceae*, which includes three distinct genera: *Arcobacter, Campylobacter*, and *Sulfurospirillum* (Lastovica, On, & Zhang, 2014). The genus *Campylobacter* includes 31 species and 10 subspecies (http://www.bacterio.net/campylobacter.html, accessed 18.03.2018). *C. ornithocola* (Cáceres, Muñoz, Iraola, Díaz-Viraqué, & Collado, 2017), *C. pinnipediorum* subsp. *caledonicus, C. pinnipediorum* subsp. *pinnipediorum* (Gilbert et al., 2017), *C. geochelonis* (Piccirillo et al., 2016), and *C. hepaticus* (Van, Elshagmani, Gor, Scott, & Moore, 2016) are the most recent species identified.

Within the genus *Campylobacter, C. jejuni* subsp. *jejuni* and *C. coli* are most frequently associated with human illness, accounting for up to 90% of infections (Debruyne, Gevers, & Vandamme, 2008). Moreover, *C. jejuni* comprises two subspecies: *C. jejuni* subsp. *jejuni* and *C. jejuni* subsp. *doylei.*

Although the pathogenic role of *C. jejuni* subsp. *doylei* is unclear, it has been isolated in a low percentage in children and adults with diarrhea all over the world (Lastovica & Allos, 2008). The two subspecies differ biochemically and can be identified by multiplex polymerase chain reaction (PCR) based on the nitrate reductase locus (*nap*) (Miller, Parker, Heath, & Lastovica, 2007). *C. jejuni* subsp. *jejuni* will hereafter be referred to as *C. jejuni*. Moreover, other species than *C. jejuni* and *C. coli* have been also related with human infections. *C. fetus* subsp. *fetus* is related with diarrhea and bacteraemia (Lastovica, 1996; Skirrow, Jones, Sutcliffe, & Benjamin, 1993). *C. concisus* has been isolated from fecal samples and intestinal biopsies from patients with inflammatory bowel disease (IBD) (Mahendran et al., 2011; Zhang et al., 2009). *C. lari* has been also related with diarrhea, bacteraemia, and reactive arthritis (Borczyk, Thompson, Smith, & Lior, 1987; Goudswaard, Sabbe, & te Winkel, 1995; Morishita et al., 2013) as well as *C. upsaliensis* has been isolated from blood and fecal samples (Lastovica, 2006; Lastovica, le Roux, & Penner, 1989). On the other hand, other *Campylobacter* species are less frequently isolated from human samples as *C. ureolyticus* (Vandamme, Debruyne, De Brandt, & Falsen, 2010); *C. hominis* (Lawson, On, Logan, & Stanley, 2001); *C. concisus, C. curvus, C. rectus*, and *C. gracilis* isolated from gingival crevices (Ngulukun, 2017). Species isolated from animals include *C. cuniculorum* in rabbits (Zanoni, Debruyne, Rossi, Revez, & Vandamme, 2009), *C. insulaenigrae* isolated from marine mammals (Foster et al., 2004); bird-associated species such as *C. avium* (Rossi et al., 2009), *C. canadensis* (Inglis, Hoar, Whiteside, & Morck, 2007), and *C. volucris* (Debruyne et al., 2010), *C. corcagiensis* from captive lion-tailed macaques (Koziel et al., 2014), and *C. iquaniorom* from reptiles (Gilbert, Kik, Miller, Duim, & Wagenaar, 2015).

1.3 Microbiology

Campylobacter species are Gram-negative spiral, rod-shaped, or curved bacteria, motile due to the presence of a single polar flagellum, bipolar flagella. However, *C. gracilis* and *C. hominis* are nonmotile species. Moreover, at microscope *C. showae* appears as straight rods. Cells are approximately 0.2–0.8 μm wide and 0.5–5 μm long. It is nonspore-forming and in old cultures may form coccoid or spherical shapes (Man, 2011; Vandamme, Dewhirst, Paster, & On, 2005).

C. jejuni is chemoorganotrophic—carbohydrates are not used to obtain energy; amino acids or tricarboxylic acid cycle intermediates are utilized instead. *Campylobacter* species reduce fumarate to succinate, are oxidase positive (except for *C. gracilis*), and are indole negative. Except for *C. jejuni* subsp. *doylei*, campylobacters will reduce nitrate. No lecithinase or lipase activity is present, and starch, gelatine, and casein are not hydrolyzed by this genus.

All *Campylobacter* species grow under microaerobic conditions (85% N_2, 3%–5% CO_2, and 5%–10% O_2). However, certain species (*C. concisus, C. curvus*, and *C. rectus*) prefer anaerobic conditions for growth (Kaakoush, Castaño-Rodríguez, Mitchell, & Man, 2015). Thermophilic campylobacters such as *C. jejuni*, *C. coli*, *C. lari*, and *C. upsaliensis* grow optimally at 42°C, while the other species grow better at 37°C, but always above 30°C (Rovira, Cencic, Santos, Jakobsen, 2006; Kärenlampi & Hänninen, 2004). Identification of *Campylobacter* spp. is challenging due to their biochemical inertness and fastidious growth requirements. Biochemical approaches like the hippurate hydrolysis test are routinely used in the differentiation between *C. jejuni* and *C. coli*. Although some *C. jejuni* subsp. *jejuni* strains can produce negative reaction, this species hydrolyzes the hippurate while *C. coli* does not (Debruyne et al., 2008). Moreover, molecular identification such as multiplex PCR is also required to identify *Campylobacter* species based on diverse genes (Vondrakova, Pazlarova, & Demnerova, 2014; Wang et al., 2002).

1.4 Genome and Population Structure of *C. jejuni*

The whole genome of *C. jejuni* strain NCTC 11168 was first sequenced in by Parkhill et al. (2000) and further reannotated by Gundogdu et al. (2007). Afterward, other three *C. jejuni* reference strains such as RM1221, 81116, and 81-176 were also sequenced (Pearson et al., 2007). The size of *C. jejuni* genome is relatively small in comparison with other *Campylobacter* spp. genomes and indeed among other bacteria (Table 1). It has a circular chromosome with 1,641,481 base pairs (bp) in length (1.64 Mbp) with a relatively low G + C content (around 32%). From the 1654 predicted coding sequences, at least 20 probably represent pseudogenes; the average gene length is 948 bp and 94.3% of the genome codes for proteins (Parkhill et al., 2000).

C. jejuni species can be described by a pan-genome consisting of a core genome, between 866 and 1350 genes, shared by all isolates, and an accessory genome (2500–4000 genes) composed of partially shared and strain-specific genes. While the core genome is thought to be involved in vital functions for the cell, the accessory genome is composed by plasmids, integrated elements, hypervariable regions, and single or paired variable genes (Llarena, 2015).

Table 1 Bacterial Comparative Genomes

Genome	Mb	G+C (%)	References
Listeria monocytogenes	2.9	39	Glaser et al. (2001)
Salmonella Typhimurium	4.9	52	Vinuesa, Puente, Calva, Zaidi, and Silva (2016)
Escherichia coli	4.6–5.7	50.60	Engelbrecht, Putonti, Koenig, and Wolfe (2017)
Yersinia enterocolitica	4.6	47.27	Sanger Institute (2018) (https://www.sanger.ac.uk/)
Campylobacter jejuni	1.6–1.8	32	Parkhill et al. (2000)

The genome sequence of *C. jejuni* is subject to evolutionary changes, which can be mediated via mobile genetic elements, the uptake of DNA via natural transformation, and changes in hypervariable sequences. *Campylobacter* are naturally competent for DNA uptake from the environment (Wan & Taylor, 1990), contributing to its wide phenotypic and genotypic heterogeneity.

The development of new sequencing technologies has made it feasible to carry out much larger and more detailed *Campylobacter* comparative genomics to better identify genes or genomic regions associated with isolates from particular sources (Bronowski, James, & Winstanley, 2014).

2. EPIDEMIOLOGICAL AND CLINICAL ASPECT OF *CAMPYLOBACTER*

2.1 Campylobacteriosis in Humans

Among the five most relevant zoonoses causing gastrointestinal bacteria disease in the EU, campylobacteriosis has been the most commonly reported since 2007 (Fig. 1). In 2016, the number of reported confirmed cases of human campylobacteriosis was 246,307, which represents 66.3 cases per 100,000 population. This means an increase of 6.1% compared with 2015, a trend that has been observed over the last 8 years. Although the number of human campylobacteriosis cases is high, their severity in terms of reported case fatality is low (0.03%). Nonetheless, campylobacteriosis is the third most common cause of mortality among the major pathogens (EFSA, 2017). A similar situation occurs in North America and Australia.

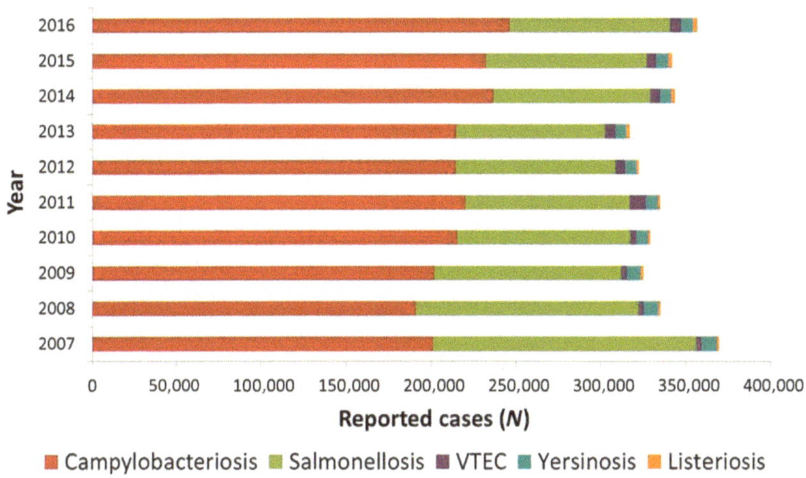

Fig. 1 Trends of the five more relevant zoonoses in EU in the period 2007–16. *Adapted from the European Centre for Disease Prevention and Control (ECDC), http://atlas.ecdc.europa.eu/public/index.aspx.*

Although epidemiological data from Africa, Asia, and the Middle East are still incomplete, these indicate that *Campylobacter* infection is endemic in these regions. However, the incidence and number of cases reported from different countries or regions within the same country may vary substantially (Kaakoush et al., 2015).

The great majority of *Campylobacter* infections are sporadic and self-limiting. Infection is characterized by watery and sometimes bloody diarrhea, fever, abdominal cramps, and vomiting (Skarp, Hänninen, & Rautelin, 2016). However, the pathogen has been associated with a wide range of gastrointestinal diseases, such as IBD, Barrett's esophagus, esophageal, and colorectal cancer and can also be responsible for nongastrointestinal problems such as Guillain–Barré syndrome (GBS) as well as bacteraemia, lung infections, brain abscesses, meningitis, or reactive arthritis among others (Kaakoush et al., 2015).

Although the infection is usually sporadic, there have been several outbreaks reported (Table 2). Calciati et al. (2012) described an outbreak of campylobacteriosis affecting 75 children in a Spanish school. Burakoff et al. (2018) reported a *C. jejuni* outbreak associated with drinking unpasteurized milk, and Koppenaal et al. (2017) concluded that an outbreak of *C. fetus* was linked to the consumption of unripened cheese products made with unpasteurized sheep's milk. Animals have been also described as sources of

Table 2 *Campylobacter* Outbreaks

Source	Species	References
Food		
Russian salad, chicken	*Campylobacter* spp.	Calciati et al. (2012)
Commercial catering serving chicken livers	*C. jejuni* and *C. coli*	Lahti, Löfdahl, Ågren, Hansson, and Olsson Engvall (2017) and Moffatt et al. (2016)
Milk	*C. jejuni*	Burakoff et al. (2018)
Cheese	*C. fetus*	Koppenaal et al. (2017)
Water	*C. jejuni*	Revez et al. (2014)
Contact with animals		
Pets	*Campylobacter* spp.	Centers for Disease Control and Prevention (https://www.cdc.gov/) (2018)
Raccoon	*C. jejuni*	Saunders, Smith, Schott, Dobbins, and Scheftel (2017)

human infections, as with the multistate outbreak multidrug-resistant *Campylobacter* infections linked to contact with pet store puppies with 113 reported cases and 23 hospitalizations along 17 states (CDC, 2018).

2.2 Reservoirs and Transmission Routes

Environmental niches and different animals are considered as important contributors to human infection; however, their particular role in the complex epidemiology of *Campylobacter* infection is still unknown (Whiley, Van den Akker, Giglio, & Bentham, 2013).

2.2.1 Reservoirs

Campylobacter spp. are considered normal microflora of the gastrointestinal tract of a number of domestic animals and birds, such as commercial broiler chickens, which are mainly considered as asymptomatic carriers (Whiley et al., 2013). Epidemiological studies have reported that poultry is the natural host for thermophilic *Campylobacter* species, and they are responsible for an estimated 80% of human campylobacteriosis. In addition, other animals such as wild birds, cattle, swine, and pets have been reported as sources of *Campylobacter* contamination (Epps et al., 2013). Nontreated water and milk have been also identified as causative of some cases of campylobacteriosis. The wide range of hosts and the high genetic variability of *Campylobacter* spp. make the tracing and attribution of the original source of infection difficult (Gölz et al., 2014; Skarp et al., 2016).

Molecular techniques such as pulsed-field electrophoresis or multilocus sequence typing (MLST), based on genetic similarity between strains from humans and reservoirs, can allow the identification of the origin of human *Campylobacter* infections (Hänninen, Perko-Mäakelä, Pitkälä, & Rautenin, 2000; Mughini et al., 2012).

2.2.2 Transmission Routes

Routes of transmission flowing through the environment, farm animals and wild animals through to humans interact in complex ways. These interactions are driven by factors such as the defecation of wild birds or farm animals, presence of pets, water flow, climatic conditions, and other complex ecological parameters (Bronowski et al., 2014). Nonvertebrae vectors, such as flies (Hald, Skovgard, Pedersen, & Bunkenborg, 2008), beetles (Skov et al., 2004), and slugs (Sproston et al., 2010) have been also identified as *Campylobacter* carriers and may act as transmission vectors.

Horizontal transmission of *Campylobacter* in the farm environment represents the usual route of transmission there. Once *Campylobacter* is introduced into a chicken flock, it spreads rapidly and results in colonization of the intestinal tracts of the majority of chickens within 1 week. Once colonized, chickens remain colonized until slaughter (Ingresa-Capaccioni et al., 2015). During slaughter and subsequent steps, *Campylobacter* can be spread through the plant environment, finally contaminating the whole poultry food chain and ultimately reaching consumers (García-Sánchez et al., 2017; Melero, Juntunen, Hänninen, Jaime, & Rovira, 2012).

Human exposure to risk occurs through direct contact with animals or through contaminated food by either consumption of undercooked meat or due to cross-contamination from raw meat or environmental reservoirs to ready-to-eat food (Skarp et al., 2016). Other possible routes of transmission include drinking raw milk and untreated water as well as practices like swimming in natural waters (Fajó-Pascual, Godoy, Ferrero-Cáncer, & Wymore, 2010; Kapperud et al., 2003). Although it is not common, person-to-person transmission is recognized as another potential route (Kaakoush et al., 2015).

All of the above factors have a role in the transmission of *Campylobacter* from farm to fork. Additionally, international travel as has been considered one of the most important risk factors for campylobacteriosis. However, in many cases, the direct link between a specific source and the human infection remains unknown (Domingues, Pires, Halasa, & Hald, 2012; Kaakoush et al., 2015).

3. PERSISTENCE ALONG POULTRY FOOD CHAIN

Despite the theoretical vulnerability of the thermophilic campylobacters to harsh environmental conditions, they are responsible for the most cases of bacterial diarrheic disease. Several studies have demonstrated the persistence of *C. jejuni* genotypes isolated in the farm along the poultry food chain (Damjanova et al., 2011; Gruntar, Biasizzo, Kusar, Pate, & Ocepek, 2015; Melero et al., 2012). Therefore, knowledge of the sources of *Campylobacter* contamination through the poultry food chain and its behavior can contribute to the general goal of reducing campylobacteriosis (EFSA, 2017). In this section, the risk factors that might contribute to the occurrence and persistence of *C. jejuni* along the main steps of the poultry food chain—farm, slaughterhouse/processing plant, and retail—will be briefly discussed.

3.1 Farm

The prevalence of *Campylobacter* spp. in broiler chicken flocks is highly variable in the EU, ranging from 2% to 100% depending on the Member State (EFSA, 2010a). It has been suggested that controlling *Campylobacter* in primary broiler production is expected to have a greater impact in public health benefits than the control of the pathogen in subsequent steps in the poultry chain. However, despite several years of research and numerous studies, the epidemiology of *Campylobacter* spp. in broiler primary production is not fully understood, and still is considered as a major problem (Battersby, Walsh, Whyte, & Bolton, 2017). Moreover, many of these studies have produced contradictory results; this confirms the complexity of this issue and the implication of multiple risk factors associated with survival and persistence of *Campylobacter* in the farm environment.

These risk factors might be divided into different sources of *Campylobacter* in broiler farms such as (1) vertical transmission, (2) animals, (3) humans, (4) farm environment, and (5) water (Agunos, Waddell, Léger, & Taboada, 2014). The relative importance of each of these risk factors for flock positivity remains unknown but will probably vary from farm to farm.

Vertical transmission: This risk factor does not appear to be an important risk factor for colonization of broiler chickens with *Campylobacter* (EFSA, 2011).

Colonization of chickens with *Campylobacter* happens around 7 days of life (Gibbens, Pascoe, Evans, Davies, & Sayers, 2001; Marotta et al., 2015), and the colonization of the whole flock occurs before 2 weeks of age (Hansson, Pudas, Harbom, & Engvall, 2010; Ingresa-Capaccioni et al., 2015). After infection, *Campylobacter* rapidly colonizes the two ceca to a high level and leads to fecal shedding. This high-level of shedding combined with the coprophagic behavior of chickens means that the bacterium is able to pass rapidly through the entire flock in just a few days once the first bird in a broiler flock becomes colonized (Chaloner et al., 2014; Marotta et al., 2015). Age has been identified as a risk factor for *Campylobacter* colonization in broilers at slaughter (Bouwknegt et al., 2004). An EU baseline survey indicates that prevalence of *Campylobacter* colonization of broiler batches increases each 10 days of age (EFSA, 2010b). Overall, the maximum prevalence of *Campylobacter* in broilers is reached between days 21 and 42 of the growth cycle.

Animals: The presence of *Campylobacter* has been investigated in adjacent broilers or layers, in other domestic farm animals such as cattle, sheep, or pigs, in cats or dogs, and in pests and wild animals that share the same farm environment or are in close proximity. Several studies proposed other farm animals as a possible reservoir for *Campylobacter* on farms (Ellis-Iversen et al., 2012; Zweifel, Scheu, Keel, Renggli, & Stephan, 2008). Cattle seem to be the most frequent nonbroiler source of *Campylobacter*. However, only in a few studies it has been observed that isolates from other domestic animals match with those isolated from broiler flocks (Agunos et al., 2014). Moreover, several studies have identified rodents (Sommer, Heuer, Sørensen, & Madsen, 2013) or flies (Borck Höng et al., 2016; Hald et al., 2008) as possible contamination vectors. Some of these studies identified the same genotypes both in the contamination vectors and within the broiler flock. However, those genotypes were only the same when the broiler flocks were present. The prevalence of *Campylobacter* among wildlife and especially wild birds, commonly present in farms, has been also confirmed. Although in many cases *Campylobacter* spp. has been isolated from those animals, again, those isolates were largely unrelated with those of the broiler flocks.

Human activity: The contribution of people related with the farm activity has also been investigated as a risk factor in the *Campylobacter* transmission. Cross-contamination between farmers entering broiler houses and birds of the flock has been detected, but in many cases reasonable doubts arise about the direction of this contamination (farmer-flock or flock-farmer). One of the most problematic operations in broiler farm management is "thinning" or partial depopulation of birds, which takes place around 30–35 days of bird age. During this operation a high number of people enter the broiler houses. Once more, contradictory data are obtained regarding the influence of this activity on flock contamination by *Campylobacter*. Several authors described a statistically significant risk associated with thinning (Allen, Burton, et al., 2008; Allen, Weaver, et al., 2008; Bouwknegt et al., 2004), whereas others questioned the importance of this procedure as a risk factor, since at the time when depopulation is carried out the birds are at the age in which there is a greater risk of already being contaminated by *Campylobacter* (Havelaar et al., 2007; Russa, Bouma, Vernooij, Jacobs-Reitsma, & Stegeman, 2005).

Farm environment: In this term is included the in-house environment and the surroundings of the broiler houses in the farm. *Campylobacter* is widely present in the farm surrounding environment once a flock becomes positive, persisting for several weeks and in some occasions even before bird placement (Hansson, Vagsholm, Svensson, and Olsson Engvall, 2007; Johnsen, Kruse, & Hofshagen, 2006). Several studies reported that free-range chickens show a higher prevalence than flocks grown conventionally (McCrea et al., 2006; Ring, Zychowska, & Stephan, 2005). However, Huneau-Salaun, Denis, Balaine, and Salvat (2007) have recently questioned this, since in their study birds were already infected with *Campylobacter* prior to their release. Crates used during catching of birds in broiler houses before slaughter have been described as another possible source of *Campylobacter* contamination due to the presence of the pathogen even after cleaning and disinfection (Allen, Burton, et al., 2008; Allen, Weaver, et al., 2008; Melero et al., 2012; Slader et al., 2002). Poor maintenance (Cardinale, Tall, Gueye, Cisse, & Salvat, 2004) and deficiencies in cleaning and disinfection of broiler housing (Battersby et al., 2017) are described as the two main in-house environment sources of carry-over between flocks. There are clear evidences of the presence of *Campylobacter* in the environment surroundings of houses, even from day 0 of broiler placement, and the prevalence in outdoor samples was relatively constant throughout the grow-out period. Nevertheless, none of the studies has been able to demonstrate the direction of the contamination between flock and environment (Agunos et al., 2014).

Water: *Campylobacter* is able to survive in water for weeks. Water treatment failure, use of unchlorinated water sources from public suppliers or from wells, or contamination of on-farm water reservoirs may enable the delivery of live *Campylobacter* to poultry houses (EFSA, 2011). Although water in house drinkers appears to be almost always contaminated by *Campylobacter*, in most of the cases there cannot be assurance that the bacteria isolated came from broiler contamination instead of from the water itself. Nontreated water has been identified several times as a source of *Campylobacter*. Rivers, ponds, and especially puddles located near the broiler houses have been described as possible sources of contamination.

Normally, *Campylobacter* infections in animals are considered asymptomatic. However, recent studies have reported that this infection can lead to diarrhea and inflammatory damage in the birds (Humphrey et al., 2014) causing lack of welfare and lesions of footpad dermatitis (Alpigiani et al., 2017). Moreover, *Campylobacter* infection could interfere with intracellular Ca^{2+} signaling and nutrient absorption in the small intestine with consequences on intestinal function, performance, and *Campylobacter* colonization itself (Awad et al., 2015). These data suggest that *Campylobacter* might be not a merely harmless commensal, as it was previously thought.

In summary, at farm level is important to improve biosecurity measures to prevent the spread of *Campylobacter* within the farm, and more importantly to the further steps in the poultry food chain. According to an EFSA report a reduction by 3 log 10-units in the numbers of *Campylobacter* in the intestines at slaughter would reduce the public health risk by at least 90% (EFSA, 2011). For more detailed information dealing with the risk factor at farm level, read the following reviews (Agunos et al., 2014; EFSA, 2011).

3.2 Slaughter and Processing Plant

Once broilers reach the desired age and weight, feed and water are usually withdrawn several hours before the birds are caught, loaded, and transported to processing plants for slaughter. Contamination with *Campylobacter* may increase significantly during those operations, as birds disseminate contamination present in the houses environment during catching and loading of the birds into the crates (Slader et al., 2002). Crates are a source of cross-contamination, and high numbers of *Campylobacter*, up to 7 log 10 CFU/crate, have been usually detected, even after washing and sanitizing (Allen, Burton, et al., 2008; Melero et al., 2012). In that respect, Newell et al. (2001) found the same subtype of *Campylobacter* in a previous negative flock that was present on crates used to transport the broilers to the slaughterhouse. This contamination could be acquired during transportation or in the waiting time in the processing plant before slaughter. Proximity within the crowded crates helps to spread *Campylobacter* present in the feathers and feces among birds. Accordingly, it is important to minimize transportation and holding time before slaughter for microbiological, product quality, economical, and animal welfare reasons (EFSA, 2011).

At the slaughter line, positive poultry flocks can carry a high load of *Campylobacter*, around 7 log 10 CFU/g, both on the outside, on the feathers and legs, as well as on the inside in the gastrointestinal tract (Seliwiorstow, Baré, Van Damme, Uyttendaele, & De Zutter, 2015). In consequence, two critical points for poultry meat contamination by *Campylobacter* in the slaughter line are the plucking/defeathering and the evisceration steps. Therefore, carcasses are contaminated by their own farm/flock genotype (Gruntar et al., 2015). A *Campylobacter* colonized batch was about 30 times more likely to yield a *Campylobacter*-contaminated carcass (EFSA, 2011). Moreover, several studies found that poultry meat from negative broiler flocks may be contaminated if the previous slaughtered flock was positive (Allen et al., 2007; Miwa, Takegahara, Terai, Kato, & Takeuchi, 2003). However, it has been shown that negative flocks may be also contaminated by strains that did not generally originate from the predominating strains recovered from the ceca of the previous positive flocks (Elvers, Morris, Newell, & Allen, 2011). In that sense, the slaughter environment may play a role as a source of cross-contamination. Several authors described the presence of *Campylobacter* after cleaning and disinfection of slaughter equipment and surfaces (García-Sánchez et al., 2017; Melero et al., 2012; Peyrat, Soumet, Maris, & Sanders, 2008a, 2008b). The latter authors described the persistence of the same *C. jejuni* genotype in the abattoir environment for at least 21 days.

The prevalence of *Campylobacter* at slaughter and in the processing plant is variable, and according to several authors the average will be around 80% (Damjanova et al., 2011; Marotta et al., 2015). However, according to the last EFSA report in 2017, the percentage of positive samples in the EU was 29.35% at slaughterhouse and 12.29% in processing plant (EFSA, 2017).

Several strategies have been proposed to reduce the presence of *Campylobacter* at this step of the poultry food chain. The less costly is to improve the GMP/HACCP during slaughtering and processing, especially by enhancing the cleaning and disinfection procedures. Automatic slaughtering lines are built with very complex equipment that is difficult to clean properly.

3.3 Retail

The prevalence of *Campylobacter* spp. in retail ranges from 2% to almost 90% depending on the EU country and the type of poultry product (EFSA, 2017). The UK Food Standards Agency corroborated that more than half of fresh chicken products, bought in retail shops and produced in the United Kingdom, tested positive for *Campylobacter* in the period between 2016 and 2017 (Food Quality News, 2017). Those data agree with others given by several authors that even raises the range from 90% to 100% (Marotta et al., 2015), and also with data obtained from South Korea ranging from 50% to 100% depending on the type of market where products were bought (Wei et al., 2016). In that sense, evaluation of poultry meats at retail is critical, as they really enter the consumers' kitchens, where cross-contamination can occur between fresh poultry and ready-to-eat products, through cooking utensils or manipulation, which constitutes a serious risk to consumers' health (Cook, Odumeru, Lee, & Pollari, 2012; Luber, Brynestad, Topsch, Scherer, & Bartelt, 2006). At this step, a high diversity of *Campylobacter* genotypes has been found in fresh poultry products, especially in those that are sold without packaging in small retail shops (Melero et al., 2012). In general, this increase in the variability of genotypes is mainly due to cross-contamination between meat products from different origin and animal species that are found together at the store counter, and to the handling of those products by retailers. It is known that *Campylobacter* is unable to grow in foodstuffs; however, it is able to persist and survive. Packaging has been proven to have a protective, but limited, effect on *Campylobacter* reduction. Several gas compositions have been proposed to reduce its presence on poultry products. Due to the microaerophilic condition of *Campylobacter*, an atmosphere rich in O_2 (>70%) has been suggested as the most appropriate, since oxygen in high concentrations might be toxic and as a consequence able to reduce the presence of the pathogen (Melero, Vinuesa, Diez, Jaime, & Rovira, 2013). However, some aerotolerant or even hyperaerotolerant *Campylobacter* strains have been recently isolated (Oh, McMullen, Chui, & Jeon, 2017). Accordingly, it has been suggested to use high CO_2 (>50%) for modified atmosphere packaging (MAP). Nevertheless, a rich CO_2 gas composition favors the development of some spoilage bacteria like lactic acid bacteria. One way to combine the effect of the different gas compositions, in order to reduce the presence of *Campylobacter*, and to delay the pernicious effect of the spoilage bacteria, is to use MAP compositions with medium levels of gases such as using 40%:30%:30% (CO_2:O_2:N_2) (Meredith et al., 2014).

4. PATHOGENESIS AND VIRULENCE FACTORS

Although several putative virulence and survival factors may be important for *Campylobacter* pathogenesis, the relevance of these particular genes and the proteins they encode is generally poorly understood. Host colonization by *Campylobacter* requires motility and chemotaxis, adhesion, invasion, and toxin production.

Virulence factors are considered to be important for the induction of gastroenteritis. The clinical and epidemiological characteristics of the disease provide clues to the molecular mechanisms that play a role in *C. jejuni* infection. Some genes have been recognized as responsible for the pathogenicity expression; for instance, *flaA* (flagellin gene), *cadF* (adhesin gene), *racR*, and *dnaJ* were selected as pathogenic genes responsible for adherence and colonization, *virB11, ciaB*, and *pldA* as pathogenic genes responsible for invasion, and *cdtA*, *cdtB*, and *cdtC* as pathogenic genes responsible for the expression of cytotoxin production (Bolton, 2015; Dasti, Tareen, Lugert, Zautner, & Groß, 2010; Datta, Niwa, & Itoh, 2003; Zhang et al., 2016).

4.1 Motility

Motility is essential for escaping from stressful environments, and the associated genes are usually upregulated under such conditions (Guerry, 2007). The motility system in *Campylobacter* requires flagella and a chemosensory system that drives flagellar movement based on environmental conditions. The corkscrew shape and the presence of flagella in *Campylobacter* are suitable for swimming through the mucus layer that covers the epithelial lining of the intestine, allowing this pathogen to efficiently reach its favored colonization site, the inner mucus layer of the intestine. The axial part of the flagellum is composed of a hook-basal body and the extracellular filament structural components. The hook-basal body includes (i) a base embedded in the cytoplasm and inner membrane of the cell, (ii) the surface localized hook, and (iii) the periplasmic rod and associated ring structures. This rod is connected to the proteins of the motor that provides energy for the movement of the flagellum. This system is composed by a high number of proteins with different roles. Among them, the principal flagellum filament proteins are the major flagellin subunits FlaA, and the minor subunit FlaB, encoded by *flaA* and *flaB* genes, respectively (Bolton, 2015). Other important protein is CheY, which is a response regulator needed for flagella rotation (Yao, Liu, Wang, Zhang, & Shen, 2017).

The bacterial flagellum is one of the most important virulence factors and is also associated with adhesion and invasion. In that sense, apart from serving to confer movement, the flagellum of *C. jejuni* has components homologous to the classical Type III secretion systems (T3SS) that serves to transport nonflagellar proteins, playing a central role in *C. jejuni* pathogenesis. T3SS are complex macromolecular structures, which allow Gram-negative bacteria to secrete proteins across the inner and outer membranes, without a periplasmic intermediate, acting as a "molecular syringe" (Cornelis, 2006). Several proteins have been proposed to be exported via the flagellum such as CiaB, CiaC, CiaI, FlaC, and FspA (Neal-McKinney & Kronkel, 2012).

In addition to their role in mobility, flagellins are major bacterial proteins that can modulate host responses via Toll-like receptor 5 (TLR5) or other pattern recognition receptors. TLR5 usually initiates a powerful host response that provides crucial signals for maintaining intestinal immune homeostasis. However, *C. jejuni* escapes TLR5 recognition because its flagellin protein has a structure that clearly differs from other bacterial flagellins that do activate this system (Zoete, Keestra, Wagenaar, & Van Putten, 2010).

4.2 Adhesion

The ability of *C. jejuni* to adhere to the host gastrointestinal tract by binding to epithelial or other cells is a prerequisite for colonization. This action is mediated by several adhesins located on the bacterial surface and is essential to trigger the disease (Konkel, Garvis, Tipton, Anderson, & Cieplak, 1997; Lin, Michel, & Zhang, 2002). *Campylobacter* adhesion to fibronectin is mediated by CadF, a 37-kDa fibronectin-binding outer membrane protein. Several studies with mutants have revealed that the lack of this protein avoids colonization by *Campylobacter* (Monteville, Yoon, & Konkel, 2003; Ziprin, Young, Stanker, Hume, & Konkel, 1999). Moreover, other proteins have been identified in the colonization process, such as the autotransporter CapA, the periplasmic-binding protein PEB1, and the surface-exposed lipoprotein JlpA (Bolton, 2015). It has been perceived that a correlation exists between the severity of clinical symptoms in infected individuals and the degree to which *C. jejuni* isolates adhere to cultured cells (Dasti et al., 2010; Fauchere et al., 1986).

4.3 Invasion

The invasion ability of *C. jejuni* is an important pathogenicity-associated factor. The clinical presentation of acute campylobacteriosis is consistent with cellular invasion. The key to host cell invasion and survival is a set of proteins called *Campylobacter* invasion antigens (Cia), which are delivered to the cytosol of host cells via a flagellar T3SS (Barrero-Tobon & Hendrixson, 2012). In that sense, flagellar mutants had significantly reduced its invasion ability (Konkel et al., 1997). There are three Cia proteins: CiaB related with adherence to the target cells, CiaC required for full invasion of INT-407 cells, and CiaI which has been reported to play a crucial role in intracellular survival. More recently, a fourth protein, CiaD, has been identified as an important factor required for maximal invasion of the host cells (Samuelson et al., 2013). Moreover, CiaB mutants have reduced their invasion ability by decreasing significantly the adherence and the potential invasiveness. Other proteins, such as FlaC, IamA, CeuE, HtrA, VirK, and FspA, have been suggested to have a role in cell host invasion, although the proper mechanisms are still poorly understood (Bolton, 2015).

4.4 Toxin Production

Campylobacter, like other Gram-negative bacteria, produces a cytolethal distending toxin encoded by the *cdtABC* operon. While *cdtA* and *cdtC* are involved with binding and internalization into the host cell, *cdtB* encodes the enzymatically active/toxic subunit. The interaction between the three proteins conforms a tripartite CDT holotoxin, which is necessary for the delivery of the toxin. In that way, CdtB is translocated into the host cell membrane and causes cell cycle arrest in the G2/M phase resulting in cell death (Dasti et al., 2010; Koolman, Whyte, Burgess, & Bolton, 2016).

CDT activity can differ somewhat depending on the eukaryotic cell types affected, showing three types of pathways: (1) in epithelial cells, endothelial cells, and keratinocytes undergo G_2 cell cycle arrest, cellular distension, and death; (2) in fibroblasts undergo G_1 and G_2 arrest, cellular distension, and death; and (3) in immune cells undergo G_2 arrest followed by apoptosis. As a result of these actions, CDT contributes to pathogenesis by inhibiting both cellular and humoral immunity, as mentioned, via apoptosis of immune response cells (Smith & Bayles, 2006). Moreover, cytotoxic activity of the *C. jejuni* CDT is dependent on its endocytosis. The toxin could be blocked by changes occurring at the level of the microtubules and actin filaments; therefore, it is unable to reach the nucleus avoiding the DNA damage and the alteration of the cell cycle (Méndez-Olvera, Bustos-Martínez, López-Vidal, Verdugo-Rodriguez, & Martínez-Gómez, 2016).

4.5 Carbohydrate Structures

Four different classes of carbohydrate structures such as lipooligosaccharides (LOS), capsular polysaccharides (CPS), O- and N-linked glycans can be found on the surface of the *Campylobacter* cell. The LOS molecule is formed with a core oligosaccharide and lipid A, and has been associated with different activities including immune evasion, host cell adhesion, invasion, and protection from complement-mediated killing. Addition of sialyl groups to the LOS molecule increases invasive potential and reduces immunogenicity of *C. jejuni* strains (Bolton, 2015). Sialylated LOS of *C. jejuni* are capable of mimicking human antigens, like those involved in the appearance of GBS and Miller Fisher syndrome. The majority of patients with GBS have had an antecedent infection with *C. jejuni* strains with LOS belonging to the locus class A (Revez & Hänninen, 2012).

On the other hand, CPS have been described to be associated with many functions, such as protecting bacteria from adverse environmental conditions like increasing resistance to desiccation, biofilm formation, and contribution to virulence in the gastrointestinal tract (Nachamkin, Szymanski, & Blaser, 2008).

C. jejuni has shown a remarkable diversity in gene encoding for CPS and LOS. Further characterization of these gene clusters established 11 classes for CPS and 18 for LOS. This structural variation of the CPS and LOS may represent important strategies for evading the immune response of *C. jejuni*. The high variation in the CPS and LOS gene has been related to the existence of multiple mechanisms including (i) lateral gene transfer, (ii) gene inactivation, duplication, deletion, and fusion, and (iii) phase variable homopolymeric tracts (Richards, Lefébureа, Pavinski-Bitara, & Stanhope, 2013).

Additionally, the N-linked glycosylation system of *C. jejuni* is responsible for posttranslational modification of over 60 periplasmic proteins, including flagellin. This activity is encoded by the pgl multigene locus present in *C. jejuni*. N-linked glycosylation of surface proteins facilitates immune evasion and protects *C. jejuni* against gut proteases. Contrary to the widespread of N-linked glycosylation, O-linked glycosylation is only limited to the flagellin subunits (Bolton, 2015).

4.6 Iron Uptake System

For many microorganisms, iron acquisition is essential for colonization and infection of the host. Iron is a cofactor in many proteins involved in metabolism and basic cellular pathways in both pathogens and their hosts. Under aqueous aerobic conditions at physiological pH, iron is predominantly present as Fe^{3+}. To acquire essential iron, bacteria produce and secrete siderophores with high affinity and selectivity for Fe^{3+} to mediate its uptake into the cell (Miller, Williams, & Ketley, 2009). *C. jejuni* is not capable of synthesizing siderophores itself; however, it possesses an uptake system that is able to use siderophores from competing species. This strategy gives a competitive advantage to *C. jejuni*, taking into account the large number of genes dedicated to iron uptake, regulation, and homeostasis in its relatively small genome (Parkhill et al., 2000). Nevertheless, comparative genomics found variations in iron uptake genes among the sequenced strains.

Several ferric iron uptake systems have been proposed for *Campylobacter* being the enterochelin system one of the most used. This is mediated by CfrA receptor outer membrane protein and the binding-protein-dependent inner membrane ABC transporter system encoded by the *ceuBCDE* genes. *C. jejuni* can use iron to growth taken from host sources such as haem-containing compounds and transferrin proteins. Ferrous iron (Fe^{2+}) diffuses through the outer membrane and only requires a transport protein across the cytoplasm membrane encoded by the gene *feoB* (Miller et al., 2009). Most of the genes involved in iron uptake are primarily regulated by the protein Fur.

5. SURVIVAL STRATEGIES OF *CAMPYLOBACTER* SPP.

Campylobacter are fastidious microaerophillic, unable to multiply outside a host, and generally unable to grow in atmospheric levels of oxygen. Nonetheless, they can adapt and survive in the environment, exhibiting aerotolerance and resistance to starvation. The survival time depends on the species and the environmental conditions, including temperature, light, biotic interactions, oxygen, and nutrient concentrations. Many genes and biochemical pathways are involved in survival strategies (Bolton, 2015; Bronowski et al., 2014; Zhang et al., 2016).

5.1 Biofilms

A biofilm is a polymeric matrix synthesized by aggregates of microbial cells from the same or different species that is attached to different types of surfaces (Teh, Lee, & Dykes, 2014). This structure allows the microorganisms involved to survive better in hostile environments. *C. jejuni*, as other bacteria, is able to form biofilms both in vitro and on processing surfaces made of different materials such as plastic, stainless steel, or glass, among others found in the poultry food chain (Gunther & Chen, 2009; Teh et al., 2014). However, biofilm structure and its consistency are strain and environmental dependent due to differences in gene content between strains, different expression of the genes involved in the synthesis of biofilms and those related with survival in the environment (Buswell et al., 1998; Joshua, Guthrie-Irons, Karlyshev, & Wren, 2006). So far, genes described as involved in the process include those responsible for cell motility (*flaA, flaB, flaC, flaG, fliA, fliS,* and *flhA*), cell surface modifications (*peb4, pgp1,* and *waaF*), quorum sensing (*luxS*), and stress response (*ppk1, spoT, cj1556, csrA, cosR, cprS*). Studies with mutants have revealed that surface proteins flagella and quorum sensing appear to be required for maximal biofilm formation (Bronowski et al., 2014; Turonova et al., 2015).

Furthermore, biofilms confer upon *C. jejuni* protection from stressful conditions that it has to withstand, both in the processing environment and during host infection. Indeed, resistance to antimicrobial agents such as antimicrobial compounds and detergents and disinfectants might be increased in these biofilms (Melo et al., 2017; Teh et al., 2014).

5.2 Stress Responses

Campylobacter must overcome a wide range of harsh and stressful conditions from farm to consumer, and even the transition through the gastrointestinal tracts of humans. Particularly, this microaerophilic foodborne pathogen must survive in atmospheric conditions prior to the initiation of infection or stresses in the food industry such as cleaning and disinfection procedures (Melero et al., 2012; Peyrat et al., 2008a, 2008b).

Reactive oxygen species (ROS), such as superoxide anion, hydrogen peroxide, and hydroxyl radical, can induce DNA and protein damage in bacteria. In order to avoid the toxicity effect of ROS, *Campylobacter* activates and/or increases the activity of the antioxidant defense system. Among this, superoxide dismutase (SodB), alkyl hydroperoxide reductase (AhpC), and a catalase (KatA) play an important role. Although other regulators like SoxRS and OxyR commonly present in other Gram-negative bacteria are not present in *C. jejuni,* this bacterium could deal with oxidative stress due to the presence of other regulators such as the peroxide-sensing regulator PerR, the ferric uptake regulator Fur, and the LysR-type transcriptional regulator *Cj1000* (Koolman et al., 2016).

5.3 VBNC and Coccoid Forms of *Campylobacter*

Rollins and Colwell (1986) described the viable but nonculturable (VBNC) state as a survival mechanism used by *C. jejuni*. In this state, the pathogen can grow under stressful conditions such as lack of nutrients, suboptimal growth temperatures, oxygen tension, pH, osmolartiy changes, and high pressure conditions. *C. jejuni* is able to survive in this state due to the entrance into a state of minimal metabolic activity (Jackson et al., 2009; Nachamkin et al., 2008).

During this state, the pathogen suffers some morphological changes, reducing in size and change to coccoid form. The capacity of some strains to enter into this dormancy state might explain the reason why some genotypes are more persistent in some niches and environmental sources (Bronowski et al., 2014). After a period of resuscitation, the culturability is restored and therefore infectivity also. The importance of this state lies in its role as a possible reservoir of infection and consequent implication for public health.

6. ANTIMICROBIAL RESISTANCE

Antimicrobial resistance in emerging and reemerging farmborne has increased over the last years; for instance, in poultry or pig farms it is considered as growing problem. Therefore, prevention of zoonoses must be a priority from farm to fork. This prevention might start at farm level with the concept of "*One Health*" where actors such as veterinarians, epidemiologists, and public health workers must cooperate to work in the same direction by reducing the antibiotics supply and therefore, possible resistance development. Welfare management and using restrictive antimicrobial measures are needed to control the spread of antibiotic resistance elements in the food chain (Cantas & Suer, 2014).

In veterinary medicine, the use of antibiotics leads to the selection of resistant bacteria in commensal microbiota (Cerf, Carpentier, & Sanders, 2009). Antimicrobial resistance in bacteria, including *Campylobacter*, originating from food of animal origin, has become in recent years an alarming situation in both developed and developing countries, and a significant concern for public health (EFSA, 2017).

6.1 Antibiotic Resistance

Campylobacter is exposed to a wide range of classes of veterinary antibiotics because it is a commensal of many animal species. Among these classes, quinolones as ciprofloxacin or enrofloxacin have been involved in high resistances in farms and food chain products. Moreover *Campylobacter* has a natural competence and hypervariable genomic sequences, conferring a considerable genomic plasticity that might confer these resistances (Iovine, 2013).

They are likely inherently resistant to cloxacillin, nafcillin, oxacillin, sulfamethoxazole, trimethoprim, and vancomycin. However, other types of resistance might be a result occurring during therapeutic antimicrobial drug use in humans and animals (Fouts et al., 2005; Llarena, 2015). *Campylobacter* pathogens have evolved multiple mechanisms for antimicrobial resistance, including (i) synthesis of antibiotic-inactivating/modifying enzymes (e.g., β-lactamase), (ii) alteration or protection of antibiotic targets (e.g., mutations in *gyrA* or 23S rRNA genes), (iii) active extrusion of drugs out of bacterial cells through drug efflux transporters (e.g., CmeABC), and (iv) reduced permeability to antibiotics due to unique membrane structures. Some of the resistance-associated traits are endogenous to *Campylobacter*, whereas others are acquired by mutation or genetic transfer (Luangtongkum et al., 2010; Nachamkin et al., 2008).

6.1.1 Multidrug Efflux Pump System

Resistance to bile salts, heavy metals, and a broad range of other antimicrobial agents is often mediated by the *Campylobacter* multidrug efflux pump (CME). It is encoded by the *cmeABC* operon, consisting of a periplasmic fusion protein (CmeA), an inner membrane efflux transporter belonging to the resistance-nodulation-cell division superfamily (CmeB), and an outer membrane protein (CmeC). The expression is modulated by CmeR, a transcriptional repressor, possibly by inhibiting the *cj0561c* gene, which encodes a putative periplasmic protein. CmeABC contributes to the intrinsic resistance of *C. jejuni* to a broad range of structurally unrelated (Lin et al., 2002).

6.1.2 Quinolones

According to the European Food Safety Authority (EFSA), very high resistance levels to ciprofloxacin were reported in human *Campylobacter* isolates from all European State Members except Denmark and Norway. Eleven out of 17 reporting countries had levels of ciprofloxacin resistance in *C. coli* between 80% and 100% with increasing trends in 2013–15 in two Member States (MSs), and increasing trends of fluoroquinolone resistance was observed for *C. jejuni* in five MSs. The level of acquired resistance to fluoroquinolones can no longer be considered appropriate for routine empirical treatment of human *Campylobacter* infection (EFSA, 2017). Therefore, other human treatment drugs as macrolides (erythromycin or/and azithromycin) have been required, and probably soon fluoroquinolones might become disused.

Many studies have shown a clear positive association between the use of fluoroquinolone in poultry production and increased resistance among chicken and human *Campylobacter* isolates (Luangtongkum et al., 2010).

Resistance to quinolones in *Campylobacter* is mediated by a single point mutation in the quinolone resistance determining region of the gene *gyrA* and also by the increased activity of the CmeABC efflux pump (Iovine, 2013). There are several different single *gyrA* modifications reported to be associated with fluoroquinolone resistance in *Campylobacter* species: Thr86Ile, Asp90Asn, Thr86Lys, Thr86Ala, Thr86Val, and Asp90Tyr. However, the most frequently observed mutation in quinolone resistant *Campylobacter* is the C257T change in the *gyrA* gene, which leads to the Thr86Ile substitution in the gyrase and confers the high-level resistance to this group of antimicrobials (Wieczorek & Osek, 2013).

6.1.3 Tetracycline

Tetracycline resistances in *Campylobacter* have mediated by the ribosomal protection protein TetO encoded by the *tet(O)* gene. This protein recognizes an open A site on the bacterial ribosome and binds it in such a manner that it induces a conformational change that results in the release of the bound tetracycline molecule (Luangtongkum et al., 2010).

Exactly how each pathway contributes to tetracycline entry in *Campylobacter* is not completely clear. According to Iovine (2013) two are the mechanisms of tetracycline resistance: (i) alteration of tetracycline's ribosomal target and (ii) multidrug efflux pump. Moreover, in most strains, the *tet(O)* gene is plasmid encoded; however, some isolates do have a chromosomally encoded copy of the gene (Avrain, Vernozy-Rozand, & Kempf, 2004).

6.1.4 Aminoglycoside

Antibiotics belonged to this class include: gentamicin, kanamycin, amikacin, neomycin, tobramycin, and streptomycin. Mainly, aminoglycosides have two ways to exert antimicrobial activity: (i) interference with the translocation of the nascent peptide chain from the ribosomal A site to the P site leading to premature termination and (ii) interference with proofreading, leading to incorporation of incorrect amino acids and dysfunctional protein. However, the main mechanism of aminoglycoside resistance in *C. jejuni* is via aminoglycoside-modifying enzymes (AphA, AphD, AadE, aacA, Sat) which are usually plasmidborne (pCG8245). Additionally, contribution of efflux is not clear (Iovine, 2013; Yao et al., 2017).

6.1.5 Macrolide

According to EFSA studies, macrolides resistance in *Campylobacter* has increased in the last years, and it is frequently detected in many European Union Members at high levels (EFSA, 2017). Historically, the incidence of resistance to macrolides has been low, especially in *C. jejuni*, even though there are several mechanisms by which *Campylobacter* can acquire resistance to these antimicrobial agents. There are four main ways involved in *Campylobacter* resistances: (i) target mutations in 23S rRNA genes, (ii) target mutations in ribosomal proteins, (iii) ribosomal methylation encoded by *erm* (B), and (iv) efflux through CmeABC and possibly others (Bolinger & Kathariou, 2017).

The third way above has recently been described in a single isolate of *C. coli* from broilers in Spain. This is the first report of *erm(B)* in *Campylobacter* in Europe. The isolate showed high-level erythromycin resistance (MIC $\geq$ 1024 mg/L erythromycin), and the *erm(B)* gene was located within a multidrug resistance island containing five antimicrobial resistance genes. Moreover, it was resistant to nalidixic acid, ciprofloxacin, tetracyclines, and streptomycin and susceptible to gentamicin (EFSA, 2017).

Macrolides interrupt protein synthesis in the bacterial ribosome by targeting the 50S subunit and inhibit bacterial RNA-dependent protein synthesis. Nucleotides 2058 and 2059 in 23S rRNA can act as key contact sites for macrolide binding. This leads to conformational changes in the ribosome and subsequent termination of the elongation of the peptide chain. The chromosome of *Campylobacter* contains three copies of the 23S rRNA gene. In erythromycin-resistant strains, generally all copies carry macrolide resistance-associated mutations, but the coexistence of wild-type alleles does not seem to affect the resistance level (Wieczorek & Osek, 2013).

Resistant in *Campylobacter* strains with the A2074G or A2075G mutation has been observed as well as mutations in the ribosomal proteins L4 (G74D) and L22 (insertions at position 86 or 98). Additionally, the synergy between the CmeABC efflux pump and mutations has also shown to confer macrolide resistance in *C. jejuni* and *C. coli*. The target mutations and active efflux confer resistance in *Campylobacter* not only to macrolides (erythromycin, clarithromycin, azithromycin, and tylosin) but also to ketolides (telithromycin) (Luangtongkum et al., 2010).

7. CONTROL STRATEGIES AND LEGISLATION

Nowadays *Campylobacter* infections have become one of the major concerns in public health all around the world, affecting equally developed and developing countries, and the number of campylobacteriosis cases are still increasing year by year. Moreover, movement of food product, especially from poultry, due to the international trade of goods and the movement of travelers between countries help to expand such concerns. Epidemiological studies using molecular typing techniques like MLST found the same *Campylobacter* genotype in different geographical locations, even widely separated ones. In the EU a total annual cost of €2.4 billion due to campylobacteriosis and its sequelae has been calculated (EFSA, 2011). The same report states that broiler meat may account for 20%–30% of campylobacteriosis cases in the EU, and 50%–80% of the chicken reservoir is contaminated (broilers as well as laying hens). Those data demand that some preventive measures and interventions along the poultry/chicken food chain, together with a new legislative framework, are needed to achieve a drastic reduction in the presence of *Campylobacter* in those products to increase consumer protection.

7.1 Control Measures in Poultry

Due to the high plasticity and adaptation level shown by *Campylobacter* to different environmental conditions, and its high genetic variability, it seems difficult to rely on only one strategy to reduce its presence in the poultry food chain. On the contrary, it seems than only an approach based on the barrier concept can achieve the necessary control of this pathogen. In that sense, several preventive measures and interventions have been proposed in the different steps of the poultry food chain.

At farm level, several strategies have been suggested. For instance, the application of strict biosecurity measures can efficiently reduce the risk of *Campylobacter* colonization and infection of the flocks. These measures should include at least: (1) a strict control of established accesses to minimize the entry of unauthorized people; (2) hygiene barriers to avoid entering of wild birds, rodents, and insects, especially flies using flying screens and the presence of other farm animals and pets in the proximity of the broiler houses; (3) access to treated water supply (chlorination); and (4) cleaning and disinfection of the whole plant and of all the equipment between flocks, as well as change of footwear and the use of footpaths before entering in the plant. Other strategies can include: the avoidance or better control of discontinuous thinning, reducing the slaughter age, the use of natural feed additives, the addition of organic acids in drinking water, and the use of bacteriocins or vaccination (EFSA, 2011). However, results of the application of those different strategies are still not conclusive.

Several strategies have been proposed to reduce the presence of *Campylobacter* at the slaughter/processing plant step. The least costly is to improve the GMP/HACCP during slaughtering and processing, especially by enhancing cleaning and disinfection procedures. Normally, slaughter productivity is enhanced in comparison with the accessibility of cleaning the equipment used in the slaughter process. In that sense, slaughter automatic lines are built with very complex equipment, making its thorough cleaning difficult. An effort should be made to improve hygienic design of slaughter equipment in order to avoid the growth or persistence of bacteria. Good manufacturing practices aimed to prevent leakage of intestinal contents during evisceration, detection, and reprocessing of poultry carcasses highly contaminated with fecal matter or cloacal plugging should be taken into account, especially in colonized flocks. However, those measures only decrease *Campylobacter* carcasses contamination by less than 2 logs.

Postslaughter interventions using chemical or physical methods might be applied as well. A risk reduction between 50% and 90% in *Campylobacter* presence in broiler carcasses can be obtained if they are freezing for 2–3 days, or by application of hot water or chemical carcass decontamination. This risk reduction can be increased over 90% if freezing period extends to 2–3 weeks. Currently in the EU, chemical decontamination, using organic acids solutions, chlorine dioxide, or trisodium phosphate, is not allowed. Moreover, a 100% reduction can be achieved by irradiation or cooking broiler carcasses or meat. However, irradiation is not well accepted by consumers, and cooking changes the sensory appearance from fresh chicken meat into a cooked product. Other interventions such as crust freezing or application of steam alone or combined with ultrasounds have also been proposed, although they show some practical limitations (EFSA, 2011).

At retail level, cross-contamination between different meats and due to handling by retailers should be avoided. In that sense, strict cleaning and disinfection procedures, keeping the adequate refrigeration temperature in the counters and proper packaging, might limit cross-contamination and therefore reduce the presence of *Campylobacter* in chicken products.

Warning labels, with food safety warnings and handling instructions on all fresh poultry packaging, may also assist better consumer handling to avoid cross-contamination. When preparing poultry products at home, the consumer must take care to avoid cross-contamination between chicken meat and other kitchen utensils or hands. Moreover, poultry products must be cooked properly. Consumers must take into account that washing chicken prior to cooking is a potential risk of cross-contamination and this practice must be avoided.

7.2 Other Measures

Although chicken meat has been designated as the main responsible for the transmission of *Campylobacter* to humans, it is not responsible for 100% of the cases of campylobacteriosis. This fact suggests that there must be other sources of contamination. Almost 20% of the campylobacteriosis cases detected in the EU in 2016 were diagnosed in children under 4 years, which is strange as it is very unlikely that they eat uncooked poultry meat. In that sense, it is important to avoid drinking untreated water or milk or swallowing water while swimming, and washing hands thoroughly, always before handling food or eating, and especially after having contact with animals and pets or after children play in playgrounds or gardens. Nevertheless, further epidemiological studies should be done to get insights into the different sources and transmission routes to avoid exposure of consumers to *Campylobacter*.

7.3 A Brief Note About Legislation

With the aim to reduce the number of campylobacteriosis cases in Europe, the EU has recently amended Regulation 2073/2005 by including a maximum contamination level of *Campylobacter* spp. in broiler carcasses of 1000 CFU/g at slaughter (European Regulation 1495/2017). In order to simplify and facilitate the application of the legislation, EFSA proposed to use the same sampling approach as for the process hygiene criteria set for *Salmonella* in poultry carcasses. Additionally, the international standard ISO 10272-2 has been adopted as a reference method for verifying compliance with the criterion for *Campylobacter* in poultry carcasses. With this new legislation, EFSA estimates that a public health risk reduction from the consumption of broiler meat of more than 50% could be achieved.

REFERENCES

Agunos, A., Waddell, L., Léger, D., & Taboada, E. (2014). A systematic review characterizing on-farm sources of *Campylobacter* spp. for broiler chickens. *PLoS One*, *9*(8), e104905.

Allen, V. M., Bull, S. A., Corry, J. E. L., Domingue, G., Jørgensen, F., Frost, J. A., et al. (2007). *Campylobacter* spp. contamination of chicken carcasses during processing in relation to flock colonization. *International Journal of Food Microbiology*, *113*, 54–61.

Allen, V. M., Burton, C. H., Wilkinson, D. J., Whyte, R. T., Harris, J. A., Howell, M., et al. (2008). Evaluation of the performance of different cleaning treatments in reducing microbial contamination of poultry transport crates. *Poultry Science*, *49*, 233–240.

Allen, V. M., Weaver, H., Ridley, A. M., Harris, J. A., Sharma, M., Emery, J., et al. (2008). Sources and spread of thermophillic *Campylobacter* spp. during partial depopulation of broiler chicken flocks. *Journal of Food Protection*, *71*, 264–270.

Alpigiani, I., Abrahantes, J. C., Michel, V., Huneau-Salaün, A., Chemaly, M., Keeling, L. J., et al. (2017). Associations between animal welfare indicators and *Campylobacter* spp. in broiler chickens under commercial settings: A case study. *Preventive Veterinary Medicine*, *147*, 186–193.

Avrain, L., Vernozy-Rozand, C., & Kempf, I. (2004). Evidence for natural horizontal transfer of tetO gene between *Campylobacter jejuni* strains in chickens. *Journal of Applied Microbiology*, *97*, 134–140.

Awad, W. A., Smorodchenko, A., Hess, C., Aschenbach, J. R., Molnár, A., Dublecz, K., et al. (2015). Increased intracellular calcium level and impaired nutrient absorption are important pathogenicity traits in the chicken intestinal epithelium during *Campylobacter jejuni* colonization. *Applied Microbiology and Biotechnology*, *99*, 6431–6441.

Barrero-Tobon, A. M., & Hendrixson, D. R. (2012). Identification and analysis of flagellar coexpressed determinants (Feds) of *Campylobacter jejuni* involved in colonization. *Molecular Microbiology*, *84*, 352–369.

Battersby, T., Walsh, D., Whyte, P., & Bolton, D. (2017). Evaluating and improving terminal hygiene practices on broiler farms to prevent *Campylobacter* cross-contamination between flocks. *Food Microbiology*, *64*, 1–6.

Bolinger, H., & Kathariou, S. (2017). The current state of macrolide resistance in *Campylobacter* spp: Trends and impacts of resistance mechanisms. *Applied and Enviromental Microbiology*, *83*, 416–417.

Bolton, D. J. (2015). *Campylobacter* virulence and survival factors. *Food Microbiology*, *48*, 99–108.

Borck Höng, B., Sommer, H. M., Larsen, L. S., Sorensen, A. I. V., David, B., Hofshagen, M., et al. (2016). Farm specific risk factors for *Campylobacter* colonisation in Danish and Norwegian broilers. *Preventive Veterinary Medicine*, *130*, 137–145.

Borczyk, A., Thompson, S., Smith, D., & Lior, H. (1987). Waterborne outbreak of *Campylobacter laridis*-associated gastroenteritis. *Lancet*, *1*, 164–165.

Bouwknegt, M., van de Giessen, A. W., Dam-Deisz, W. D., Havelaar, A. H., Nagelkerke, N. J., & Henken, A. M. (2004). Risk factors for the presence of *Campylobacter* spp. in Dutch broiler flocks. *Preventive Veterinary Medicine*, *62*, 35–49.

Bronowski, C., James, C. E., & Winstanley, C. (2014). Role of environmental survival in transmission of *Campylobacter jejuni*. *FEMS Microbiology Letters*, *356*, 8–19.

Burakoff, A., Brown, K., Knutsen, J., Hopewell, C., Rowe, S., Bennett, C., et al. (2018). Outbreak of fluoroquinolone-resistant *Campylobacter jejuni* infections associated with raw milk consumption from a herdshare dairy—Colorado, 2016. *Morbidity and Mortality Weekly Report*, *67*, 146–147.

Buswell, C. M., Herlihy, Y. M., Lawrence, L. M., Mcguiggan, J. T., Marsh, P. D., Keevil, C. W., et al. (1998). Extended survival and persistence of *Campylobacter* spp.

in water and aquatic biofilm and their detection by immunofluorescent antibody and rRNA staining. *Applied and Environmental Microbiology, 49*, 733–745.

Butzler, J. P. (2004). *Campylobacter*, from obscurity to celebrity. *Clinical Microbiology and Infection, 10*, 868–876.

Butzler, J. P., Dekeyser, P., Detrain, M., & Dehaen, F. (1973). Related vibrio in stools. *Journal of Pediatrics, 82*, 493–495.

Cáceres, A., Muñoz, I., Iraola, G., Díaz-Viraqué, F., & Collado, L. (2017). *Campylobacter ornithocola* sp. nov., a novel member of the *Campylobacter lari* group isolated from wild bird faecal samples. *International Journal of Systematic and Evolutionary Microbiology, 67*, 1643–1649.

Calciati, E., Lafuente, S., De Simó, M., Balfagon, P., Bartolomé, R., & Caylà, J. (2012). A *Campylobacter* outbreak in a Barcelona school. *Enfermedades Infecciosas y Microbiología Clínica, 30*(5), 243–245.

Cantas, L., & Suer, K. (2014). Review: The important bacterial zoonoses in "One Health" concept. *Frontiers in Public Health, 2*, 1–8.

Cardinale, E., Tall, F., Gueye, E. F., Cisse, M., & Salvat, G. (2004). Risk factors for *Campylobacter* spp. infection in senegalese broiler-chicken flocks. *Preventive Veterinary Medicine, 64*, 15–25.

Centers for Disease Control and Prevention (CDC). (2018). *Multistate outbreak of multidrug-resistant* Campylobacter *infections linked to contact with pet store puppies*. Available https://www.cdc.gov/campylobacter/outbreaks/puppies-9-17/index.html [accessed 26.03.2018].

Cerf, O., Carpentier, B., & Sanders, P. (2009). Test for determining in-use concentrations of antibiotics and disinfectants are based on entirely different concepts: "Resistance" has different meanings. *International Journal of Food Microbiology, 136*, 247–254.

Chaloner, G., Wigley, P., Humphrey, S., Kemmett, K., Lacharme-Lora, L., Humphrey, T., et al. (2014). Dynamics of dual infection with *Campylobacter jejuni* strains in chickens reveals distinct strain-to-strain variation in infection ecology. *Applied and Environmental Microbiology, 80*, 6366–6372.

Cook, A., Odumeru, J., Lee, S., & Pollari, F. (2012). *Campylobacter, Salmonella, Listeria monocytogenes*, verotoxigenic *Escherichia coli*. Prevalence, enumeration and subtypes on retail chicken breast with and without skin. *Journal of Food Protection, 75*, 34–40.

Cornelis, G. R. (2006). The type III secretion injectisome. *Nature Reviews. Microbiology, 4*, 811–825.

Damjanova, I., Jakab, M., Farkas, T., Meszaros, J., Galantai, Z., Turcsanyi, I., et al. (2011). From farm to fork follow-up of thermotolerant campylobacters throughout the broiler production chain and in human cases in a Hungarian county during a ten-months period. *International Journal of Food Microbiology, 150*, 95–102.

Dasti, J. I., Tareen, A. M., Lugert, R., Zautner, A. E., & Groß, U. (2010). *Campylobacter jejuni*: A brief overview on pathogenicity-associated factors and disease-mediating mechanisms. *International Journal Medicine of Microbiology, 300*, 205–211.

Datta, S., Niwa, H., & Itoh, K. (2003). Prevalence of 11 pathogenic genes of *Campylobacter jejuni* by PCR in strains isolated from humans, poultry meat and broiler and bovine faeces. *Journal of Medical Microbiology, 52*, 345–348.

Debruyne, L., Broman, T., Bergstrom, S., Olsen, B., On, S. L., & Vandamme, P. (2010). *Campylobacter volucris* sp. nov., isolated from black-headed gulls (*Larus ridibundus*). *International Journal of Systematic and Evolutionary Microbiology, 60*, 1870–1875.

Debruyne, L., Gevers, D., & Vandamme, P. (2008). Taxonomy of the family *Campylobacteraceae*. In *Campylobacter* (3rd ed., pp. 3–25): American Society of Microbiology.

Dekeyser, P., Gossuin-Detrain, M., Butzler, J. P., & Sternon, J. (1972). Acute enteritis due to related vibrios: First positive stool cultures. *Journal of Infectious Disease, 125*, 390–392.

Domingues, A. R., Pires, S. M., Halasa, T., & Hald, T. (2012). Source attribution of human campylobacteriosis using a meta-analysis of case-control studies of sporadic infections. *Epidemiology and Infection, 140*, 970–981.

Doyle, L. P. (1948). The etiology of swine dysentery. *American Journal of Veterinary Research, 9*, 50–51.

Ellis-Iversen, J., Ridley, A., Morris, V., Sowa, A., Harris, J., Atterbury, R., et al. (2012). Persistent environmental reservoirs on farms as risk factors for *Campylobacter* in commercial poultry. *Epidemiology and Infection, 140*, 916–924.

Elvers, K. T., Morris, V. K., Newell, D. G., & Allen, V. M. (2011). Molecular tracking, through processing, of *Campylobacter* strains colonizing broiler flocks. *Applied and Environmental Microbiology, 77*, 5722–5729.

Engelbrecht, K. C., Putonti, C., Koenig, D. W., & Wolfe, A. J. (2017). Draft genome sequence of *Escherichia coli* K-12 (ATCC 29425). *Genome Announcements, 5*, e00574-17.

Epps, S. V. R., Harvey, R. B., Hume, M. E., Phillips, T. D., Anderson, R. C., & Nisbet, D. J. (2013). Foodborne *Campylobacter*: Infections, metabolism, pathogenesis and reservoirs. *International Journal of Environmental Research and Public Health, 10*, 6292–6304.

European Food Safety Authority. (2017). The European Union summary report on trends and sources of zoonoses, zoonotic agents and food-borne outbreaks in 2016. *EFSA Journal, 15*, 5077. https://doi.org/10.2903/j.efsa.2017.5077.

European Food Safety Authority (EFSA). (2010a). Analysis of the baseline survey on the prevalence of *Campylobacter* in broiler batches and of *Campylobacter* and *Salmonella* on broiler carcasses in the EU, 2008, part A: *Campylobacter* and *Salmonella* prevalence estimates. *EFSA Journal, 8*, 1503.

European Food Safety Authority (EFSA). (2010b). Analysis of the baseline survey on the prevalence of *Campylobacter* in broiler batches and of *Campylobacter* and *Salmonella* on broiler carcasses, in the EU, 2008; part B: Analysis of factors associated with *Campylobacter* colonisation of broiler batches and with *Campylobacter* contamination of broiler carcasses; and investigation of the culture method diagnostic characteristics used to analyse broiler carcass samples. *EFSA Journal, 8*(8), 1552.

European Food Safety Authority. Panel on Biological Hazards (BIOHAZ). (2011). Scientific on *Campylobacter* in broiler meat production: Control options and performance objectives and/or targets at different stages of the food chain. *EFSA Journal, 9*, 2013–2105.

Fajó-Pascual, M., Godoy, P., Ferrero-Cáncer, M., & Wymore, K. (2010). Case-control study of risk factors for sporadic campylobacter infections in northeastern Spain. *European Journal of Public Health, 20*, 443–448.

Fauchere, J. L., Rosenau, A., Veron, M., Moyen, E. N., Richard, S., & Pfister, A. (1986). Association with HeLa cells of *Campylobacter jejuni* and *Campylobacter coli* isolated from human feces. *Infection and Immunology, 54*, 283–287.

Food Quality News. (2017). *More than half of chickens positive for* Campylobacter. https://www.foodqualitynews.com/Article/2017/10/19/FSA-Campylobacter-in-chicken. Accessed 25 February 2018.

Foster, G., Holmes, B., Steigerwalt, A. G., Lawson, P. A., Thorne, P., Byrer, D. E., et al. (2004). *Campylobacter insulaenigrae* sp. nov., isolated from marine mammals. *International Journal of Systematic and Evolutionary Microbiology, 54*, 2369–2373.

Fouts, D. E., Mongodin, E. F., Mandrell, R. E., Miller, W. G., Rasko, D. A., Ravel, J., et al. (2005). Mayor structural differences and novel potential virulence mechanisms from the genomes of multiple *Campylobacter* species. *PLoS Biology, 3*, 15.

García-Sánchez, L., Melero, B., Jaime, I., Hänninen, M. L., Rossi, M., & Rovira, J. (2017). *Campylobacter jejuni* survival in a poultry processing plant environment. *Food Microbiology, 65*, 185–192.

Gibbens, J. C., Pascoe, S. J. S., Evans, S. J., Davies, R. H., & Sayers, A. R. (2001). A trial of biosecurity as a means to control *Campylobacter* infection of broiler chickens. *Preventive Veterinary Medicine, 48*, 85–99.

Gilbert, M. J., Kik, M., Miller, W. G., Duim, B., & Wagenaar, J. A. (2015). *Campylobacter iguaniorum* sp. nov., isolated from reptiles. *International Journal of Systematic and Evolutionary Microbiology, 65*, 975–982.

Gilbert, M. J., Miller, W. G., Leger, J. S., Chapman, M. H., Timmerman, A. J., Duim, B., et al. (2017). *Campylobacter pinnipediorum* sp. nov., isolated from pinnipeds, comprising *Campylobacter pinnipediorum* subsp. *pinnipediorum* subsp. nov. and *Campylobacter pinnipediorum* subsp. *caledonicus* subsp. nov. *International Journal of Systematic and Evolutionary Microbiology*, *67*, 1961–1968.

Glaser, P., et al. (2001). Comparative genomic of Listeria species. *Science*, *294*, 849–852.

Gölz, G., Rosner, B., Hofreuter, D., Josenhans, C., Kreienbrock, L., Löwenstein, A., et al. (2014). Relevance of *Campylobacter* to public health-the need for a One Health approach. *International Journal of Medicine and Microbiology*, *304*, 817–823.

Goudswaard, J., Sabbe, L., & te Winkel, W. (1995). Reactive arthritis as a complication of *Campylobacter lari* enteritis. *Journal of Infection*, *31*, 171–176.

Gruntar, I., Biasizzo, M., Kusar, D., Pate, M., & Ocepek, M. (2015). *Campylobacter jejuni* contamination of broiler carcasses: Population dynamics and genetic profiles at slaughterhouse level. *Food Microbiology*, *50*, 97–101.

Guerry, P. (2007). *Campylobacter* flagella: Not just for motility. *Trends Microbiology*, *15*, 456–461.

Gundogdu, O., Bentley, S. D., Holden, M. T., Parkhill, J., Dorrell, N., & Wren, B. W. (2007). Re-annotation and re-analysis of the *Campylobacter jejuni* NCTC11168 genome sequence. *BioMed Central Genomics*, *8*, 162.

Gunther, N. W., & Chen, C. Y. (2009). The biofilm forming potential of bacterial species in the genus *Campylobacter*. *Food Microbiology*, *26*, 44–51.

Hald, B., Skovgard, H., Pedersen, K., & Bunkenborg, H. (2008). Influxed insects as vectors for *Campylobacter jejuni* and *Campylobacter coli* in Danish broiler houses. *Poultry Science*, *87*, 1428–1434.

Hänninen, M. L., Perko-Mäakelä, P., Pitkälä, A., & Rautenin, H. (2000). A three-year study of Campylobacter jejuni genotypes in humans with domestically acquired infections and in chicken samples from the Helsinki area. *Journal of Clinical Microbiology*, *38*, 1998–2000.

Hansson, I., Pudas, N., Harbom, B., & Engvall, E. O. (2010). Within-flock variations of Campylobacter loads in caeca and on carcasses from broilers. *International Journal of Food Microbiology*, *141*, 51–55.

Hansson, I., Vagsholm, I., Svensson, L., & Olsson Engvall, E. (2007). Correlations between *Campylobacter* spp. prevalence in the environment and broiler flocks. *Journal and Applied of Microbiology*, *103*, 640–649.

Havelaar, A. H., Mangen, M. J., de Koeijer, A. A., Bogaardt, M. J., Evers, E. G., Jacobs-Reitsma, W. F., et al. (2007). Effectiveness and efficiency of controlling *Campylobacter* on broiler chicken meat. *Risk Analysis*, *27*, 831–844.

Humphrey, S., Chaloner, G., Kemmett, K., Davidson, N., Williams, N., Kipar, A., et al. (2014). *Campylobacter jejuni* is not merely a commensal in commercial broiler chickens and affects bird welfare. *MBio*, *5*, 1–7.

Huneau-Salaun, A., Denis, M., Balaine, L., & Salvat, G. (2007). Risk factors for *Campylobacter* spp. colonization in French free-range broiler-chicken flocks at the end of the indoor rearing period. *Preventive Veterinary Medicine*, *80*, 34–48.

Inglis, G. D., Hoar, B. M., Whiteside, D. P., & Morck, D. W. (2007). *Campylobacter canadensis* sp. nov., from captive whooping cranes in Canada. *International Journal Medicine and Microbiology*, *57*, 2636–2644.

Ingresa-Capaccioni, S., González-Bodí, S., Jiménez-Trigos, E., Marco-Jiménez, F., Catalá, P., Vega, S., et al. (2015). Comparison of different sampling types across the rearing period in broiler flocks for isolation of *Campylobacter* spp. *Poultry Science*, *94*, 766–771.

Iovine, N. M. (2013). Resistance mechanisms in *Campylobacter jejuni*. *Virulence*, *4*, 230–240.

Jackson, D. N., Davis, B., Tirado, S. M., Duggal, M., van Frankenhuyzen, J. K., Deaville, D., et al. (2009). Survival mechanisms and culturability of *Campylobacter jejuni* under stress conditions. *Antonie van Leeuwenhoek*, *96*, 377–394.

Johnsen, G., Kruse, H., & Hofshagen, M. (2006). Genetic diversity and description of transmission routes for *Campylobacter* on broiler farms by amplified-fragment length polymorphism. *Journal of Applied Microbiology, 101*, 1130–1139.

Jones, F. S., Orcutt, M., & Little, R. B. (1931). Vibrios (*V. jejuni* n. sp.) associated with intestinal disorders in cows and calves. *Journal of Experimental Microbiology, 81*, 163–168.

Joshua, G. W. P., Guthrie-Irons, C., Karlyshev, V., & Wren, B. W. (2006). Biofilm formation in *Campylobacter jejuni*. *Microbiology, 152*, 387–396.

Kaakoush, N. O., Castaño-Rodríguez, N., Mitchell, H. M., & Man, S. M. (2015). Global epidemiology of Campylobacter infection. *Clinical Microbiology Reviews, 28*, 687–720.

Kapperud, G., Espeland, G., Wahl, E., Walde, A., Herikstad, H., Gustavsen, S., et al. (2003). Factors associated with increased and decreased risk of Campylobacter infection: A prospective case-control study in Norway. *American Journal of Epidemiology, 158*, 234–242.

Kärenlampi, R., & Hänninen, M. L. (2004). Survival of *Campylobacter jejuni* on various fresh produce. *International Journal of Food Microbiology, 97*, 187–195.

Kist, M. (1986). Who discovered *Campylobacter jejuni/coli*? A review of hitherto disregarded literature. *Zentralbl Bakteiology Mikrobiology Hygiene, 261*, 177–186.

Konkel, M. E., Garvis, S. G., Tipton, S. L., Anderson, D. E., Jr., & Cieplak, W., Jr. (1997). Identification and molecular cloning of a gene encoding a fibronectin-binding protein (CadF) from *Campylobacter jejuni*. *Molecular Microbiology, 24*, 953–963.

Koolman, L., Whyte, P., Burgess, C., & Bolton, D. (2016). Virulence gene expression, adhesion and invasion of *Campylobacter jejuni* exposed to oxidative stress (H_2O_2). *International Journal of Food Microbiology, 220*, 33–38.

Koppenaal, H., Groenendijk, F., van den Berge, M., Verkade, E., Verduin, K., Zomer, A. L., et al. (2017). Outbreak of Campylobacter fetus infection after consumption of unpasteurized sheep's milk cheeses: How to trace the source? *Nederlands Tijdschrift voor Geneeskunde, 161*, 1704.

Koziel, M., O'Doherty, P., Vandamme, P., Corcoran, G. D., Sleator, R. D., & Lucey, B. (2014). *Campylobacter* corcagiensis sp. nov., isolated from feces of captive lion-tailed macaques (*Macaca silenus*). *International Journal of Systematic and Evolutionary Microbiology, 64*, 2878–2883.

Lahti, E., Löfdahl, M., Ågren, J., Hansson, I., & Olsson Engvall, E. (2017). Confirmation of a Campylobacteriosis outbreak associated with chicken liver paté using PFGE and WGS. *Zoonoses and Public Health, 64*, 14–20.

Lastovica, A. J. (1996). Campylobacter/Helicobacter bacteraemia in Cape Town, South Africa, 1977–1995. In D. G. Newell, J. M. Ketley, & R. A. Feldman (Eds.), *Campylobacters, helicobacters and related organisms* (pp. 475–479). New York: Plenum.

Lastovica, A. J. (2006). Emerging *Campylobacter* spp: The tip of the iceberg. *Clinical of Microbiology Newsletters, 28*, 49–56.

Lastovica, A. J., & Allos, B. M. (2008). Clinical significance of *Campylobacter* and related species other than *Campylobacter jejuni* and *Campylobacter coli*. In *Campylobacter* (3rd ed., pp. 123–149): American Society of Microbiology.

Lastovica, A. J., le Roux, E., & Penner, J. L. (1989). "*Campylobacter upsaliensis*" isolated from blood cultures of pediatric patients. *Journal of Clinical Microbiology, 27*, 657–659.

Lastovica, A. J., On, S. L., & Zhang, L. (2014). The family Campylobacteraceae. In *The prokaryotes* (pp. 307–335): Springer Berlin Heidelberg.

Lawson, A. J., On, S. L. W., Logan, J. M. J., & Stanley, J. (2001). *Campylobacter* hominis sp. nov. from the human gastrointestinal tract. *International Journal of Systematic and Evolutionary Microbiology, 51*, 651–660.

Levi, A. J. (1946). A gastroenteritis outbreak probably due to a bovine strain of Vibrio. *The Yale Journal of Biology and Medicine, 18*, 243.

Lin, J., Michel, L. O., & Zhang, Q. (2002). CmeABC functions as a multidrug efflux system in *Campylobacter jejuni*. *Antimicrobial Agents Chemotherapy*, *46*, 2124–2131.

Llarena, A. K. (2015). *Population genetics and molecular epidemiology of* Campylobacter jejuni. PhD Thesis. ISSN 2342-5423 (p. 12).

Luangtongkum, T., Jeon, B., Han, J., Plummer, P., Logue, C. M., & Zhang, Q. (2010). Antibiotic resistance in *Campylobacter*: Emergence, transmission and persistence. *Future Microbiology*, *4*, 189–200.

Luber, P., Brynestad, S., Topsch, D., Scherer, K., & Bartelt, E. (2006). Quantification of *campylobacter* species cross-contamination during handling of contaminated fresh chicken parts in kitchens. *Applied and Environmental Microbiology*, *72*, 66–70.

Mahendran, V., Riordan, S., Grimm, M., Tran, T., Major, J., Kaakoush, N., et al. (2011). Prevalence of *Campylobacter* species in adult Crohn's disease and the preferential colonization sites of *Campylobacter* species in the human intestine. *PLoS One*, *6*, e25417.

Man, S. M. (2011). The clinical importance of emerging *Campylobacter* species. *Nature Reviews: Gastroenterology & Hepatology*, *8*, 669–685.

Marotta, F., Garofolo, G., Di Donato, G., Aprea, G., Platone, I., Cianciavicchia, S., et al. (2015). Population diversity of *Campylobacter jejuni* in poultry and its dynamic of contamination in chicken meat. *BioMed Research International*, *2015*, 85984.

McCrea, B. A., Tonooka, K. H., VanWorth, C., Boggs, C. L., Atwill, E. R., & Schrader, J. S. (2006). Prevalence of *Campylobacter* and *Salmonella* species on farm, after transport, and at processing in specialty market poultry. *Poultry Science*, *85*, 136–143.

Melero, B., Juntunen, P., Hänninen, M. L., Jaime, I., & Rovira, J. (2012). Tracing population diversity of *Campylobacter jejuni* in poultry and its dynamic of contamination in chicken meat strains along the poultry meat production chain from farm to retail by pulsed-field gel electrophoresis, and the antimicrobial resistance of isolates. *Food Microbiology*, *32*, 124–128.

Melero, B., Vinuesa, R., Diez, AM., Jaime, I., & Rovira, J. (2013). Application of protective cultures against *Listeria monocytogenes* and *Campylobacter jejuni* in chicken products packaged under modified atmosphere. *Poultry Science*, *92*, 1108–1116. https://doi.org/10.3382/ps.2012-02539.

Melo, R. T., Mendonca, E. P., Monteiro, G. P., Siqueira, M. C., Pereira, C. B., Peres, P. A. B. M., et al. (2017). Intrinsic and extrinsic aspects on *Campylobacter jejuni* biofilms. *Frontiers Microbiology*, *18*, 1332.

Méndez-Olvera, E. T., Bustos-Martínez, J. A., López-Vidal, Y., Verdugo-Rodriguez, A., & Martínez-Gómez, D. (2016). Cytolethal distending toxin from *Campylobacter jejuni* requires the cytoskeleton for toxic activity. *Jundishapur Journal of Microbiology*, *9*, 35591.

Meredith, H., Valdramidis, V., Rotabakk, B. T., Sivertsvik, M., McDowell, D., & Bolton, D. J. (2014). Effect of different modified atmospheric packaging (MAP) gaseous combinations on *Campylobacter* and the shelf-life of chilled poultry fillets. *Food Microbiology*, *44*, 196–203. https://doi.org/10.1016/j.fm.2014.06.005.

Miller, W. G., Parker, C. T., Heath, S., & Lastovica, A. J. (2007). Identification of genomic differences between *Campylobacter jejuni* subsp. *jejuni* and *C. jejuni* subsp. *doylei* at the nap locus leads to the development of a *C. jejuni* subspeciation multiplex PCR method. *BioMed Centre Microbiology*, 7(1), 11.

Miller, C. E., Williams, P. H., & Ketley, J. M. (2009). Pumping iron: Mechanisms for iron uptake by *Campylobacter*. *Microbiology*, *155*, 3157–3165.

Miwa, N., Takegahara, Y., Terai, K., Kato, H., & Takeuchi, T. (2003). *Campylobacter jejuni* contamination on broiler carcasses of *C. jejuni*-negative flocks during processing in a Japanese slaughterhouse. *International. Journal of Food Microbiology*, *84*, 105–109.

Moffatt, C. R., Greig, A., Valcanis, M., Gao, W., Seemann, T., Howden, B. P., et al. (2016). A large outbreak of *Campylobacter jejuni* infection in a university college caused by chicken liverpâté, Australia, 2013. *Epidemiology and Infection*, *144*, 2971–2978.

Monteville, M. R., Yoon, J. E., & Konkel, M. E. (2003). Maximal adherence and invasion of INT 407 cells by *Campylobacter jejuni* requires the CadF outer membrane protein and microfilament reorganization. *Microbiology*, *149*, 153–165.

Morishita, S., Fujiwara, H., Murota, H., Maeda, Y., Hara, A., & Horii, T. (2013). Bloodstream infection caused by *Campylobacter lari*. *Journal of Infection and Chemotherapy*, *19*, 333–337.

Mughini, G., Smid, J. H., Wagenaar, J. A., de Boer, A. G., Havelaar, A. H., Friesema, I. H., et al. (2012). Risk factors for campylobacteriosis of chicken ruminants and environmental origin: A combined case control and source attribution analysis. *PLoS One*, *7*, 42599.

Nachamkin, I., Szymanski, C., & Blaser, M. (2008). *Campylobacter* (3rd ed.). Washington, DC: ASM Press, ISBN: 978-1-55581-437-3.

Neal-McKinney, J. M., & Kronkel, M. E. (2012). The Campylobacter jejuni CiaC virulence protein is secreted from the flagellum and delivered to the cytosol of host cells. *Frontiers in Cellular and Infection Microbiology*, *2*, 1–15. article 31.

Newell, D. G., Shreeve, J. E., Toszeghy, M., Domingue, G., Bull, S., Humphrey, T., et al. (2001). Changes in the carriage of Campylobacter strains by poultry carcasses during processing in abattoirs. *Applied and Environmental Microbiology*, *67*, 2636–2640.

Ngulukun, S. (2017). Taxonomy and physiological characteristics of Campylobacter spp. In *Campylobacter* (3rd ed., pp. 41–60). Washington, DC: ASM Press, ISBN: 978-1-55581-437-3.

Oh, E., McMullen, L. M., Chui, L., & Jeon, B. (2017). Differential survival of hyper-aerotolerant *Campylobacter jejuni* under different gas conditions. *Frontiers in Microbiology*, *8*, 1–8. https://doi.org/10.3389/fmicb.2017.00954.

Parkhill, J., Wren, B. W., Mungall, K., Ketley, J. M., Churcher, C., Basham, D., et al. (2000). The genome sequence of the food-borne pathogen *Campylobacter jejuni* reveals hypervariable sequences. *Nature*, *10*(403), 665–668.

Pearson, B. M., Gaskin, D. J., Segers, R. P., Wells, J. M., Nuijten, P. J., & van Vliet, A. H. (2007). The complete geneome sequence of *Campylobacter jejuni* strain 81116 (NCTC 11828). *Jounal of Bacteriology*, *189*, 8402–8403.

Peyrat, M. B., Soumet, C., Maris, P., & Sanders, P. (2008a). Phenotypes and genotypes of campylobacter strains isolated after cleaning and disinfection in poultry slaughterhouses. *Veterinary Microbiology*, *128*, 313–326.

Peyrat, M. B., Soumet, C., Maris, P., & Sanders, P. (2008b). Recovery of *Campylobacter jejuni* from surfaces of poultry slaughterhouses after cleaning and disinfection procedures: Analysis of a potential source of carcass contamination. *International Journal of Food Microbiology*, *124*, 188–194.

Piccirillo, A., Niero, G., Calleros, L., Pérez, R., Naya, H., & Iraola, G. (2016). *Campylobacter geochelonis* sp. nov. isolated from the western Hermann's tortoise (*Testudo hermanni* hermanni). *International Journal of Systematic and Evolutionary Microbiology*, *66*, 3468–3476.

Revez, J., & Hänninen, M. L. (2012). Lipooligosaccharide locus classes are associated with certain *Campylobacter jejuni* multilocus sequence types. *Journal of Clinical and Microbiology Infection Disease*, *31*, 2203–2209.

Revez, J., Llarena, A. K., Schott, T., Kuusi, M., Hakkinen, M., Kivistö, R., et al. (2014). Genome analysis of *Campylobacter jejuni* strains isolated from a waterborne outbreak. *BioMed Central Genomics*, *15*, 768.

Richards, V. P., Leféburea, T., Pavinski-Bitara, P. D., & Stanhope, M. J. (2013). Comparative characterization of the virulence gene clusters (lipooligosacharide [LOS] and capsular polysaccharide [CPS]) for *Campylobacter coli*, *Campylobacter jejuni* subsp. *jejuni* and related *Campylobacter* species. *Infection and Genetic Evolution*, *14*, 200–213.

Ring, M., Zychowska, M. A., & Stephan, R. (2005). Dynamics of *Campylobacter* spp. spread investigated in 14 broiler flocks in Switzerland. *Avian Diseases*, *49*, 390–396.

Rollins, D. M., & Colwell, R. R. (1986). Viable but non-culturable stage of *Campylobacter jejuni* and its role in survival in the natural aquatic environment. *Applied and Environmental Microbiology*, *52*, 531–538.
Rossi, M., Debruyne, L., Zanoni, R. G., Manfreda, G., Revez, J., & Vandamme, P. (2009). *Campylobacter avium* sp. nov., a hippurate-positive species isolated from poultry. *International Journal of Systematic and Evolutionary Microbiology*, *59*, 2364–2369.
Rovira, J., Cencic, A., Santos, E. M., & Jakobsen, M. (2006). Biological hazards. In P. A. Luning, F. Devlieghere, & R. Verhé (Eds.), *Safety in the agrifood chain* (pp. 67–143). Wageningen, The Netherlands: Wageningen Academic Publishers.
Russa, A. D., Bouma, A., Vernooij, J. C., Jacobs-Reitsma, W., & Stegeman, J. A. (2005). No association between partial depopulation and Campylobacter spp. colonization of Dutch broiler flocks. *Letters of Applied Microbiology*, *41*, 280–285.
Samuelson, D. R., Eucker, T. P., Bell, J. A., Dybas, L., Dybas, L., Mansfield, L. S., et al. (2013). The *Campylobacter jejuni* CiaD effector protein activates MAP kinase signaling pathways and is required for the development of disease. *Cell Communication and Signaling*, *11*, 79.
Sanger Institute. (2018). (accessed 26.03.2018). Available in website http://www.sanger.ac.uk.
Saunders, S., Smith, K., Schott, R., Dobbins, G., & Scheftel, J. (2017). Outbreak of Campylobacteriosis associated with raccoon contact at a wildlife rehabilitaton centre, Minnesota, 2013. *Zoonoses and Public Health*, *64*, 222–227.
Sebald, M., & Veron, M. (1963). Teneur en bases da l'AND et classification des vibrions. *Annales de L'institut Pasteur (Paris)*, *105*, 897–910.
Seliwiorstow, T., Baré, J., Van Damme, I., Uyttendaele, M., & De Zutter, L. (2015). *Campylobacter* carcass contamination throughout the slaughter process of *Campylobacter*-positive broiler batches. *International Journal of Food Microbiology*, *194*, 25–31.
Skarp, C. P. A., Hänninen, M.-L., & Rautelin, H. I. K. (2016). Campylobacteriosis: The role of poultry meat. *Clinical Microbiology and Infection*, *22*, 103–109.
Skirrow, M. B. (1977). *Campylobacter* enteritis: A "new" disease. *British Medical Journal*, *2*, 9–11.
Skirrow, M. B., Jones, D. M., Sutcliffe, E., & Benjamin, J. (1993). *Campylobacter* bacteraemia in England and Wales, 1981. *Epidemiology and Infection*, *119*, 563–567.
Skov, M. N., Spencer, A. G., Hald, B., Petersen, L., Nauerby, B., Carstensen, B., et al. (2004). The role of litter beetles as potential reservoir for *Salmonella enterica* and thermophilic campylobacter spp. between broiler flocks. *Avian Diseases*, *48*, 9–18.
Slader, J., Domínguez, G., Jorgensen, F., McAlpine, K., Owen, R. J., Bolton, F. J., et al. (2002). Impact of transport crate reuse and of catching and processing on *Campylobacter* and *Salmonella* contamination of broiler chickens. *Applied and Environmental Microbiology*, *68*, 713–719.
Smith, J. L., & Bayles, D. O. (2006). The contribution of cytolethal distending toxin to bacterial pathogenesis. *Critical Reviews in Microbiology*, *32*, 227–248.
Smith, T., & Taylor, M. S. (1919). Some morphological and biological characters of the spirilla (Vibrio fetus, n. sp.) associated with disease of the fetal membranes in cattle. *The Journal of Experimental Medicine*, *30*, 299–312.
Sommer, H. M., Heuer, O. E., Sørensen, A. I. V., & Madsen, M. (2013). Analysis of factors important for the occurrence of Campylobacter in Danish broiler flocks. *Preventive Veterinary Medicine*, *111*, 100–111.
Sproston, E. L., Ogden, I. D., MacRae, M., Forbes, K. J., Dallas, J. F., Sheppard, S. K., et al. (2010). Multi-locus sequence types of *Campylobacter* carried by flies and slugs acquired from local ruminant faeces. *Journal of Applied Microbiology*, *109*, 829–838.
Teh, A. H. T., Lee, S. M., & Dykes, G. A. (2014). Does *campylobacter jejuni* form biofilms in food-related environments? *Applied and Environmental Microbiology*, *80*, 5154–5160.

Turonova, H., Briandet, R., Rodrigues, R., Hernould, M., Hayek, N., Stintzi, A., et al. (2015). Biofilm spatial organization by the emerging pathogen *Campylobacter jejuni*: Comparison between NCTC 11168 and 81-176 strains under microaerobic and oxygen-enriched conditions. *Frontiers Microbiology, 6*, 1–11.

Van, T. T. H., Elshagmani, E., Gor, M. C., Scott, P. C., & Moore, R. J. (2016). *Campylobacter* hepaticus sp. nov., isolated from chickens with spotty liver disease. *International Journal of Systematic and Evolutionary Microbiology, 66*, 4518–4524.

Vandamme, P. (2000). Taxonomy of the family *Campylobacteraceae*. In I. Namchamkin & M. J. Blaser (Eds.), *Campylobacter* (pp. 3–27). Washington, DC: ASM Press.

Vandamme, P., Debruyne, L., De Brandt, E., & Falsen, E. (2010). Reclassification of Bacteroides ureolyticus as *Campylobacter* ureolyticus comb. nov., and emended description of the genus *Campylobacter*. *International Journal of Systematic and Evolutionary Microbiology, 60*, 2016–2022.

Vandamme, P., Dewhirst, F. E., Paster, B. J., & On, S. L. W. (2005). Campylobacteraceae. In G. M. Garrity, D. J. Brenner, N. R. Krieg, & J. T. Staley (Eds.), *Bergey's manual of systematic bacteriology: Vol. 2* (pp. 1147–1160). New York: Springer Science.

Veron, M., & Chatelain, R. (1973). Taxonomic study of the genus *Campylobacter* and designation of the genotype strain for the type species, *Campylobacter fetus*. *International Journal of Systematic Bacteriology, 23*, 122–134.

Vinuesa, P., Puente, J. L., Calva, E., Zaidi, M. B., & Silva, C. (2016). Complete genome sequence of *Salmonella* enterica Serovar *Typhimurium* strain SO3 (sequence type 302) isolated from a baby with meningitis in Mexico. *Genome Announcement, 4*, 231–285.

Vinzent, R., Dumas, J., & Picard, N. (1947). Septicemia grave au cours de la grossesse, due a un vibrion. *Bulletin de l'Académie Nationale de Médecine, 131*, 90.

Vondrakova, L., Pazlarova, J., & Demnerova, K. (2014). Detection, identification and quantification of *Campylobacter jejuni, coli* and *lari* in food matrices all at once using multiplex PCR. *Gut Pathogens, 6*, 12.

Wan, Y., & Taylor, D. E. (1990). Natural transformation in Campylobacter species. *Journal of Bacteriology, 172*, 949–955.

Wang, G., Clark, C. G., Taylor, T. M., Pucknell, C., Barton, C., Price, L., et al. (2002). Colony multiplex PCR assay for identification and differentiation of. *Campylobacter jejuni, C. coli, C. lari, C. upsaliensis*, and *C. fetus* subsp. *fetus*. *Journal of Clinical Microbiology, 40*, 4744–4747.

Wei, B., Cha, S.-Y., Yoon, R. H., Kang, M., Roh, J. H., Seo, H. S., et al. (2016). Prevalence and antimicrobial resistance of *Campylobacter* spp. from duck in South Korea. *Food Control, 62*, 63–68.

Whiley, H., Van den Akker, B., Giglio, S., & Bentham, R. (2013). The role of environmental reservoirs in human campylobacteriosis. *Interantional Journal of Environmental Research Public Health, 8*, 5886–5907.

Wieczorek, K., & Osek, J. (2013). Antimicrobial resistance mechanisms among *Campylobacter*. *Biomedical Research International, 2013*, 340605.

Yao, H., Liu, D., Wang, Y., Zhang, Q., & Shen, Z. (2017). High prevalence and predominance of the aph(2′)-if gene conferring aminoglycoside resistance in *Campylobacter*. *Antimicrobial Agents and Chemotherapy, 61*, 1–9.

Zanoni, R. G., Debruyne, L., Rossi, M., Revez, J., & Vandamme, P. (2009). *Campylobacter cuniculorum* sp. nov., from rabbits. *International Journal of Systematic and Evolutionary Microbiology, 59*, 1666–1671.

Zhang, T., Luo, Q., Chen, Y., Li, T., Wen, G., Zhang, R., et al. (2016). Molecular epidemiology, virulence determinants and antimicrobial resistance of *Campylobacter* spreading in retail chicken meat in Central China. *Gut Pathogens, 8*, 48.

Zhang, L., Man, S. M., Day, A. S., Leach, S. T., Lemberg, D. A., Dutt, S., et al. (2009). Detection and isolation of Campylobacter species other than *C. jejuni* from children with Crohn's disease. *Journal of Clinical Microbiololgy*, *47*, 453–455.

Ziprin, R. L., Young, C. R., Stanker, L. H., Hume, M. E., & Konkel, M. E. (1999). The absence of ceca colonization of chicks by mutant of Campylobacter jejuni not expressing bacterial fibronectin-binding protein. *Avian Disease*, *43*, 586–589.

Zoete, M. R., Keestra, A. M., Wagenaar, J. A., & Van Putten, J. P. M. (2010). Reconstitution of a functional Toll-like receptor 5 binding site in *Campylobacter jejuni* flagellin. *The Journal of Biological Chemistry*, *285*, 12149–12158.

Zweifel, C., Scheu, K. D., Keel, M., Renggli, F., & Stephan, R. (2008). Occurrence and genotypes of *Campylobacter* in broiler flocks, other farm animals, and the environment during several rearing periods on selected poultry farms. *International Journal of Food Microbiology*, *125*, 182–187.

FURTHER READING

Abuoun, M., Manning, G., Cawthraw, S., Ridley, A., Ahmed, I. H., Wassenaar, T. M., et al. (2005). Cytolethal distending toxin (CDT)-negative *Campylobacter jejuni* strains and anti-CDT neutraliszing antibodies are induced during human infection but not during colonization in chickens. *Infection and Immunity*, *73*, 3053–3062.

Barker, C. S., Meshcheryakova, I. V., Kostyukova, A. S., Freddolino, P. L., & Samatey, F. A. (2017). An intrinsically disordered linker controlling the formation and the stability of the bacterial flagellar hook. *BioMed Central Biology*, *15*, 1–14.

Battersby, T., Whyte, P., & Bolton, D. J. (2016). The pattern of *Campylobacter* contamination on broiler farms; external and internal sources. *Journal of Applied Microbiology*, *120*, 1108–1118.

Facciolà, A., Riso, R., Aventuoso, E., Visalli, G., Delia, S. A., & Laganà, P. (2017). *Campylobacter*: Form microbiology to prevention. *Journal of Preventive Medicine and Hygiene*, *58*, 79–92.

Vandamme, P. (2009). *Campylobacter* avium sp. nov., a hippurate positive species isolated from poultry. *International Journal of Systematic and Evolutionary Microbiology*, *59*, 2364–2369.

FSC
www.fsc.org
MIX
Papier | Fördert gute Waldnutzung
FSC® C083411

Kolibri 360 GmbH
Ferdinand-Jühlke-Straße 7
99095 Erfurt, Deutschland
produktsicherheit@kolibri360.de